PRINCIPLES *of* CARDIOVASCULAR RADIOLOGY

PRINCIPLES *of* CARDIOVASCULAR RADIOLOGY

Stuart J. Hutchison, MD, FRCPC, FACC, FAHA

Clinical Professor of Medicine

University of Calgary

Division of Cardiology

Departments of Cardiac Sciences and Radiology

Foothills Medical Center

Calgary, Canada

ELSEVIER
SAUNDERS

1600 John F. Kennedy Blvd.
Ste 1800
Philadelphia, PA 19103-2899

PRINCIPLES OF CARDIOVASCULAR RADIOLOGY   ISBN: 978-1-4377-0405-1

Notice

Knowledge and best practice in this field are constantly changing. As new research and experience broaden our understanding, changes in research methods, professional practices, or medical treatment may become necessary.

Practitioners and researchers must always rely on their own experience and knowledge in evaluating and using any information, methods, compounds, or experiments described herein. In using such information or methods they should be mindful of their own safety and the safety of others, including parties for whom they have a professional responsibility.

With respect to any drug or pharmaceutical products identified, readers are advised to check the most current information provided (i) on procedures featured or (ii) by the manufacturer of each product to be administered, to verify the recommended dose or formula, the method and duration of administration, and contraindications. It is the responsibility of practitioners, relying on their own experience and knowledge of their patients, to make diagnoses, to determine dosages and the best treatment for each individual patient, and to take all appropriate safety precautions.

To the fullest extent of the law, neither the Publisher nor the authors, contributors, or editors, assume any liability for any injury and/or damage to persons or property as a matter of products liability, negligence or otherwise, or from any use or operation of any methods, products, instructions, or ideas contained in the material herein.

Library of Congress Cataloging-in-Publication Data

Hutchison, Stuart J.
 Principles of cardiovascular radiology / Stuart J. Hutchison.—1st ed.
   p. ; cm.
 Includes index.
 ISBN 978-1-4377-0405-1 (pbk. : alk. paper)
 1. Heart—Imaging—Handbooks, manuals, etc. 2. Heart—Diseases—Diagnosis—
 Handbooks, manuals, etc. I. Title.
   [DNLM: 1. Cardiovascular Diseases—radiography—Handbooks. 2. Radiography,
 Thoracic—methods—Handbooks. WG 39]
   RC683.5.I42H88 2011
   616.1'0757—dc22   2011013110

Acquisitions Editor: Natasha Andjelkovic
Editorial Assistant: Bradley McIlwain
Publishing Services Manager: Pat Joiner-Myers
Project Manager: Marlene Weeks
Design Direction: Steven Stave

Printed in China.

Last digit is the print number: 9 8 7 6 5 4 3 2 1

To my Liam James, Noel Keith, and Cindy. Your gifts of love, time, and belief can only ever be repaid in kind.

Good readers are almost as rare as good authors.

William Heberden
(1710–1801)

PREFACE

Despite continuing advances in cardiovascular imaging technology, the chest radiograph rightly retains its place as a key cardiac diagnostic tool and as a simple means of following disease progression and treatment effect. Over the 2 decades since writing the original handbook version of this text, it has been my impression that proficiency with the chest radiograph has not withstood the test of time well and has suffered under the distraction of other newer forms of imaging.

The chest radiograph yields clinically useful information in the management of many patients and may often yield clinically unsuspected information. The incremental information provided by the radiographic depiction of the pulmonary parenchyma and pleura to that of clinical assessment is highly relevant and contributory toward the optimal assessment and management of the cardiology patient population.

In writing this book to encourage development during cardiology fellow training, my goal was threefold:

1. To provide a systematic approach to the review of frontal and lateral chest radiographs
2. To foster an appreciation of radiographic signs of disease
3. To impart an awareness of the typical radiographic findings of common and interesting acquired and congenital cardiovascular diseases

As well, I wanted to maintain the practical nature of the handbook on which this book is based while integrating some intriguing and unusual topics for the sake of interest. The origin of the handbook was my set of study notes from when I was a resident in training, a short 2 decades ago. I initially wrote a set of notes so as to not lose track of the many "pearls" that I had been taught while in training, and therein is the intended spirit of the book—the development, especially of cardiology trainees, and, I hope as well, of other trainees and of those in established practice in the care of patients with cardiovascular disease.

ACKNOWLEDGMENTS

To my former mentors and colleagues at McGill University, especially Jim Stewart, MD, whose disciplined clinical excellence and proficiency with the chest radiograph were inspiring examples of insight into disease, clinical reasoning, and the utility of diagnostic imaging in clinical medicine, and John H. Burgess, MD, whose superb clinical acumen, alacrity, and analytical approach were as inspiring. I am indebted to both of them for their openness and generosity in communicating their knowledge, their encouragement, and as well for their wonderful example as physicians that set the standard that I sought to live up to.

WITH SINCERE APPRECIATION

Abdulelah al-Mobeirek, MD; Nanette Alvarez, MD; Natasha Andjelkovic, PhD; Jehangir Appoo, MD; Graham Boag, MD; John H. Burgess, MD; Patrick Champagne, MD; Kanu Chatterjeee, MD; Anson Cheung, MD; Robert J. Chisholm, MD; Paul Chong, MD; Michael S. Connelly, MD; Frank Dicke, MD; Tracy Elliot, MD; Bahaa Fadel, MD; Marie Faughnan, MD; Jason Field; Bryan Har, MD; Joyce Harder, MD; Eric Herget, MD; Ross Hill, MD; Eric Horlick, MD; Jonathon Howlett, MD; Michael Kanakos, MD; Bruce Klanke; Anne Lennehan; Vince Lo, BSc, PT; Carmen Lydell, MD; J. H. MacGregor, MD; Brad McIlwain; Naeem Merchant, MD; Juan-Carlos Monge, MD; David Patton, MD; Susan Pioli; Bill Parmley, MD; Tim Prieur, MD; Mark Rabinovitch, MD; Myra Rudakewich, MSc; Rob Sevick, MD; Gordon Snell; James A. Stewart, MD; Glen Summer, MD; Inga Tomas; John Webb, MD; Joel Wolkowicz, MD; Jason Wong, MD; and Sayeh Zielke, MBA, MD.

Stuart J. Hutchison, MD, FRCPC, FARC, FAHA

CONTENTS

First Things First

General points to uphold in the approach to the chest radiograph, before reviewing the film for cardiovascular detail, include the following:
■ Review the indication for the radiograph
· ■ Avoid cases of mistaken identity. Confirm the identity of the patient.
■ The accuracy of the conclusions is based on the quality of the radiograph.
  ■ Was the inspiration adequate?
  ■ Was the patient well centered? If the patient's body was significantly rotated, be wary of interpreting mediastinal contours that would be projected differently.
  ■ Was the penetration/exposure optimal for the purposes of examining the heart? If it was not optimal, adjust the windowing as needed to review the heart, devices within the heart, the aorta, and the lungs.
■ When possible, review serial chest radiographs.

INDICATIONS FOR CHEST RADIOGRAPHY

Chest radiography is indicated for all patients admitted to hospital because of a cardiovascular diagnosis and can arguably be said to be indicated at the initial assessment of all outpatients evaluated for suspected cardiovascular diagnoses. The ability of the chest radiograph to estimate heart size, image pulmonary vascular and aortic findings, lung parenchymal and pleural disease, and chest wall pathology contributes to the management of cardiovascular disease patients with many diagnoses such as the following:
❏ Coronary artery disease
❏ Congestive heart failure
❏ Valvular heart diseases
❏ Prosthetic heart valves
❏ Myopathic diseases
❏ Pericardial diseases
❏ Aortic diseases
❏ Hypertension
❏ Congenital heart and vascular diseases
❏ Chest pain syndromes
❏ Post–cardiovascular surgery
❏ Post–thoracic aortic endografting
❏ Suspected cardiovascular trauma

Additional reasons to perform chest radiography at initial assessment include the relatively high frequency of pulmonary disease in the adult cardiovascular patient and the ability of the chest radiograph to image some of these forms of pathology. Adverse change in clinical status and need to assess treatment effect should also prompt chest radiography. Hence, a liberal strategy for the use of chest radiography is appropriate because, in general, the modality is often underused; thus proficiency with its use and interpretation (outside of radiology) is often suboptimal.

Review of the indication for imaging helps establish an approach and awareness of various possible complications or associations.

Standard chest radiography includes a frontal (posteroanterior [PA]) radiograph and a lateral radiograph. The frontal radiograph is taken with the patient's back toward the incident x-rays to minimize the amplification of the size of the heart shadow. The two radiographs are complementary and confirmatory to each other. To have PA and lateral radiographs taken, the patient must be able to stand or lean against a screen with his or her arms abducted. PA and lateral radiographs are taken in radiology facilities. It is not possible to routinely take high-quality PA and lateral radiographs with portable x-ray equipment. The quality and amount of information offered by PA and lateral radiographs make them more useful than portable radiographs, and they are far and away the first choice whenever possible. Therefore chest radiography should include PA and lateral radiographs, except for critically ill, unstable, or suspected unstable patients.

Portable radiographs are taken with the patient sitting in bed (preferable) or lying in bed (often the only option for critically ill patients) with the radiograph plate behind the patient's back. The x-ray–generating equipment is facing the patient, either at the foot of the bed or over the bed; hence, the incident x-ray beams enter the patient in an anteroposterior (AP) fashion. Consequently, the size of the heart shadow is exaggerated. Sicker patients who have portable AP radiographs, rather than standard PA and lateral radiographs, are often unable to take a deep breath or sit erect (or even upright), which alters many factors such as alignment/projection and the lung volume/ratio of the heart size to the chest width. Hence, the technical quality of portable x-rays is usually far lower than that of standard radiographs for a combination of reasons. Nonetheless, portable chest radiographs are extremely useful for verification of chest tube and catheter placement and for following the clinical course of pulmonary edema, pulmonary parenchymal diseases, and pleural effusions.

AVOID CASES OF MISTAKEN IDENTITY: CONFIRM THE IDENTITY OF THE PATIENT AND THE RADIOGRAPH

With the advent of flat panel digital radiography came improvement in image speed of access, quality, and organization of radiographic image archiving. Digital archiving/networking systems have greatly reduced the frequency of cases of mistaken identity that arose in the radiograph-based era where a film could have been left in the wrong folder and been associated with the wrong time, date, or patient.

When reviewing a radiograph, whether digital or film, the identity of the radiograph and the patient needs to be confirmed, and the technical adequacy of the radiographs needs to be assured. Therefore, it is mandatory to confirm that the PA and lateral radiographs being reviewed have the correct information for each of the following:
- Patient name
- Patient hospital ID number/code
- Date
- Time

THE ACCURACY OF THE CONCLUSIONS IS BASED ON THE QUALITY OF THE RADIOGRAPH

Was the Inspiration Adequate?
An inadequate inspiration results in a chest radiograph with higher diaphragms, a wider carinal angle, an exaggerated cardiopericardial silhouette (CPS)-to-chest ratio, and less aerated lungs with more visible markings. Standard cardiac and pulmonary radiographic criteria are predicated on normal ("adequate") inspiration (Fig. 1-1). To determine adequacy, find the anterior end of the first thoracic rib (just below the medial ends of the clavicles). The right diaphragm should be at, or below, the level of the anterior end of the sixth rib, and at, or below, the level of the posterior end of the tenth rib.

Was the Patient Well Centered?
Failure to achieve optimal centering will result in the heart not being viewed in the usual PA or AP projection, and consequently the three-dimensionally complex heart, as well as its complex vascular pedicle, will have nonstandard and, therefore, difficult to understand, silhouettes (Fig. 1-2).

Posteroanterior Chest Radiograph
Was the patient well centered (not rotated)? Standard chest position is indicated by alignment of posterior and anterior chest structures. To determine this, place your thumbs on the medial ends of the clavicles; the midline spinous vertebral processes should appear in the middle, centered between your thumbs. Unless there is a deviation of the trachea caused by displacement or traction by thoracic structures, the tracheal air column should also appear centered over the midline spinous vertebral processes (between your thumbs). Rotation of the head alone may also occur, projecting the upper tracheal air column to the side, but not the lower part of the air column or the clavicular heads asymmetrically to the spinous processes (Graphic 1-1; Figs. 1-3 and 1-4).

Lateral Chest Radiograph
Rotation is suggested by asymmetric projection of ribs posterior to the spine.

Was the Penetration/Exposure Optimal?
For cardiovascular purposes, adequate exposure reveals detail of the lungs and some detail of the lungs and some detail of the thoracic vertebrae.

The Electrocardiogram and Other Surface Leads
Electrocardiographic leads are often present on cardiac patients undergoing chest radiography. If they are grouped over the heart, it facilitates interpretation of pulmonary and pleural disease findings. However, it can make understanding the course of endocardial pacer wires and catheters within the heart complex and sometimes ambiguous, and it may partially obscure valve prostheses (Fig. 1-5).

WHEN POSSIBLE, REVIEW SERIAL CHEST RADIOGRAPHS

When reviewing a patient's chest radiograph, try to obtain and review at least the previous set of radiographs, and, if possible, the admission and preadmission radiography history. In sequence, compare the frontal and then the lateral radiographs. There are at least two reasons to compare current radiographs with previous radiographs:
1. Disease progression and treatment effect may be appreciated.
2. What may be subtle and missed on one chest radiograph may have been more apparent (because of a chance difference in technique) on another (Fig. 1-6).

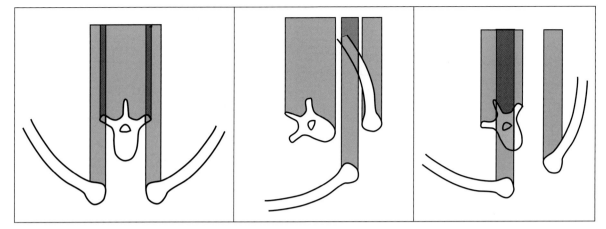

Graphic 1-1. Rotation as seen on a frontal chest radiograph. *Left schematic:* The projection of the heads of the clavicles is symmetrical with respect to that of the vertebral column—correct/optimal alignment. *Middle and right schematics:* Differing degrees of rotatation, denoted by nonsymmetric projection of the clavicle heads with respect to the vertebral column.

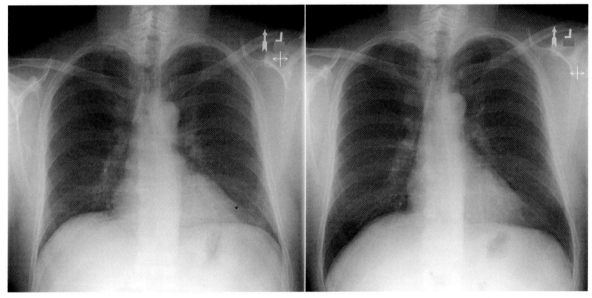

Figure 1-1. Differing depths of inspiration and the perception of heart size on the posteroanterior (PA) chest radiograph. With an average depth of inspiration (*left*), the heart appears to be borderline dilated. With a deep inspiration (*right*), the heart size is more convincingly normal. With the deeper inspiration, the heart is falling more steeply down the diaphragm (as the diaphragm has steepened) and has rotated clockwise (posteriorly) into the chest, reducing the PA silhouette.

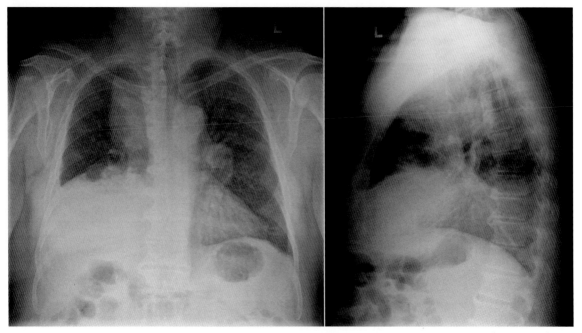

Figure 1-2. The right hemidiaphragm is markedly elevated, due to paralysis resulting from phrenic nerve disruption from bronchogenic carcinoma. The cardiopericardial silhouette is incompletely defined; with this limited and suboptimal visualization of the heart, conclusions about the heart should also be limited.

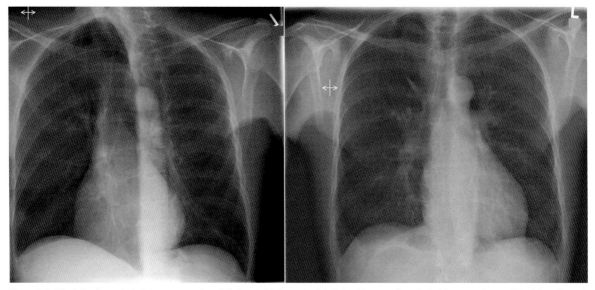

Figure 1-3. The left radiograph depicts severe rotation of the heart with the patient's left shoulder away from the incident x-ray beams. The right radiograph has correct alignment. As the projection of the heart rotates, the contours of the cardiopericardial silhouette and the appearance of the pulmonary vasculature alter.

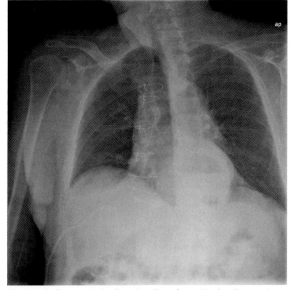

Figure 1-4. Severe rotation (intentionally performed to view the percutaneous drain into a liver abscess) markedly alters the appearance of the heart and the mediastinum. Note the hiatus hernia with an air-fluid level.

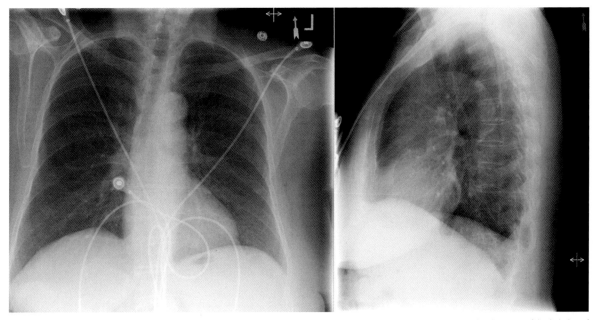

Figure 1-5. On the posteroanterior chest radiograph, coils of the electrocardiogram leads have been laid over the heart, to the detriment of the imaging of the heart itself.

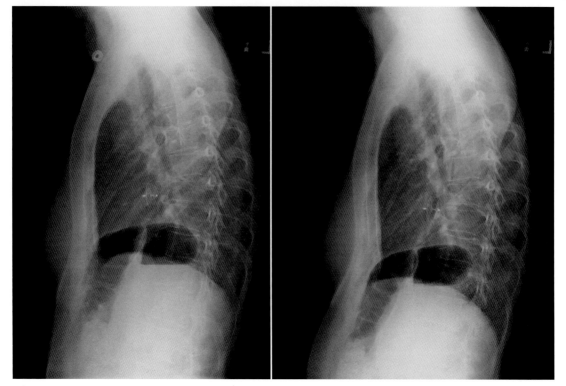

Figure 1-6. Lateral chest radiographs of a patient with an atrial septal defect occluder device. The phalanges of the device are fairly well seen nearly on the left film and, due to a small difference of alignment, almost perfectly tangentially seen on the right film, simplifying the recognition.

The Frontal Chest Radiograph

CARDIOVASCULAR SILHOUETTES

Cardiovascular structures that are visible on the chest radiograph owe their visibility to being bordered by air-inflated lung. The difference in radiographic attenuation of aerated lung versus the cardiac or vascular structure results in an often very well-defined visually apparent boundary. The greater the attenuation difference of the two tissues that form an interface, the greater the radiographic definition of the interface and the greater the clarity and distinction of the silhouette. Hence, the border of a cardiac chamber against lung is readily apparent. Such a margin of a cardiac or vascular structure is referred to as "border forming" and results in a silhouette, many of which are recognizable. Think of Alfred Hitchcock, whose unique silhouette became his logo.

Conversely, if the other walls of the cardiac chamber are adjacent to other cardiac chambers of equal attenuation, then the boundary of the two cannot be determined by the chest radiograph. Hence, non–border-forming regions of the heart are inapparent radiographically. Alternative imaging modalities, particularly the tomographic ones (echocardiography, computed tomography, and magnetic resonance imaging), are the most reliable means of measuring true chamber dimensions.

Accumulation of high attenuation tissue adjacent to the heart (consolidated lung, pleural effusion, intrathoracic mass) results in loss of silhouettes and their usefulness as signs.

It is through the understanding of which cardiac or vascular structure is responsible for which specific silhouette curves on the chest radiograph that one achieves an understanding of which cardiac or vascular structure is enlarged or displaced and therefore causing the curvature. Hence, a comprehensive understanding of which cardiac or vascular structure is enlarged or displaced and therefore causing the curvature is an essential prerequisite to reading and understanding chest radiographs, because interpretation of the chest radiograph is based on silhouette recognition. Although silhouette recognition as a means of identification can never be as obvious and accurate as having full tomographic rendering, it is surprisingly useful, and more rapidly and widely available than tomographic methods such as echocardiography, cardiac MRI, or cardiac CT.

Normal Right-Sided Silhouettes
From superior to inferior, the silhouettes are (Graphic 2-1; Fig. 2-1) as follows:

❒ **Superior vena cava:** The superior vena cava normally forms most of the right superior border of the cardiovascular structures in the chest.
❒ **Azygous arch:** The distal arch of the azygous vein, where it arches anteriorly at and over the right tracheobronchial angle, is often behind the superior vena cava and, unless enlarged, is not readily visible in normal patients (see Graphic 2-1). Normally, it is less than 1.0 cm in size with the patient standing, and less than 1.3 cm in size with the patient supine. The size of the azygous vein is determined by the central venous pressure. In 5% of the population, the azygous vein resides more laterally and superiorly in the azygous fissure.
❒ **Right pulmonary artery:** The diverging right pulmonary artery crosses the border formed by the superior vena cava.
❒ **Right pulmonary veins:** The converging right pulmonary veins are inferior to the right pulmonary arteries.
❒ **Right atrium:** The right atrium normally forms a well defined border and appears as a gentle, nearly flat curve. Most of the right inferior border of the cardiopericardial silhouette (CPS) is formed by the right atrium.

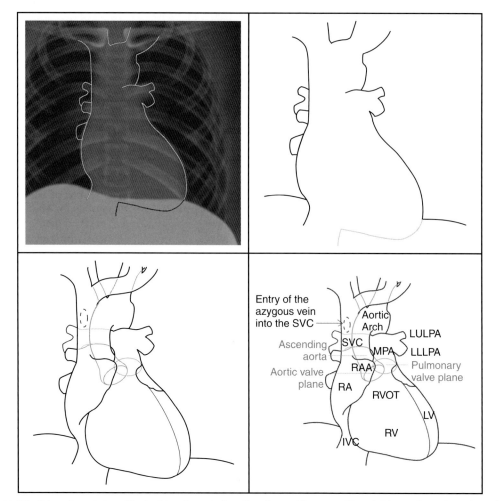

Graphic 2-1. Schematic renderings of the frontal cardiac projection silhouettes, and the responsible underlying cardiac and vascular anatomy.

❐ **Inferior vena cava:** A small portion of the inferior vena cava is usually revealed on the frontal radiograph, but generally only with deep inspiration.

❐ **Right cardiophrenic junction** (where the cardiac silhouette joins the diaphragmatic silhouette): This may be formed by either the inferior vena cava, or, more commonly, by a fat pad.

Normal Left-Sided Silhouettes

From superior to inferior, the silhouettes are (see Graphic 2-1) as follows:

❐ **Left subclavian artery:** The left subclavian artery forms the border of the left superior mediastinum as seen on the chest radiograph. The curve should be gentle and gradual. If the left subclavian artery has an exaggerated curve, underlying possibilities include elongation/dilation from hypertension, from hypertension secondary to coarctation of the aorta, and atherosclerosis. If the contour in the vicinity of the left subclavian artery is more vertical and straight than usual, then persistence of a left superior vena cava is likely.

❐ **Aortic "knob":** The "knob" of the aorta is a term that refers to the distal aortic arch/proximal descending aorta that resides below the left subclavian artery. The term is obviously a misnomer because there is not normally a protruding "knob" to the aorta, but the term is forgivingly used. This silhouette is visible on every normal chest radiograph. The normal diameter of the aorta averages 2 cm in this region but may be up to 3 cm in larger individuals. The trachea is mildly displaced to the right side by the arch of the aorta. A small bump or nipple is evident on the lateral aspect of the aortic "knob" in a minority of patients; this is caused by the left superior intercostal vein. Prominence of this vein results from elevated central venous pressure (Graphic 2-2).

❐ **Aortic pulmonary window:** Beneath the aortic "knob," and above the pulmonary artery, there is normally an abrupt indentation with the inferior margin aorta forming the upper border and the superior margin of the pulmonary artery forming the lower border. Within this space (the aorticopulmonary window), multiple important structures reside—the ductus/ligamentum arteriosus, the left recurrent

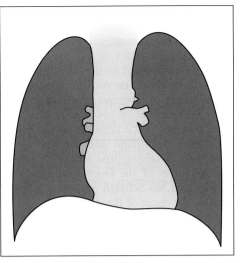

Graphic 2-2. The location of the left superior intercostal vein may be apparent on a frontal radiograph as a nipple-shaped silhouette on the lateral aspect of the aortic arch.

laryngeal nerve, and the ductus lymph node(s), as well as fat. Compromise of this space (by enlargement of the aorta, the left atrium lymph nodes, or a ductal diverticulum) may result in compression of the left recurrent laryngeal nerve. Aerated lung between the aortic arch and main pulmonary artery is a sign of absence of the pericardium.

❒ **Main pulmonary artery:** Inferior to the aortico-pulmonary window is the main pulmonary artery, which is well-defined against the left lung. The main pulmonary artery arches over the left main bronchus, slightly above the level of the left pulmonary artery bifurcation. Normally, the silhouette of the left side of the main pulmonary artery is slightly convex.

❒ **Left atrial appendage:** On the frontal radiograph, the only portion of the left atrium that can normally be seen is a small portion of the left atrial appendage. The appendage lies under the main pulmonary artery and above the CPS border formed by the left ventricle. Normally, the curvature of the appendage is mildly concave, because it is normally nearly empty (Fig. 2-2). Straightening or bulging of the left atrial appendage silhouette strongly suggests left atrial enlargement/dilation but also may be caused by the presence of mass lesions.

❒ **Left ventricle (LV):** Most of the left border of the heart is normally formed by the left ventricle, although only 10% of the frontal CPS area is normally occupied by the left ventricle. The left ventricular border runs as a smooth continuation of the border formed by the left atrial appendage. Lengthening of the left ventricular border is consistent with lengthening of the left ventricle, a sign of enlargement.

❒ **Left cardiophrenic junction** (where the cardiac silhouette joins the diaphragmatic silhouette) is usually formed by the left ventricle and is less commonly formed by a fat pad (Fig. 2-3).

Normal Non–Border-Forming Structures on the Frontal Chest Radiograph

❒ **Right ventricle:** The right ventricle is not CPS border-forming on the frontal chest radiograph, although it typically occupies 70% of the anterior projection of the heart.

❒ **Left atrial body (left atrial appendage excluded):** The body of the left atrium is posterior and therefore does not form an edge border of the CPS, but it is evident in most individuals as a silhouette medial to the right atrial border. The reason that the left atrium forms a silhouette separate from the right atrial silhouette is that both structures abut lung tissue, with the left atrium lying posteriorly and superiorly, and the right atrium lying laterally, anteriorly, and inferiorly, as each atrium protrudes separately posteriorly in a slightly bulbous fashion.

❒ **Ascending aorta:** Normally, the lateral border of the ascending aorta lies medially to the lateral border of the superior vena cava, and is therefore not radiographically apparent. When the root and/or ascending aorta dilate, however, they may assume the lateral border and overlay the right hilum, obscuring it. This is an important sign of ascending aortic enlargement.

SIGNS OF CARDIAC CHAMBER ENLARGEMENT ON THE FRONTAL CHEST RADIOGRAPH

The following discussion about particular radiographic signs and their association with specific chamber enlargement is predicated on enlargement of solely or primarily one chamber or structure. When any chamber enlarges substantially, the position, orientation, and radiographic appearance of the other chambers, and even blood vessels, may be altered. Hence, displacement of a cardiac border does not necessarily imply enlargement of the adjacent chamber. When more than one cardiac chamber enlarges substantially, the positions and orientations of all of the cardiac chambers may become altered in a more complex fashion. Many forms of heart disease, particularly valvular and myopathic, result in multi-chamber enlargement.

Consider the case of right heart enlargement from an atrial septal defect. Enlargement of the right ventricle rotates the heart to the left (when viewed from the patient's head), causing the aortic arch to fold on itself (looking smaller on the frontal chest radiograph) and the main pulmonary trunk to rotate and appear more prominent. The enlarged right ventricle may actually assume the left heart border (which is normally formed by the left ventricle).

When assessing the chest radiograph for signs of chamber enlargement, another consideration is that chest cavity configuration may play into the

CARDIAC VALVES, VALVE PROSTHESES, AND ANNULI

Identifying a Valve or Prosthesis on the Frontal Chest Radiograph

On the PA chest radiograph, the aortic valve is projected onto the left border of the vertebral column (Graphic 2-8), and calcified aortic valve cusps may therefore be obscured by their projection onto the normally dense vertebral calcification. Calcification of the aortic valve is commonly associated with stenosis of the valve. The plane of the aortic valve is such that the valve or prosthesis is seen largely edge-on on the frontal chest radiograph. An aortic valve prosthesis with radiopaque components is often visible on the frontal chest radiograph but may be lost in the CPS shadow or the vertebral column shadow.

On the PA chest radiograph, the mitral valve is projected more inferiorly and more vertically (than the aortic valve), toward the patient's left, and is often partially (but seldom completely) obscured by the spine (and opaque CPS) unless the mitral valve calcification is uncommonly dense. The plane of the mitral orifice is such that the valve is seen face-on (en-face) in the frontal chest radiograph. It is more common for calcification to occur within the mitral annulus than within the mitral valve leaflets themselves. Mitral annular calcification (submitral calcification) is often visible to the left of the patient's spine and is seen as a reverse **C**. It is commonly associated with mild-to-moderate mitral insufficiency but only rarely with significant or severe mitral stenosis. Insertion of a mitral prosthesis into a heavily calcified mitral annulus is technically difficult. See Chapters 9 through 11 for further discussion of mechanical prosthetic valves, bioprosthetic valves, and annuloplasty rings.

"DOUBLE CONTOURS" ON THE FRONTAL CHEST RADIOGRAPH

Double contours may be seen on either the right or left sides of the CPS and are generally indicative of chamber enlargement (Fig. 2-6).

Causes of Right-Sided "Double Contours"

Causes (see Graphic 2-7) include the following:
- Superior ascending aorta (usually the upper border)
- Right ventricle (rare)
- Left atrium, normal-sized or enlarged (usually the lower border)
- Right atrium (usually the lower border)
- Right atrial appendage enlargement (very rare) usually upper border
- Inferior right pulmonary vein confluence (usually the lower border)
- Pulmonary venous varix (usually the upper border)
- Anomalous pulmonary venous return
- Pericardial cysts (usually the lower border)
- Mediastinal adenopathy
- Esophageal dilation
- Mass
- Enlarged azygous vein

Bulge on the Left Superior Cardiopericardial Silhouette (Graphic 2-9): Differential

The differential diagnosis includes the following:
- Left atrial appendage
- Main pulmonary artery
- Partial absence of the left pericardium
- Right ventricular outflow tract in the presence of valvular pulmonary stenosis or shunt
- Localized hypertrophy from hypertrophic cardiomyopathy

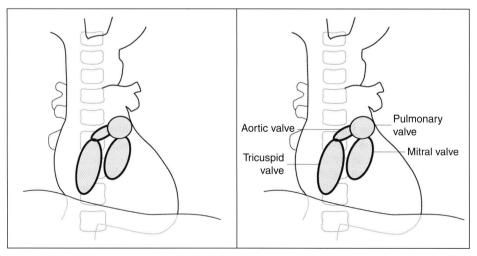

Graphic 2-8. The location of the different valve planes on the frontal projection.

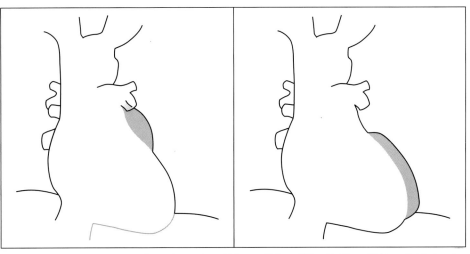

Graphic 2-9. Posteroanterior graphic representations of left upper (*left graphic*) and left lower (*right graphic*) "bulges."

- ❑ "L-transposition," or transposition of the great arteries
- ❑ Juxtaposed (on the left side) atrial appendages
- ❑ Left ventricular aneurysm
- ❑ Tumor or cyst
- ❑ Aneurysm of the left circumflex artery
- ❑ Saphenous vein bypass graft aneurysm
- ❑ Lymphadenopathy

Bulge on the Left Lower Cardiopericardial Silhouette (see Graphic 2-9): Differential

The differential diagnosis includes the following:
- ❑ Left ventricular aneurysm
- ❑ Left ventricular false aneurysm
- ❑ Left ventricular tumor
- ❑ Pericardial cyst or tumor
- ❑ Left ventricular diverticulum
- ❑ Mediastinal/lung tumor

EVIDENCE OF PRIOR THORACIC SURGERY

To establish the likelihood of previous surgery, look for incisions, clips and wires, and other surgical or post-surgical findings. The type of incision and findings may suggest or prove the type of surgery.

Right-Sided Thoracotomy

A right thoracotomy was formerly a common surgical approach to repair an atrial septal defect or to con-struct a Blalock-Taussig shunt. It was occasionally used to perform a mitral valve commissurotomy. The radiographic signs of a right thoracotomy include an absent right third rib and axillary edema (soft tissue thickening in the axilla).

Left-Sided Thoracotomy

A left thoracotomy was formerly a common surgical approach to perform a mitral valve commissurotomy or perform other mitral valve surgery. It is still occasionally used for mitral surgery. Other operations performed through a left thoracotomy include repair of the descending aorta (including aortic coarctation), patent ductus arteriosus ligation, and creation of a left-sided Blalock-Taussig shunt.

Median Sternotomy

The single most common reason to perform a median sternotomy is coronary artery bypass grafting (85%). The second most common reason is valve surgery (10%), of which nearly all is currently performed through a median sternotomy. Repair of congenital cardiac lesions, repairs of the aortic, root (aortic root/ascending aneurysm repair, dissection repair), heart and lung transplants, and pericardial surgery (other than subxiphoid approach windows) are also generally performed through a median sternotomy.

Transverse Sternotomy

A transverse sternotomy is occasionally used to per-form pericardiectomy or lung transplant.

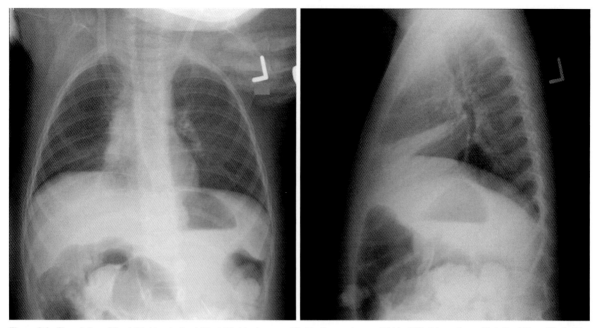

Figure 2-1. The relation of the right atrium to the right middle lobe is exemplified by the syndrome of right middle lobe collapse. Note the "silhouetting" of the right (atrial) heart border on the frontal radiograph and the triangular-shaped opacity on the lateral radiograph.

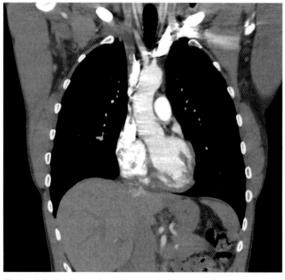

Figure 2-2. Contrast-enhanced computed tomography scan, coronal image approximately at the plane corresponding to the posteroanterior chest radiograph. The structures that generate the left mediastinum and left heart border silhouettes are apparent (from superior to inferior) as follows:
- Left subclavian artery (note the excess contrast effect and the artifacts arising from injection into a left arm vein)
- Distal aorta ("knob")
- Main pulmonary artery
- Left atrial appendage (more obvious in this case than usual)
- Left ventricular lateral anterolateral wall

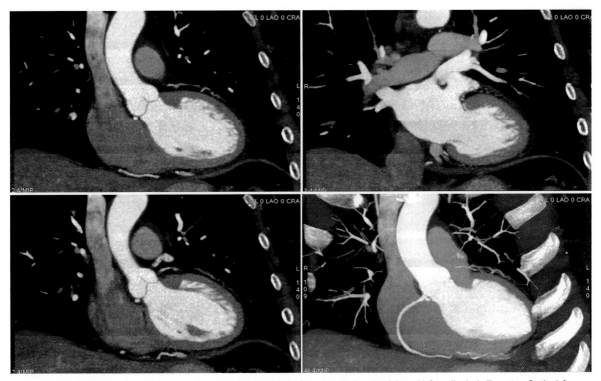

Figure 2-3. Coronal computed tomography scans revealing the right and left heart as well as the right and left mediastinal silhouettes. On the left upper image, the superior vena cava and right atrial contributions to the right-sided silhouettes are apparent, as are the aortic arch, main pulmonary artery, and left ventricle along the left heart border. The slight indentation of the left heart border at the angle between the main pulmonary artery and the left ventricle is also apparent. On the left lower image, on a slightly deeper plane, (part of) the left atrial appendage is normally present between the main pulmonary artery and the left ventricular anterolateral wall. On the right upper image, on yet a deeper plane, the body as well as the tail of the appendage can be seen, under the left upper pulmonary vein, now deep to the pulmonary artery. As well, the supradiaphragmatic portion of the inferior vena cava is also visible, now deep to the right atrial freewall. On the right lower image (thick maximum intensity projection view), the right coronary artery is seen, yielding the discrimination of the right atrium and right ventricle on the frontal plane image.

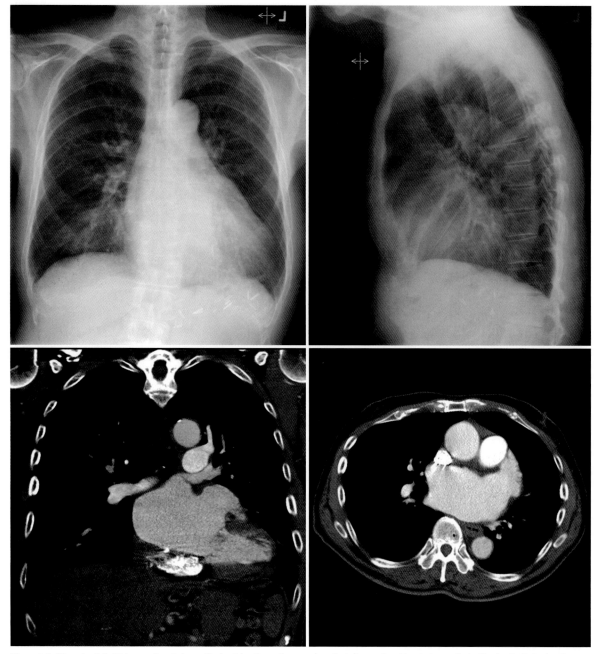

Figure 2-4.   There is a left atrial appendage bulge on the frontal radiograph, seen along the left upper heart border in a patient with mixed mitral valve disease. The contrast-enhanced computed tomography scan delineates the extent of the bulging of the left atrial appendage superiorly and laterally beyond that of the main pulmonary artery and the left ventricular border.

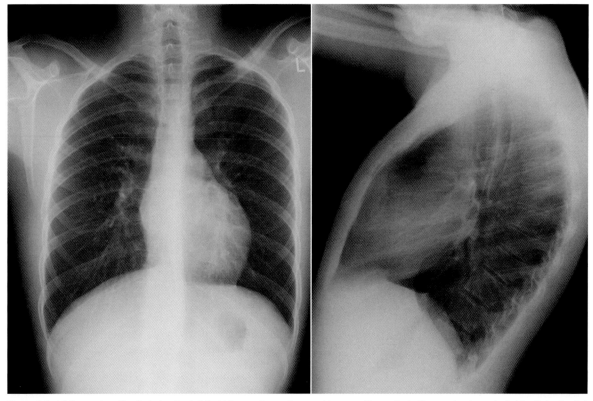

Figure 2-5. A left upper heart border bulge due to left atrial appendage enlargement is present in a patient with a previously repaired cleft mitral valve that exhibited 3+ mitral regurgitation, resulting in left atrial dilation, manifested on the chest radiographs as a left atrial appendage bulge, a double right heart border, and a posteriorly displaced left atrial contour.

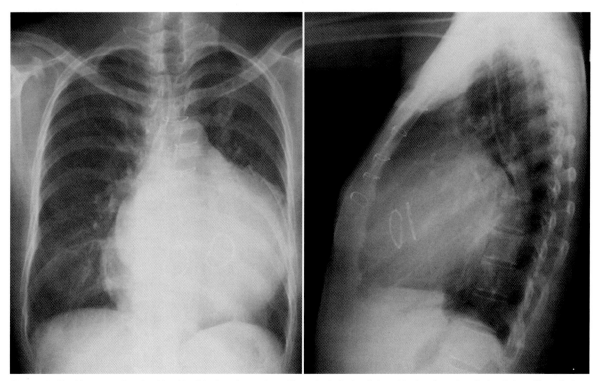

Figure 2-6. "Double contours" on the right side of the heart in a patient with repaired mitral and tricuspid valves (note the mitral and tricuspid annuloplasty rings), in addition to enlargement of the left and right atria. The upper shadow results from left atrial dilation, and the lower shadow results from right atrial dilation.

The Lateral Chest Radiograph

3

Key Points

- The lateral chest radiograph is particularly useful for the recognition of specific chamber enlargement (other than that of the right atrium) for the recognition of the valve prostheses and rings as they are projected away from the spine. Protheses and rings themselves, as well as their location and orientation, are more apparent than on the frontal radiograph, as are pleural effusions, and left lower lobe disease.
- The normal anterior and posterior border silhouettes of the heart should be familiar.

CARDIOVASCULAR SILHOUETTES ON THE LATERAL CHEST RADIOGRAPH

As with the frontal chest radiograph, it is important to be familiar with the silhouettes of the cardiopericardial silhouettes (CPS) and major vascular structures on the lateral chest radiograph. Although often ignored, the lateral chest radiograph is particularly useful for valve localization and for the left and right ventricular chamber size assessment (Graphic 3-1).

Normal Anterior Border Silhouettes

In some patients, the anterior border of the right brachiocephalic vein and superior vena cava are visible (from superior to inferior) as the first silhouette on the lateral radiograph.

- **Ascending aorta:** The anterior border of the ascending aorta is usually the first anterior silhouette on the lateral chest radiograph. However, it usually presents as a vague image because of mediastinal fat obscuring the silhouette. The arch of the aorta is usually well defined except where there are adjacent blood vessels (branch vessels and the great veins).
- **Main pulmonary artery:** A small segment of the anterior border of the main pulmonary artery above the pulmonic valve is visible as a less vertically oriented silhouette. It is not normally against the sternum. As with the ascending aorta, it is usually a vague image because of mediastinal fat obscuring the silhouette.
- **The right ventricular outflow tract:** The anterior border of the right ventricular outflow tract is seen as an inferior continuation of the pulmonary artery. The tract and the pulmonary artery cannot be radiographically distinguished.

- **The right ventricle:** The anterior portion of the right ventricle is the lowermost portion of the anterior border of the CPS. Normally, most of it is in contact with the sternum. It is for this reason that sternal and parasternal injury commonly results in right ventricular injury.

Normal Posterior Border Silhouettes

From superior to inferior, the normal silhouettes are as follows:

- **Aortic arch:** The posterior border of the arch of the aorta (outside curvature), and often the arch itself, is visible arcing posteriorly and inferiorly. The inside border is seldom visible.
- **Left pulmonary artery:** The distal portion of the main pulmonary artery and the left pulmonary artery are visible under the aorta.
- **Left atrium:** The posterosuperior and posterior borders of the left atrium form the majority of the posterior border of the CPS.
- **Left ventricle:** The normal basal posterior left ventricle may be seen as an oblique silhouette under the left atrium but does not normally project far behind the inferior vena cava. Note that the posterior border of the inferior vena cava and right atrium may be uncovered with a deep inspiration.

"Narrow anteroposterior diameter" fulfills both of the following criteria:

- Lateral chest radiograph: Measure from the posterior surface of the sternum to the anteriormost border of a thoracic vertebra. The normal dimension is greater than 8.0 cm (Fig. 3-1).
- Frontal chest radiograph: The ratio of the transverse diameter on frontal CXR to the anteroposterior diameter (as mentioned previously) is greater than 2.7.

SIGNS OF CARDIAC CHAMBER ENLARGEMENT ON THE LATERAL CHEST RADIOGRAPH

Enlargement of the Left Atrium

The normal left atrial posterior border is formed by pulmonary veins entering into segments of atrial wall and does not have a smooth and regular contour. For this reason, the normal left atrium is vaguely

20

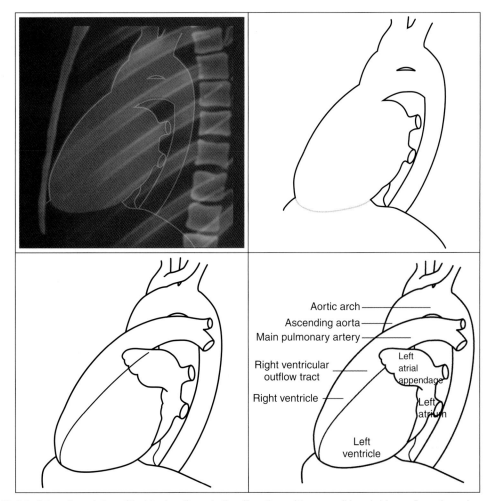

Graphic 3-1. Schematic renderings of the lateral cardiac projection silhouettes and the responsible underlying cardiac and vascular anatomy.

Aortic arch
Ascending aorta
Main pulmonary artery
Right ventricular outflow tract
Right ventricle
Left atrial appendage
Left atrium
Left ventricle

defined on the lateral chest radiograph (Fig. 3-2). An enlarged left atrium forms a more evenly rounded and smooth border and is more clearly seen on the radiograph (Graphic 3-2).

Posterior and superior displacement of the left atrium can be easily seen on the lateral chest radiograph. Be attentive for the presence of rotation of the chest (apparent because of projection of ribs posterior to the spine), which may project the left atrium to appear more posterior than it is, falsely suggesting enlargement.

Left atrial size can be measured on the lateral chest radiograph. To do this, distinct visualization of the anterior border of the right pulmonary artery is required. Measure from that border to the most posterior contour of the left atrium, as seen on the lateral chest radiograph or a barium esophagram (normal, <3.5 cm). This measurement is seldom used.

Enlargement of the Left Ventricle
(see Graphic 3-2)
The left ventricular posterior border is usually well defined because it abuts on lung and forms a "clean"

radiographic interface. The left ventricle generally enlarges laterally, inferiorly, and posteriorly. Only posterior enlargement is appreciated on a lateral chest radiograph. The degree of posterior enlargement is assessed using the relationship of the inferior vena cava (IVC) to the posterior left ventricular silhouette, known as the rule of Rigler (Graphic 3-3).

On a true lateral radiograph with deep inspiration the following details should be identified:
❑ Identify the supradiaphragmatic portion of the IVC by looking for the right hemidiaphragm.
❑ Identify the posterior border of the left ventricle.

At a height of 2 cm above the diaphragm, the posterior border of the left ventricle is normally less than 1.8 cm posterior to the IVC (2.0 cm above, 1.8 cm behind).

Potential Problems with the Rule of Rigler
Problems may include the following:
❑ The supradiaphragmatic portion of the IVC may not be visualized (poor inspiration, poor penetration).

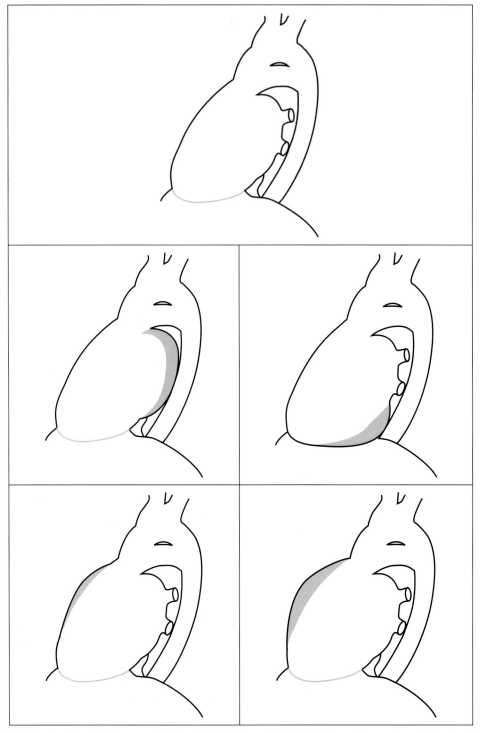

Graphic 3-2. Lateral cardiac silhouettes. *Upper graphic:* Normal. *Middle left graphic:* Left atrial dilation of the superior posterior silhouette of the heart. *Middle right graphic:* Left ventricular dilation along the posterior aspect of the cardiac silhouette. *Lower left graphic:* Slight anterior displacement of the cardiac silhouette due to right atrial dilation. *Lower right graphic:* Anterior displacement of the cardiac silhouette (against the sternum) due to right ventricular enlargement.

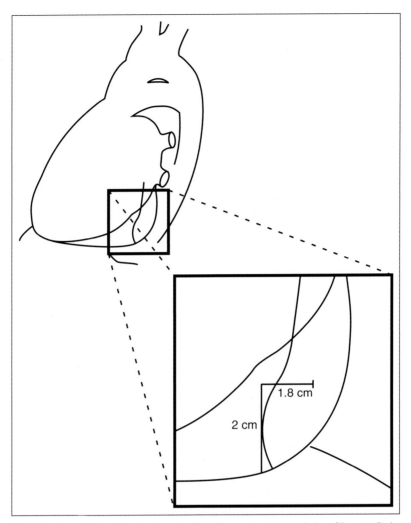

Graphic 3-3. The rule of Rigler. An enlarged left ventricle extends greater than 1.8 cm posterior to the shadow of the supradiaphragmatic inferior vena cava at a height of 2 cm above the right diaphragm.

❐ Rotation of the chest away from a transverse lateral plane may alter the projection of the left ventricular posterior border.

Enlargement of the Right Atrium

Determination of right atrial size on the lateral chest radiograph is imprecise at best. To some extent, right atrial enlargement (see Graphic 3-2) displaces the superoanterior heart border more anteriorly. Right atrial enlargement may be suggested on the lateral chest radiograph when the posterior border of the supradiaphragmatic portion of the IVC is far posterior, behind the rest of the heart.

Enlargement of the Right Ventricle

(see Graphic 3-2)
Determination of right ventricular size on the lateral chest radiograph is also imprecise at best. The size of the retrosternal air space is notoriously variable in normal people, and even more so in those with disease. The commonly quoted sign is the amount of apposition of the right ventricle to the inside of the sternum. Normally, this is less than 30% to 40% of the height of the heart. Greater apposition may occur from right ventricular enlargement anteriorly.

False Positives of Right Ventricle: Sternal Apposition Sign

False positives include the following:
❐ Narrow chest anteroposterior distance (pectus excavatum, straight back, scoliosis or kyphosis)
❐ Other structures obliterating the space (enlarged ascending aorta anterior-superior mediastinal masses, such as thymus in a young child or lymphoma)

False Negative of Right Ventricle: Sternal Apposition Sign

Chronic obstructive pulmonary disease/hyperinflation (increased retrosternal air space) is a false negative.

The sternovertebral space is normally greater than 8 cm. The space is measured from the posterior border of the sternum to the anteriormost border of the thoracic spine. When the sternovertebral space is less than 8 cm, the degree of right ventricle-to-sternum apposition cannot be reliably used to discern right ventricular size.

IDENTIFYING A VALVE OR VALVE PROSTHESIS ON THE LATERAL CHEST RADIOGRAPH (Graphic 3-4)

A line from the left mainstem bronchus (a dark circular/elliptical shadow seen end-on under the branching pulmonary artery), or from the T4–T5 vertebrae, to the sternodiaphragmatic angle localizes the mitral valve below, and the aortic valve above and anteriorly. Right anterior oblique angulation assists in detection of mitral valve calcification (in this projection, the mitral valve is projected free of vertebral calcification). On the lateral chest radiograph, the mitral valve is more vertically oriented, and the aortic valve is more horizontally oriented.

NORMALS

Several images illustrate normal chest radiographs (Figs. 3-3 to 3-11).

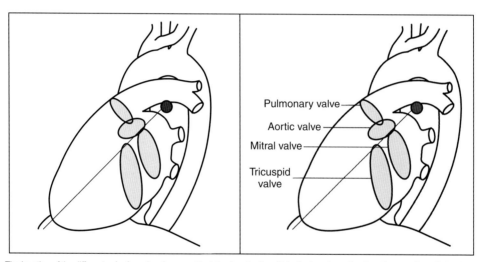

Graphic 3-4. The location of the different valve/annular planes on the lateral projection. Note the imaginary line from the usually well-visualized left mainstem bronchus to the sternodiaphragmatic angle that separates the aortic and pulmonary valves (*above*) from the mitral and tricuspid valves (*below*).

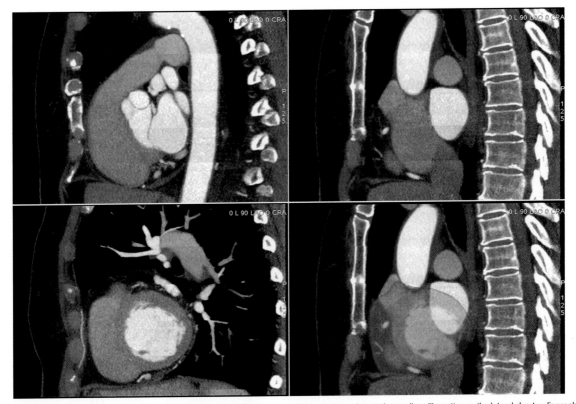

Figure 3-1. Sagittal contrast-enhanced computed tomography (CT) scans revealing anterior and posterior cardiac silhouettes on the lateral chest radiograph. In the left upper image, the anterior border is formed of the right ventricular anterior wall, the right ventricular outflow tract more superiorly, then the pulmonary valve, and the beginning of the pulmonary artery. The relatively superior position of the left atrium is also seen. In the right upper image (sagittal view to the right side), the inferior vena cava (IVC; non–contrast-enhanced because of dye injection only via the left arm veins) is seen in longitudinal depiction, rising vertically above the diaphragm. The supradiaphragmatic IVC forms an important relation to the posterior wall of the left ventricle, as the position of the IVC varies little due to its tethering by the diaphragm. As well, the left atrium above it is also seen. The left lower image is a sagittal view toward the left of midline revealing the two ventricles in cross-section. The posterior border of the left ventricle is usually nearly as well seen by chest radiography as it is by CT scanning. The right lower image is a superimposition of images with the IVC and the left ventricle depicting how little the (normal) left ventricular posterior wall extends behind the line of the supradiaphragmatic IVC.

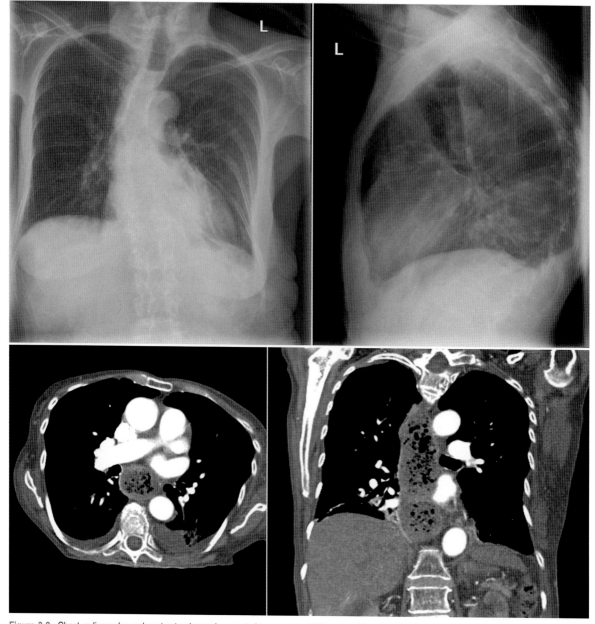

Figure 3-2. Chest radiographs and contrast-enhanced computed tomography (CT) scans. Other than borderline cardiomegaly, the cardiac silhouette in the frontal radiograph is largely unremarkable. There are infiltrates in the left lower lobe, atherosclerotic calcification of the aortic arch, and kyphoscoliosis. The lateral radiograph does not reveal a posterior silhouette of the heart at either the left atrial or left ventricular levels. The contrast-enhanced CT scans demonstrate marked dilation of the esophagus, due to retention of a large volume of food, that resulted in loss of the posterior cardiac silhouette (and aspiration pneumonia). Unsuspected esophageal carcinoma was present. The distended, food content–filled esophagus posterior to the heart, and apposed to it, eliminated the posterior silhouette of the heart on the lateral projection.

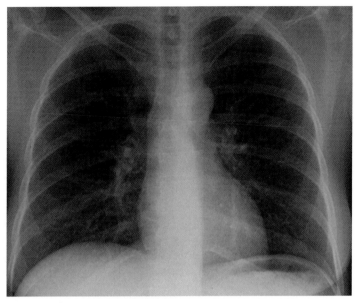

Figure 3-3. The cardiopericardial silhouette has normal contours and the cardiothoracic ratio is normal. The appearance of the pulmonary vasculature is normal. The aorta has a left-sided arch and its size and contour are normal.

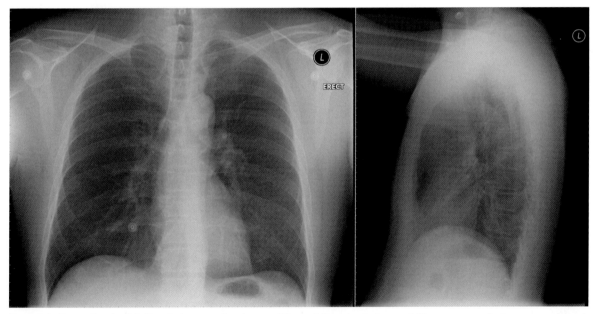

Figure 3-4. The cardiopericardial silhouette has normal contours, and the cardiothoracic ratio is normal. The appearance of pulmonary vasculature is normal. The aortic arch is left-sided, and the dimensions of the aorta and its contours are normal. No aortic intimal calcification is evident. The lateral chest radiograph again shows a normal heart size and a normal cardiopericardial silhouette. The distinction of the retrosternal air space from the anterior right ventricle and the distinction of the left ventricular posterior border from the left lower lobe are not crisp; this is a common occurrence.

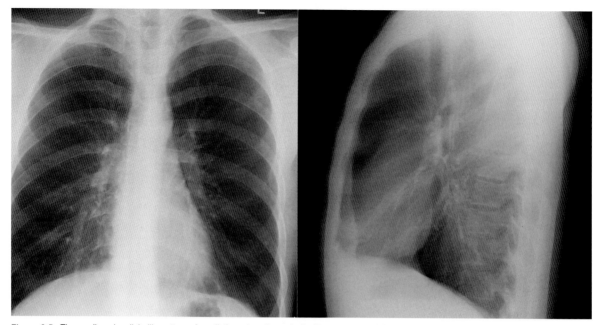

Figure 3-5. The cardiopericardial silhouette and cardiothoracic ratio on both views are normal. The aortic arch is left-sided, and the dimensions and contour of the aorta are normal. No aortic intimal calcification is evident. The appearance of pulmonary vasculature is normal. On lateral chest radiograph, the retrosternal air space and its distinction from the anterior right ventricular border is crisply defined. The left ventricular posterior border is also better defined. Because the left ventricular contour is well defined, its contour is better appreciated. Although it appears to be projecting posteriorly excessively, the supradiaphragmatic portion of the inferior vena cava denotes that the left ventricular posterior border is not posteriorly displaced, indicating enlargement.

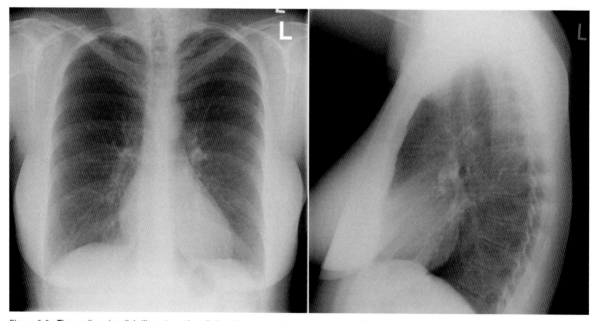

Figure 3-6. The cardiopericardial silhouette and cardiothoracic ratio in both views are normal. The aortic arch is left-sided, and the dimensions and contour of the aorta are normal. No aortic intimal calcification is evident. The appearance of pulmonary vasculature is normal.

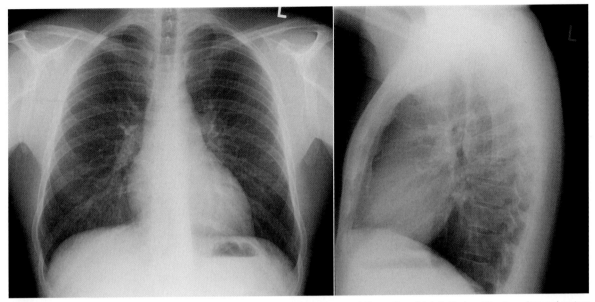

Figure 3-7. The cardiopericardial silhouette and cardiothoracic ratio on both views are normal. The aortic arch is left-sided, and the dimensions and contour of the aorta are normal. No aortic intimal calcification is evident. The appearance of pulmonary vasculature is normal.

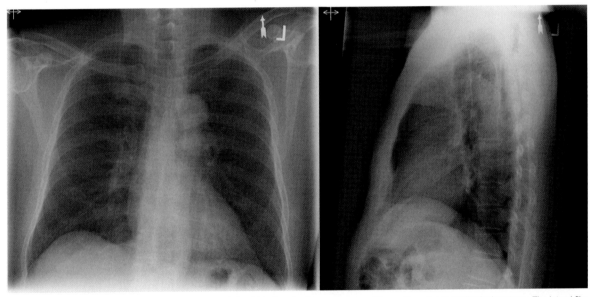

Figure 3-8. Normal chest radiographs, with rotation toward the right, changing the appearance of the aortic arch and mediastinal contours. The lateral film shows a normal cardiac silhouette.

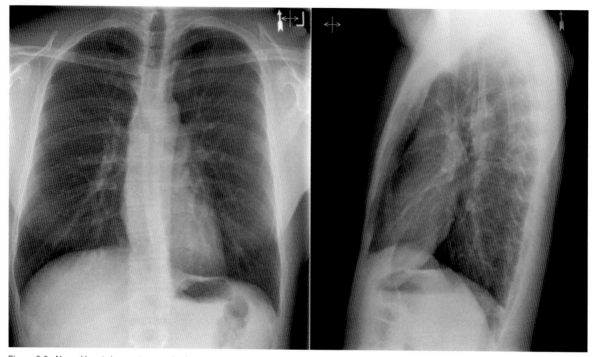

Figure 3-9. Normal heart size, contours and pulmonary vasculature in a patient with a straight back and mild scoliosis with a narrow anteroposterior dimension available for the heart.

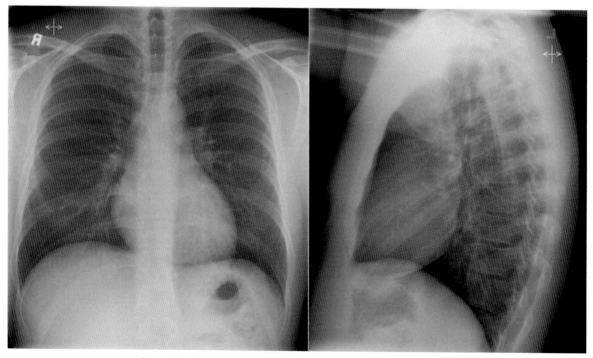

Figure 3-10. Normal cardiac and aortic contours as well as pulmonary vasculature.

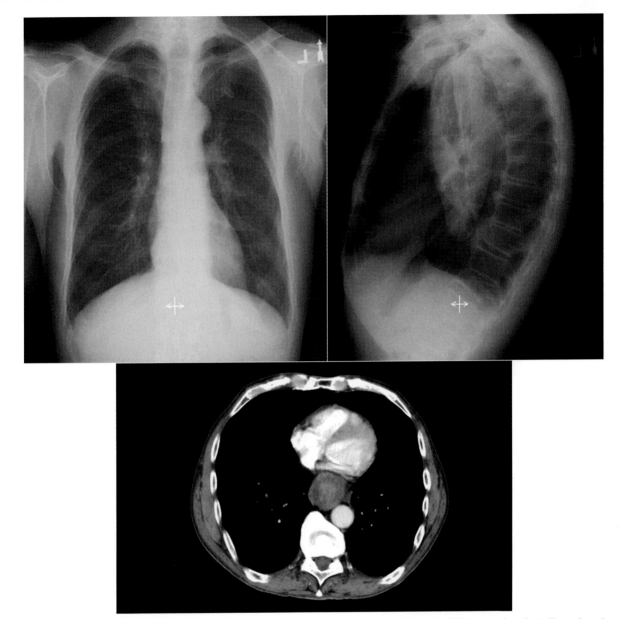

Figure 3-11. Posteroanterior and lateral chest radiographs and contrast-enhanced axial computed tomography (CT) images of a patient with esophageal dilation due to obstruction from esophageal carcinoma. On the frontal chest radiograph, note the indistinct detail of the vertebral column and aorta. On the lateral radiograph, note the exclamation mark–shaped soft tissue mass in the posterior mediastinum. The CT image reveals the marked esophageal dilation that indents on the left atrium, and which resulted in the blurred posterior silhouette of the heart on the lateral radiograph.

Assessment of Heart Size

Accurate assessment of heart size, and particularly of heart chamber size, requires the use of techniques such as echocardiography, computed tomography, or magnetic resonance imaging. However, estimates of the overall heart size are still very useful clinically, because, as a general rule, "cardiomegaly is disease."

METHODS TO ASSESS CARDIAC SIZE

Methods for assessment include the following:

❏ **Gestalt:** By integrating cardiopericardial silhouette (CPS) frontal plane area, cardiac contour, and ancillary findings, an experienced and able reader can appreciate an abnormally large CPS, with an accuracy favorable to more time-consuming measurement techniques.

❏ **Cardiothoracic ratio** (CTR; equivalent to transverse cardiac diameter divided by greatest internal chest width) (Graphic 4-1): Several numbers are used as benchmarks to determine enlargement of the CPS: 0.50, 0.55, and 0.60. Obviously, a lower cutoff value is more sensitive but less specific. Generally, 0.50 is accepted as the upper limit of normal CTR. CTR correlates poorly with height, fairly with body weight, and best with height and weight together. There is a surprisingly wide range of normal values. Chest width is not a very useful index of body build, and its use introduces another noncardiac potential error; therefore, transverse cardiac dimension alone may be a better measure. Tables are available in some radiology texts.

❏ **Frontal plane area:** This has the best correlation (vs. gestalt and CTR) with cardiac volume but is time-consuming and seldom used.

❏ **Cardiac volume:** Currently cardiac volume is assessed by echocardiography, cardiac magnetic resonance, cardiac computed tomography, or contrast ventriculography, and it is almost never quantitatively assessed from a chest radiograph. However, validated formulas are available that calculate cardiac volume from measurements of cardiac dimension along its long axis, transverse axis (posteroanterior radiograph), and depth (lateral radiograph). In routine clinical practice, they are no longer used.

PITFALLS IN THE ESTIMATION OF CARDIOPERICARDIAL SILHOUETTE SIZE

Problems include the following:

❏ **Degree of inspiration:** If the inspiration is not adequate, then the apex of the heart is more horizontal (increasing the transverse cardiac dimension) and the lungs are not full (reducing the CTR). Some patients, attempting to cooperate, make a deep inspiration and inadvertently make a Valsalva maneuver, reducing heart size, or Müller's maneuver, increasing heart size.

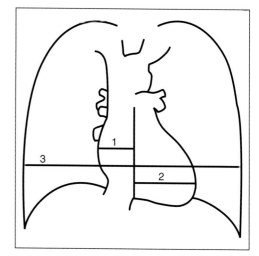

Graphic 4-1. Cardiothoracic ratio: maximal cardiac transverse diameter (1 + 2) divided by internal diameter of the chest cage (3).

- **Cardiac cycle phase:** A radiograph is randomly exposed with respect to systole and diastole. Patients with atrioventricular block (large stroke volume) may have up to 2 cm of difference in diameter between cardiac cycle phases. With a normal heart and normal heart rate, there is at most 1 cm of difference between systolic and diastolic dimensions.
- **Air in the stomach:** The "infradiaphragmatic" part of the heart (lying to the left) is revealed, and the cardiac width is therefore greater.
- **Thoracic deformities** giving a narrow mediastinal space to sternovertebral distance (normal sternovertebral distance is >8 cm), such as straight back, pectus excavatum, or severe kyphosis. All "compress" the heart, which therefore appears less dense but wider.
- **Anteroposterior versus posteroanterior:** Magnification of the CPS on an anteroposterior radiograph is inevitable (about 10% to 15%).

SMALL CARDIOPERICARDIAL SILHOUETTE: DIFFERENTIAL

The differential diagnosis includes the following:
- Normal variant
- Emphysema
- Dehydration/malnutrition (Fig. 4-1)
- Addison disease
- Constrictive pericarditis (sometimes)

ENLARGED CARDIOPERICARDIAL SILHOUETTE: DIFFERENTIAL

The differential diagnosis includes both congenital and acquired heart disease.

Acquired Heart Disease
- Pericardial disease: effusion, masses, cysts (Figs. 4-2 and 4-3)
- Cardiomyopathy
- Valvular disease
- Coronary disease with myocardial damage (Fig. 4-4)
- Hypertension

Congenital Heart Disease
- Single lesions
  - Shunts
  - Obstructions
- Complex lesions

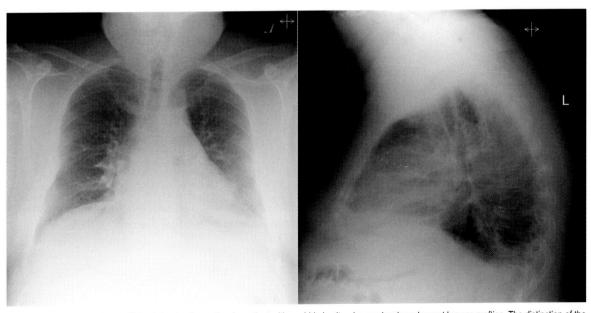

Figure 4-1. Posteroanterior and lateral chest radiographs of a patient with morbid obesity who previously underwent bypass grafting. The distinction of the cardiac silhouette is less crisp and the lung fields have their appearance influenced by the extent of superimposed soft tissue, which increases the markings. With such a body habitus, some proportion of the size of the cardiopericardial silhouette is due to adipose tissue (epicardial fat and pericardial fat and aprons).

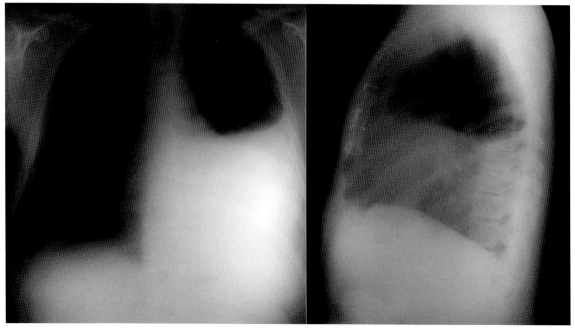

Figure 4-2. Due to the presence of a large left pleural effusion, the cardiopericardial silhouette can be neither readily nor accurately assessed.

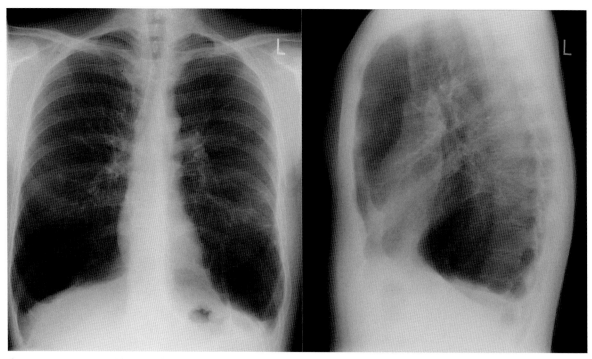

Figure 4-3. The heart was normal sized, though it appears small within this enlarged chest cavity.

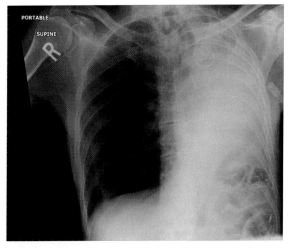

Figure 4-4. The cardiopericardial silhouette is not apparent. The position of the aortic arch is apparent only because of its calcification. There is severe leftward shift of the tracheal air column, post–left pneumonectomy. The left pleural space is replaced with organizing fluid.

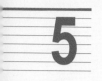

5 Pulmonary Vasculature and Pulmonary Embolism

Key Points

- To appreciate the abnormal patterns of pulmonary vasculature, it is important to be proficient with the details and nuances of normal pulmonary vasculature patterns.
- The classic patterns of abnormal pulmonary vasculature include cephalization, centralization, collateralization, lateralization, localization, generalized decreased flow, and overcirculation vascularity.
- There are radiographic signs of large and small pulmonary embolism as well as complications of pulmonary embolism, although final diagnosis resides with, usually, contrast-enhanced computed tomography scanning.
- Recognition of other right-sided heart disease associated patterns such as those of large and small pulmonary arteries, dilation of the azygous vein, and enlargement of the superior vena cava is clinically useful.

PATTERNS OF PULMONARY VASCULATURE

The influence of a cardiac lesion on the pulmonary vasculature is indicative of its hemodynamic consequence. Because the pulmonary vasculature is surrounded by air-filled lung, the pulmonary vessels are well defined. The distal one third of the intrapulmonary vessels are normally not apparent because of their small size. The arteries are normally slightly larger than their accompanying bronchi at any distance into the lung (Graphic 5-1).

Normal Pulmonary Vasculature

The left hilum is normally a couple of centimeters more carinal than the right because the left pulmonary artery is slightly raised by the left mainstem bronchus. Pulmonary arteries to the upper lobes run medial and parallel to the veins. Normally, these veins are fairly well defined. Pulmonary veins from the lower lobes run more horizontally than the pulmonary arteries and enter the hila more inferiorly than the arteries leave the hila. The dependent portions of the lung receive greater flow; hence, in the erect chest radiograph, the lower lobe vessels are greater in size than the upper lobe vessels. In fact, the apical arteries are usually only faintly visualized because in the normal individual, there is little blood flow to the lung apices. The chest radiograph of a normal individual lying flat shows equal vessel size in the lower and upper lobes, because gravitational forces increase the flow and vessel size of the posterior lower and upper lobes. Bronchial vessels are normally not visible.

Abnormal Pulmonary Vasculature Patterns

The following categories are useful, because these radiographic descriptive patterns correspond to different pathophysiologic processes. Increased vessel size is noticeable only when vessels are at least twice normal size.

Cephalization: With pulmonary venous hypertension, pulmonary veins become dilated and more visible throughout the lung fields. However, dilated upper lobe pulmonary arteries are the most apparent feature of pulmonary venous hypertension, because lower lobe vessels are constricted (i.e., narrower than the apical vessels) as a result of local vascular reflexes initiated by raised intravascular pressure (>10–15 mm Hg). To maintain pulmonary perfusion in the face of constricted lower lobe vessels, upper lobe vessels become recruited. Such a pattern strongly suggests elevated pulmonary venous pressure. It is not often seen in left-to-right intracardiac and extracardiac shunts. It is a reliable sign only for erect (nonsupine) radiographs, because, for the reasons mentioned previously, equal vessel sizes to the upper and lower lobes are to be expected in supine radiographs.

Centralization: Increased size of the main pulmonary artery and proximal pulmonary arteries with some reduction of peripheral pulmonary vessels is referred to as centralization. It is found in states of precapillary pulmonary hypertension (Figs. 5-1 to 5-8).

Collateralization: This is suggested by oligemia of the lung fields, with evidence of
- Bronchial collateralization (vessels seen in the upper and medial lung zones near their origin from the descending aorta)

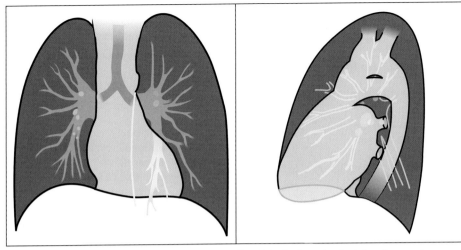

Graphic 5-1. Normal pulmonary vasculature as seen on posteroanterior and lateral chest radiographs. Centrally, a few vessels are seen end-on and are therefore rounded in shape. Vessels radiate outward from the hila and normally can be clearly followed about two thirds of the way toward the pleura.

❏ Intercostal collateralization (indicated by rib notching) (see Chapter 6)

Lateralization of flow: This is suggested by segmental oligemia and segmental preserved flow. This may be seen in the clinical setting of a pulmonary embolus (Westermark sign), or pulmonary artery anomalies (Fig. 5-9).

Localization of pulmonary vasculature: This usually indicates a pulmonary arteriovenous malformation (Figs. 5-10 to 5-12).

Generalized decreased flow: This occurs with severe congenital right-sided obstructive lesions or advanced pulmonary vascular disease. Reduced blood flow is suggested by abnormal lung lucency and small vessel size.

Overcirculation vascularity: This refers to uniform increase in prominence of central and intrapulmonary vessels. The pattern may be symmetric or asymmetric (asymmetry may be because of a congenital cause or a surgical corrective procedure). Causes of overcirculation vascularity include

❏ Left-to-right shunting
• Intracardiac (e.g., atrial septal defect, ventral septal defect)
• Extracardiac (e.g., patent ductus arteriosus, truncus, transposition, anomalous pulmonary venous return, surgical shunts, other)
❏ High flow states (e.g., hyperthyroidism, pregnancy, anemia)

Obviously, plethoric pulmonary vasculature is always due to a shunt of greater than 2:1 pulmonary-to-systemic flow ratio (Qp:Qs). A less obvious appearance may be from any hyperdynamic state.

Pulmonary Artery Sizing

The most frequent visible branch of the pulmonary arteries is the right descending pulmonary artery. This component of the pulmonary arterial system is the most visible because it is surrounded by air-filled lung and lies free of other radiopaque structures in the heart. It is usually well visualized near the right hilum, lateral and parallel to the lower lobe bronchus and is measured there.

Interlobar Pulmonary Artery

An increase in the pulmonary artery size is seen in states of increased pressure, increased flow, or turbulent flow (i.e., poststenotic dilatation, pulmonary hypertension, atrial septal defect). Normally, the diameters of the bronchi and pulmonary arteries are roughly comparable at any distance into the lung. The interlobar (right) pulmonary artery is typically silhouetted on its medial and lateral aspects on the frontal radiography and can be measured:

❏ Normal: 9–14 mm
❏ Abnormal: ≥17 mm (male or female) (<14 mm is unlikely to have significantly increased flow)
❏ Upper limit normal (males): 15 mm
❏ Upper limit normal (females): 16 mm

PULMONARY EMBOLISM

The chest radiograph is abnormal in 90% of patients with pulmonary embolism. However, the chest radiograph is never diagnostic for pulmonary embolism. The radiographic signs depend on the size of the embolism and on the presence or absence of pulmonary infarction (Figs. 5-13 to 5-27).

Large or Central Pulmonary Artery Embolism

Signs of this type of pulmonary embolism include the following:
❏ Central pulmonary artery enlargement
❏ Lucency of the affected lung

- ❑ Infarction less common
- ❑ Absent vessels
- ❑ Compensatory dilation of the nonaffected vessels
- ❑ Raised diaphragm
- ❑ Nondilated main pulmonary artery

Medium, Lobar, or Segmental Pulmonary Artery Embolism

The affected artery appears "amputated" proximally. Pulmonary infarction may occur.

Small or Peripheral Pulmonary Artery Embolism

There are seldom immediately detectable radiographic ischemic changes, although this may chronically evolve to have the findings of pulmonary hypertension.

Pulmonary Embolism with Infarction

Large acute pulmonary emboli may result in lung parenchyma infarction which results in consolidation of the involved area of the lung with blood/effusion. Pulmonary infarction is more common in the lower lobes and in the presence of pulmonary venous congestion.

Radiographic signs of pulmonary infarction include the following:

- ❑ Infarct shadow (triangular)
- ❑ "Hampton hump" is a rarely seen sign, classically a rounded cone with its base against pleura
- ❑ Cavitation (occasional finding, more common when the embolus was septic and resulted in local septic necrosis)
- ❑ Size: 0.5 to 10 cm (almost any size) but always against a pleural surface
- ❑ Usually without air bronchograms
- ❑ Rounded patchy infiltrates (50%)
- ❑ Curvilinear densities (25%)
- ❑ Pleural effusion (50%)
- ❑ Atelectasis
- ❑ Diaphragmatic elevation (17%)
- ❑ Westermark sign: segmental/lobar oligemia, usually associated with enlargement of the main pulmonary artery

Causes of Pulmonary Embolism

Causes of pulmonary embolism include the following:

- ❑ Thrombus (peripheral sources): lower and upper extremities, pelvic, renal veins, from central venous lines, pacemakers, and implantable cardiac defibrillators
- ❑ Infective endocarditis vegetations (tricuspid and pulmonic valves)
- ❑ Air
- ❑ Amnion
- ❑ Fat
- ❑ Catheter fragments
- ❑ Tumor

Large Pulmonary Artery

When enlarged, the main pulmonary artery, which is normally mildly convex, will form an accentuated bulge, and have a greater diameter.

Causes of a Large Pulmonary Artery

See Figures 5-28 to 5-33.

Volume Overload

Causes in enlarged central and peripheral vessels include the following:

- ❑ Left-to-right shunt especially when the Qp:Qs is greater than 3:1
  - Patent ductus arteriosus with or without pulmonary hypertension
- ❑ Atrial or ventricular septal defect with or without pulmonary hypertension, pulmonary valve insufficiency, hyperdynamic circulation (thyrotoxicosis, anemia, beriberi)

Pressure Overload

Causes of enlarged central vessels only include the following:

- ❑ Vasoconstriction
- ❑ Pulmonary venous hypertension
- ❑ Left-to-right shunts
- ❑ Vascular obliteration
- ❑ Thromboembolic disease, other emboli (e.g., tumor)
- ❑ Vasculitides
- ❑ Idiopathic (primary) pulmonary hypertension
- ❑ Hilar adenopathy, which should not be mistaken for enlargement of the central pulmonary arteries (Fig. 5-34)

Secondary to Left-to-right Shunts

Causes include the following:

- ❑ Atrial septal defects
- ❑ Ventricular septal defects
- ❑ Ductus arteriosus

Other

Causes include the following:

- ❑ Idiopathic dilation of the pulmonary artery (increased main pulmonary artery size with normal left pulmonary artery size)
- ❑ Valvular pulmonary stenosis, which is always associated with an increase in the size of the left pulmonary artery size ("poststenotic dilatation")
- ❑ False aneurysms of a pulmonary artery

Pseudodilation

Signs of pseudodilation include the following:

- ❑ Straight back, pectus excavatum, or severe scoliosis
- ❑ Compression, rotation, or displacement of the heart leads to this sign; gives the false impression of an enlarged pulmonary artery.

❏ Pericardial fluid, fat, cysts, or tumor
❏ Congenital absence of the pericardium

Causes of Small Central or Peripheral Pulmonary Arteries

❏ Congenital pulmonary atresia
❏ Intrauterine congenital infection: toxoplasmosis, other, rubella, cytomegalovirus, herpes simplex (TORCH), rubella
❏ Congenital lesions
  • Tetralogy of Fallot
  • Patent ductus arteriosus (may be associated with hypoplastic main pulmonary arteries)
  • Congenitally corrected transposition of the great arteries
  • Pulmonary atresia with ventral septal defect

Causes of a Large Azygous Vein

A normal azygous vein becomes smaller when the patient is in the erect position or on deep inspiration and enlarges with a Valsalva maneuver, whereas the size of an enlarged azygous lymph node does not vary itself according to changes in body position and hydrostatic forces. When greater than 1 cm in diameter, the vein is seen lateral to the superior vena cava above the right pulmonary artery on a posteroanterior radiograph (Graphic 5-2).

Causes of Increased Pressure

Obstruction of the superior or inferior vena cava increases central venous pressure without increasing right atrial pressure. Causes of central venous or right atrial pressure greater than 10 cm include the following:
❏ Tamponade
❏ Constrictive pericarditis
❏ Restrictive cardiomyopathy
❏ Right-sided heart failure

Causes of Increased Flow

The differential diagnosis is sinus venosus atrial septal defect plus right upper lobe pulmonary vein, with or without right middle lobe pulmonary vein drainage into the superior vena cava. Causes include the following:
❏ Anomalous pulmonary venous return
❏ Inferior vena cava interruption with azygous continuation
❏ Tricuspid insufficiency
❏ Portal hypertension
❏ Pregnancy
❏ Increased intravenous fluid support (e.g., trauma cases)

Causes of an Enlarged Superior Vena Cava

Volume Overload

Causes include the following:
❏ Tricuspid insufficiency
❏ Total anomalous pulmonary venous return

Obstruction (Pressure Overload)

Causes include the following:
❏ Carcinoma: bronchogenic, breast
❏ Lymphoma
❏ Fibrosing mediastinitis
❏ Constrictive pericarditis
❏ Right-sided heart mass lesion (myxoma)
❏ Right-sided heart failure
❏ Tricuspid stenosis

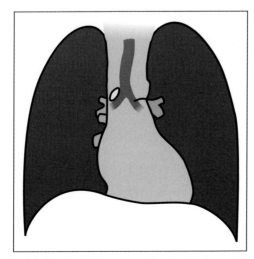

Graphic 5-2. Location of the azygous vein entry into the superior vena cava.

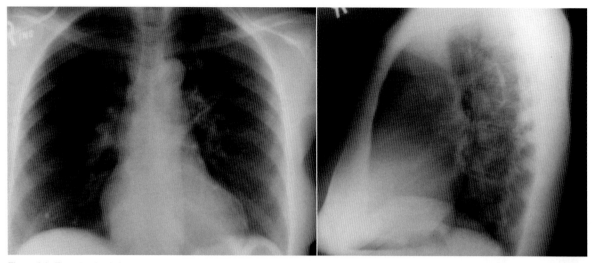

Figure 5-1. There is a borderline increase of the cardiothoracic ratio on the posteroanterior (PA) radiograph and more obvious enlargement of the heart on the lateral chest radiograph. There is some prominence of the right atrial curvature on the PA radiograph and increased apposition of the right ventricle to the sternum consistent with right ventricular enlargement on the lateral chest radiograph. The appearance of the aorta is unremarkable. The main pulmonary artery appears to be enlarged, and the interlobar pulmonary artery is clearly enlarged. In addition, there is reduced peripheral vascularity. No pleural effusions are present. Severe pulmonary hypertension was present due to recurrent thromboembolic disease.

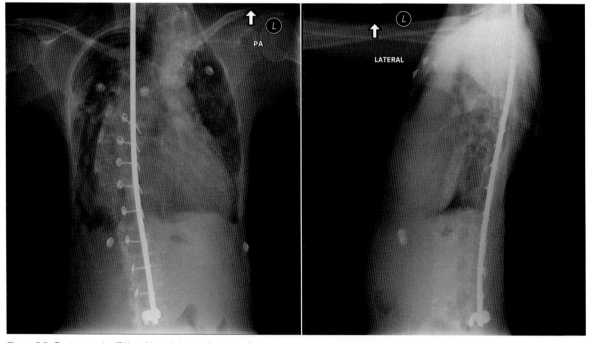

Figure 5-2. Posteroanterior (PA) and lateral chest radiographs. Spinal rods and extreme scoliosis are present. On the PA chest radiograph, cardiomegaly with ambiguous contours are apparent. The lateral chest radiograph shows that anterior postural dimension of the heart of the chest is narrow. The aorta is left-sided, and the main pulmonary artery appears to be enlarged. The remainder of the pulmonary vasculature is difficult to evaluate. There were systemic levels of pulmonary hypertension from restrictive chest disease due to childhood treatment of a neuroblastoma. There is marked enlargement of the right heart confirmed by echocardiography.

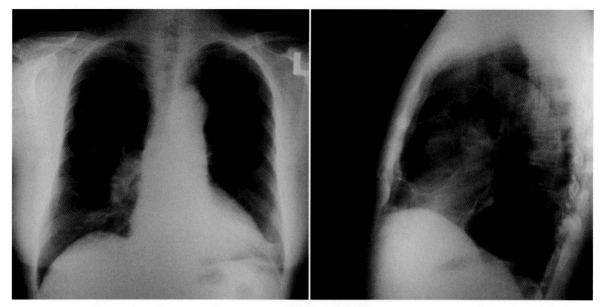

Figure 5-3. Posteroanterior (PA) and lateral chest radiographs. On the PA chest radiograph, there is no definite cardiomegaly or abnormal contours to the heart. The aorta is left-sided, and its appearance is normal. The main pulmonary artery is difficult to scrutinize, but the interlobar pulmonary artery is clearly enlarged and there is reduced peripheral pulmonary vasculature. On the lateral chest radiograph, the relation of the right ventricle to the sternum is ambiguous. There are systemic levels of pulmonary hypertension due to primary pulmonary hypertension in this adult male. There was considerable enlargement of the right heart on echocardiography, although this is not apparent on the chest radiograph.

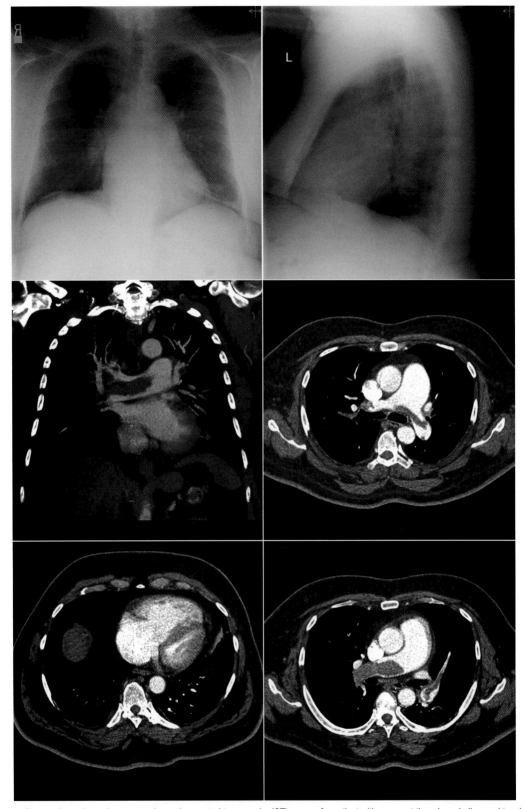

Figure 5-4. Chest radiographs and contrast-enhanced computed tomography (CT) scans of a patient with recurrent thromboembolism and terminal right-sided heart failure. Note the size of the main and central pulmonary arteries and of the right heart chambers on both the chest radiographs and the CT scans.

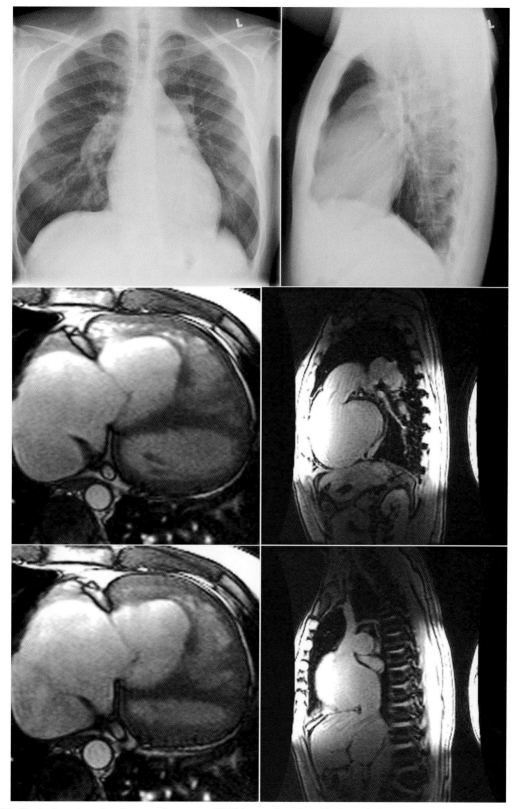

Figure 5-5. Chest radiographs and cardiac magnetic resonance (CMR) images of a patient with advanced primary pulmonary hypertension. On the radiographs, the main and central pulmonary arteries are dilated, the right ventricle is prominent, and the azygous vein may be dilated. There is rapid tapering of the pulmonary arteries ("centralization") and paucity of peripheral vessels, including veins. The CMR steady-state free precession images demonstrate the extent of right-sided chamber, main pulmonary artery, and caval and azygous vein enlargement.

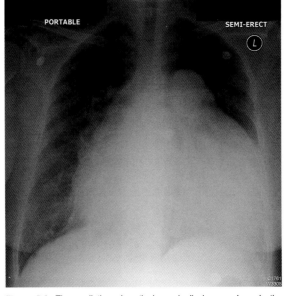

Figure 5-6. The cardiothoracic ratio is markedly increased, as is the dimension of the main pulmonary artery. There is terminal right-sided heart failure from primary pulmonary hypertension.

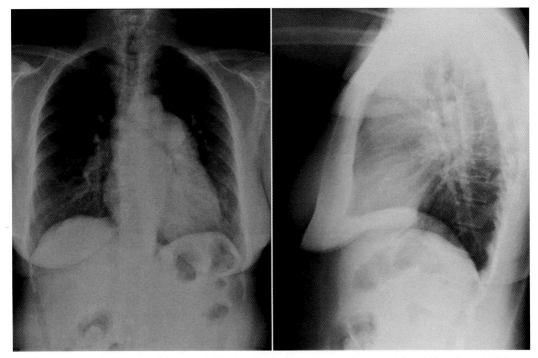

Figure 5-7. Severe pulmonary hypertension. Note the markedly enlarged main, left, and central pulmonary arteries, which are "pruned." As is seen on the lateral radiograph, the right ventricle is enlarged.

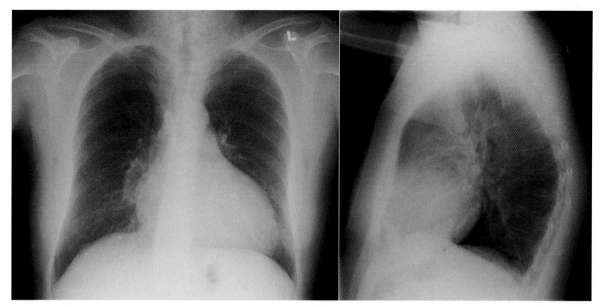

Figure 5-8. Posteroanterior (PA) and lateral radiographs in an adult male with systemic levels of pulmonary hypertension due to primary pulmonary hypertension. There is an increase of the cardiothoracic ratio, with some prominence of the right atrial curvature on the PA radiograph. There is increased apposition of the right ventricle to the sternum on the lateral chest radiograph. Some kyphosis is present. The main pulmonary artery is slightly enlarged, and the interlobar pulmonary artery is clearly enlarged.

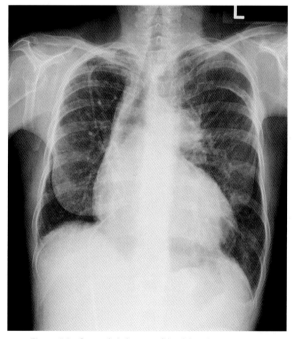

Figure 5-9. Congenital absence of the right pulmonary artery.

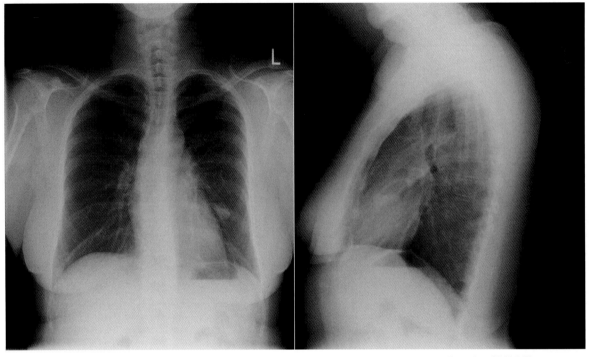

Figure 5-10. Posteroanterior (PA) and lateral chest radiographs of a patient with bilateral pulmonary arteriovenous malformations (AVMs). The appearance of AVM on the left side is rounded and nodular and projects just over the left heart border on the PA film. The appearance of AVM on the right side is more classic, with a prominent feeder pulmonary artery and draining pulmonary vein extending to and away from it.

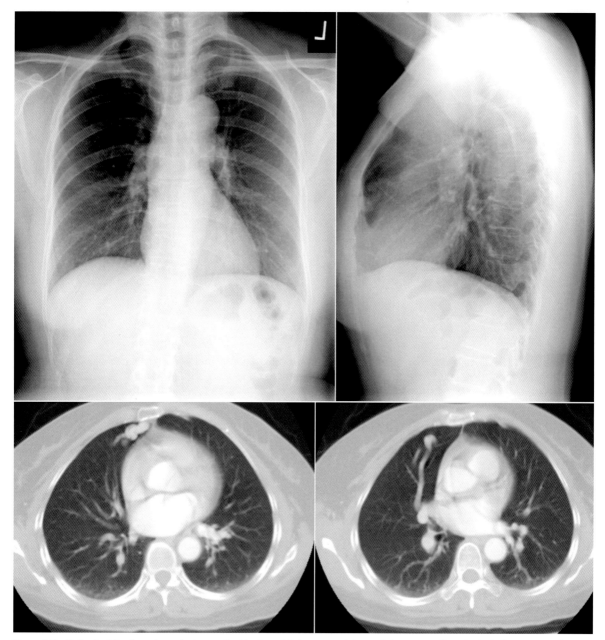

Figure 5-11. On the frontal radiograph, a pair of worm-sized feeder and drainage vessels to an arteriovenous malformation in the lingua is seen. Contrast-enhanced axial computed tomography images depict it well.

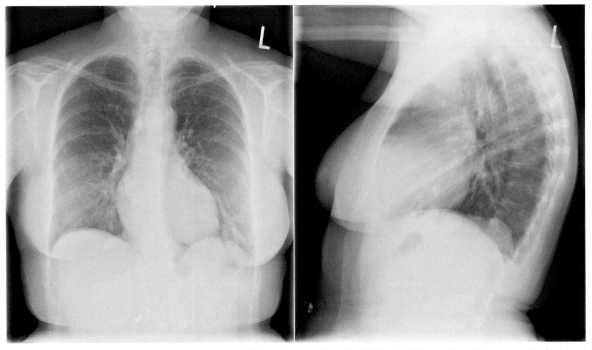

Figure 5-12. Bilateral pulmonary arteriovenous malformations (AVMs) of the lower lobes. The AVM in the left lower lobe is obvious, as are the feeder and drainage vessels.

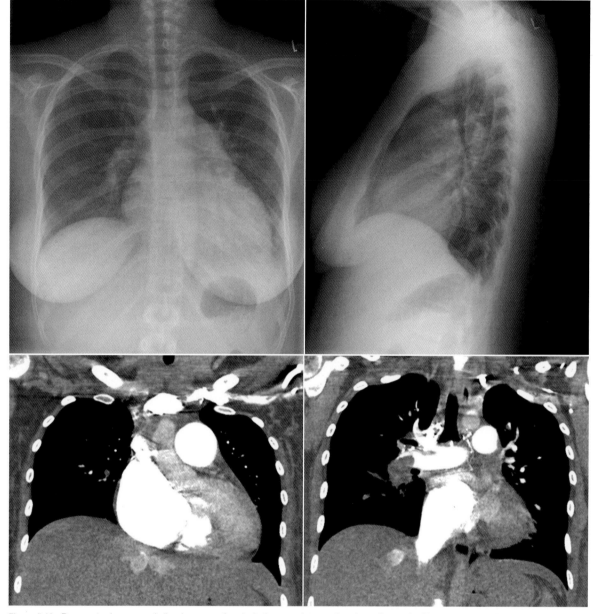

Figure 5-13. Recurrent pulmonary embolism in a young female. In the upper images, there is cardiomegaly with an accentuated right atrial contour on the posteroanterior radiograph, and dilation of the right ventricle on the lateral radiograph. There is dilation of the main pulmonary artery trunk. The superior vena cava and the azygous vein are enlarged, consistent with right-sided heart failure. The left pulmonary artery is not prominent, and only the very central part of the right pulmonary artery is prominent. In the lower images, coronal contrast-enhanced computed tomography reveals the dilation of the right atrium, cava, and main pulmonary artery, as well as extensive thrombus within the pulmonary arterial vasculature with obliteration of the left pulmonary vasculature. The reflux of contrast dye into the inferior vena cava is consistent with right-sided heart failure.

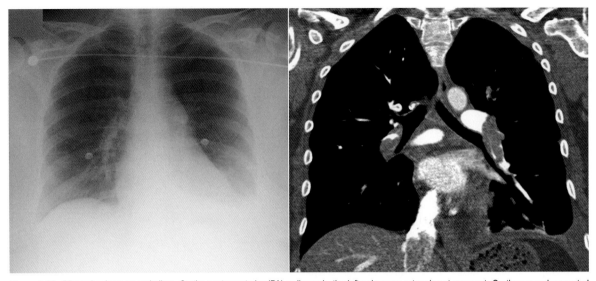

Figure 5-14. Bilateral pulmonary embolism. On the posteroanterior (PA) radiograph, the left pulmonary artery is not apparent. On the coronal computed tomography image, thrombi are seen in both the right and left pulmonary arteries, and the left pulmonary artery that is missing on the PA radiograph, is seen to be almost completely occluded/truncated by thrombus.

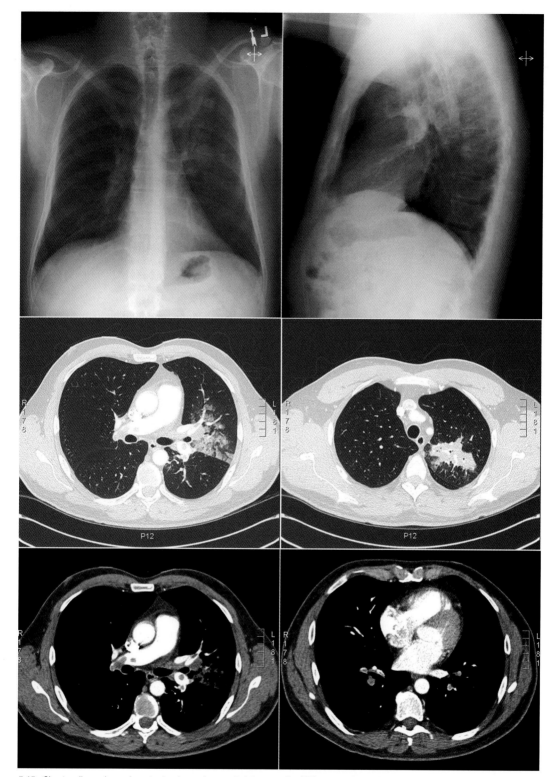

Figure 5-15. Chest radiographs and contrast-enhanced computed tomography (CT) scans of a patient with pulmonary embolism to both lungs with pulmonary infarction of the left upper lobe. This is apparent as consolidation on the chest radiographs and clearly shown to be wedge-shaped and pleural-based on the lung view CT scans. The lower contrast-enhanced CT scans show filling defects bilaterally to most vessels.

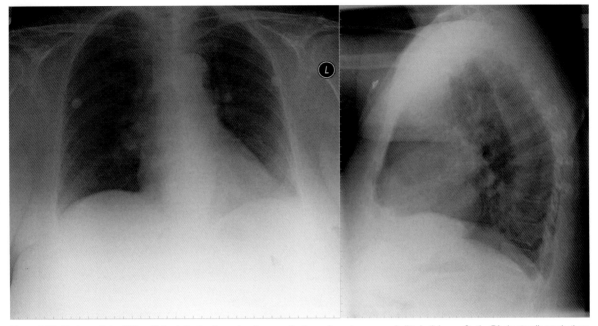

Figure 5-16. Posteroanterior (PA) and lateral chest radiographs of a case of submassive pulmonary emboli to both lungs. On the PA chest radiograph, there is no definite cardiomegaly or contour abnormality. There is oligemia of the mid and peripheral lung zones, prominently of the right lung but also of the left upper lobe. The pulmonary arteries in the hilar regions have a prominent appearance, either because of some enlargement or because of oligemia elsewhere. On the lateral chest radiograph, cardiomegaly is more obvious with increased apposition of the right ventricle against the sternum, suggesting right ventricular enlargement. Again, the pulmonary arteries and their more central branches appear enlarged.

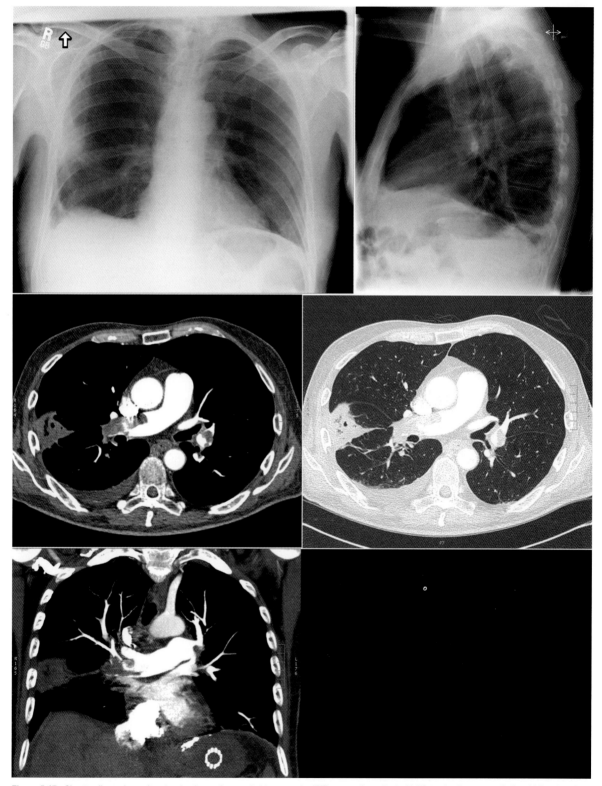

Figure 5-17. Chest radiographs and contrast-enhanced computed tomography (CT) scans of a patient with bilateral pulmonary emboli and infarction of the right lung. This is apparent as a pleural-based triangular-shaped consolidation on both the chest radiographs and CT scans. Note the thrombi in the artery leading to that segment.

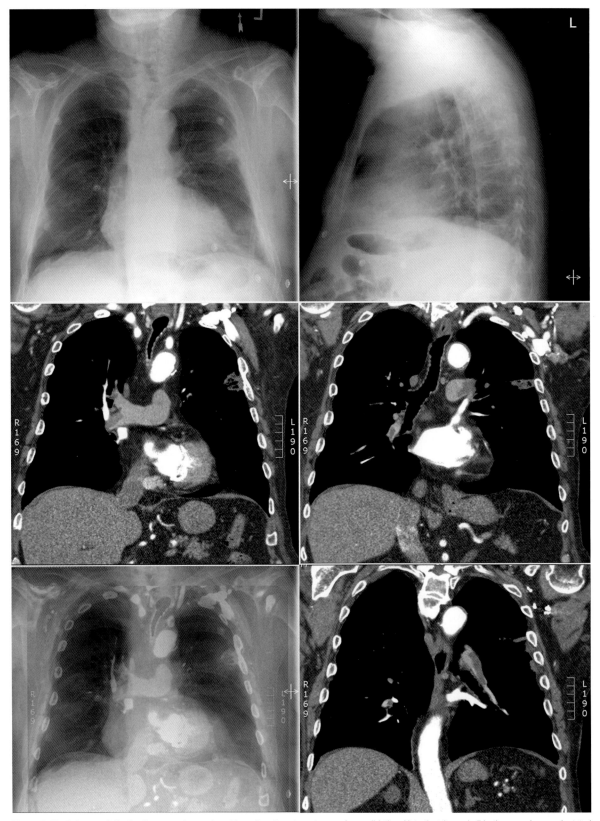

Figure 5-18. Pulmonary infarction is apparent as a pleural-based wedge-shaped area of consolidation. Note that the emboli in the vessels are orientated toward those segments seen on computed tomography (CT) scans to be infarcted. The left lower image represents the superposition of the coronal CT scan and the posteroanterior chest radiograph, showing coincidence of the area of consolidation but greater appearance on the CT scan.

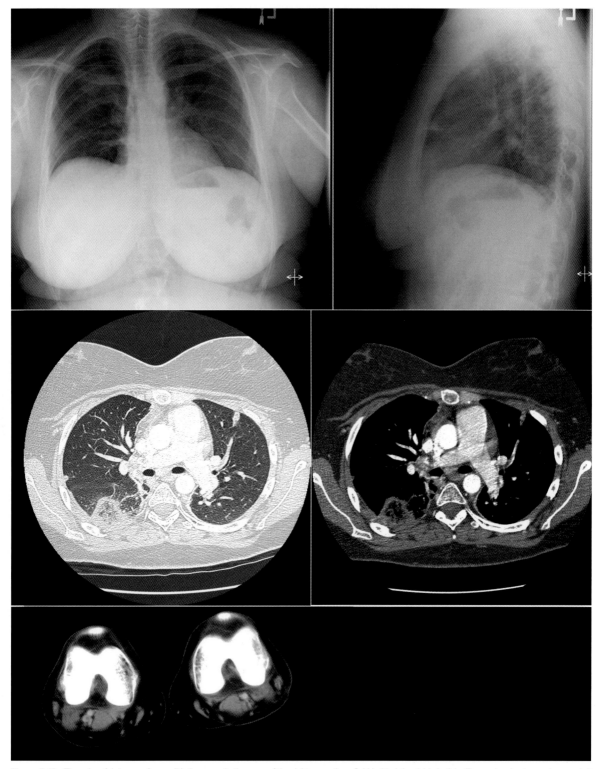

Figure 5-19. There is a faint area of consolidation seen in the area of the right upper lung field behind the right clavicle. The contrast-enhanced computed tomography (CT) angiogram demonstrates somewhat more clearly a pleural-based triangular-shaped area of pulmonary infarction than it does embolism to that area. The CT venogram at the popliteal level is less conclusive for a deep vein thrombosis.

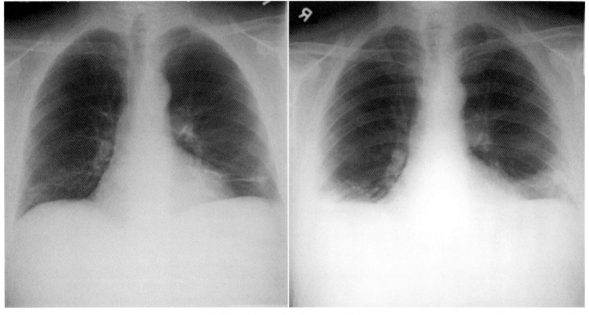

Figure 5-20. Anteroposterior chest radiographs during (left) and following (right) pulmonary infarction due to pulmonary embolism. The consolidation of the left lung and partial silhouetting over the left heart border have partially resolved.

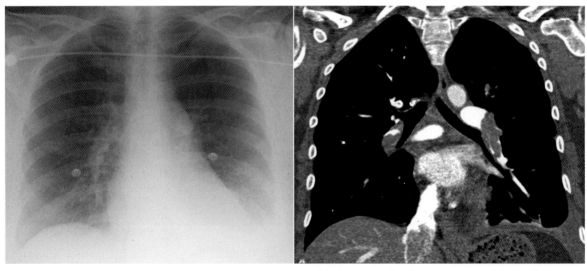

Figure 5-21. On the posteroanterior (PA) radiograph, the left pulmonary artery is minimally apparent. The left lung has less vascularity than the right lung. The contrast-enhanced computed tomography scan demonstrates bilateral pulmonary embolism, with subtotal occlusion of the left pulmonary artery, which explains why it is not apparent on the PA radiograph.

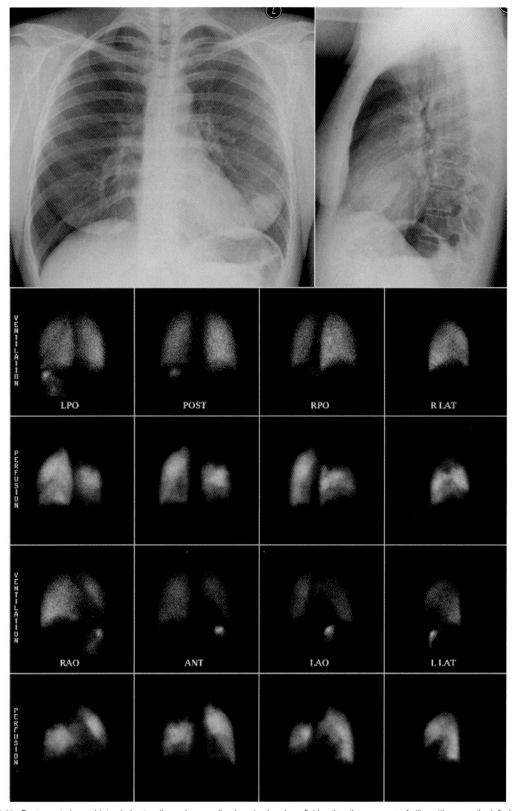

Figure 5-22. Posteroanterior and lateral chest radiographs revealing largely clear lung fields other than an area of silhouetting over the left-sided heart border. The ventilation-perfusion scans below depict normal ventilation but a perfusion defect to the left lower lobe having resulted from embolism and having led to infarction over the left-sided heart border resulting in the silhouetting of the left-sided heart border on the posteroanterior chest radiograph.

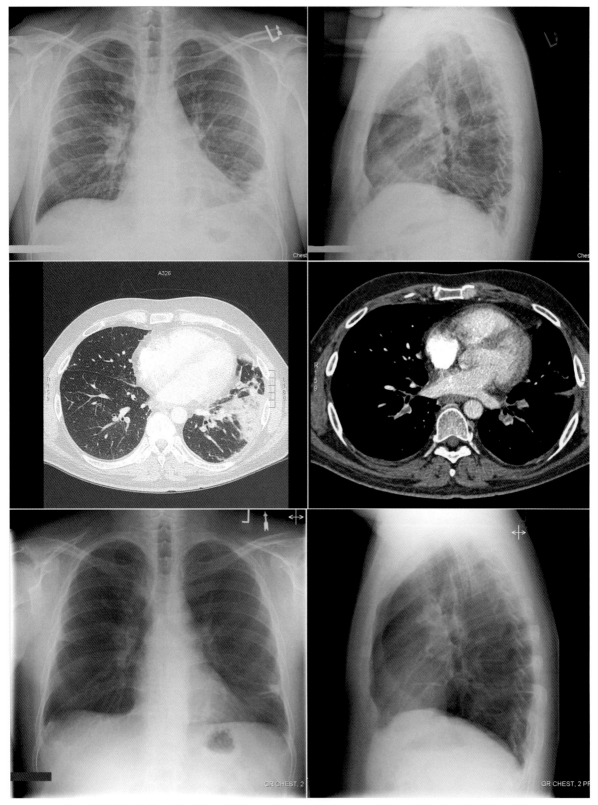

Figure 5-23. Chest radiographs and computed tomography scans of pulmonary embolism and infarction of the left lower lobe.

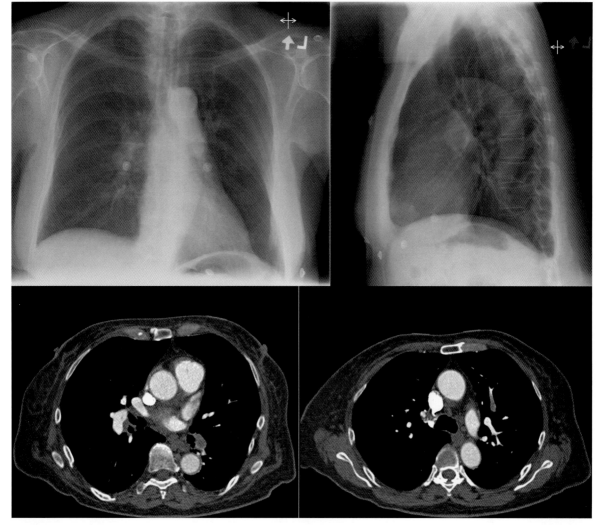

Figure 5-24. Recurrent pulmonary embolism with predominance of obstruction on the left side, resulting in segmental/lobar oligemia—Westermark sign. There is oligemia of the left lung and dilation of the main pulmonary artery, the right pulmonary artery, and interlobar arteries. The contrast-enhanced computed tomography axial images reveal the bilateral emboli, particularly heavily on the left side.

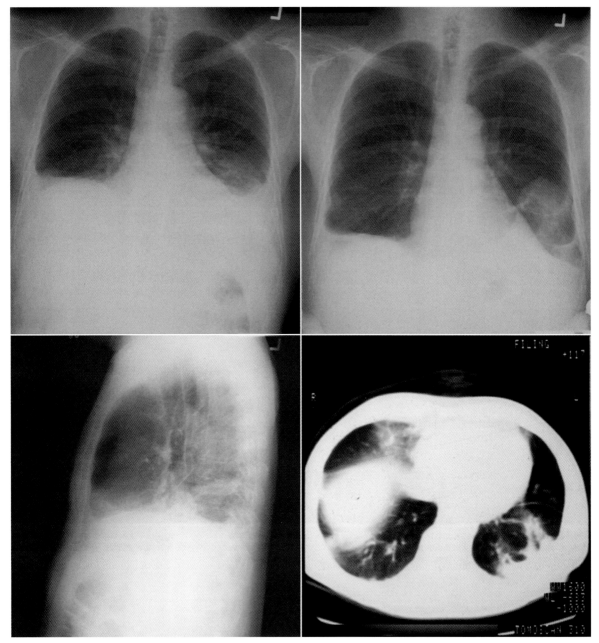

Figure 5-25. On the posteroanterior radiograph, there is an area of consolidation over the left lower lung field. On the computed tomography scan, this is seen to be due to infarction.

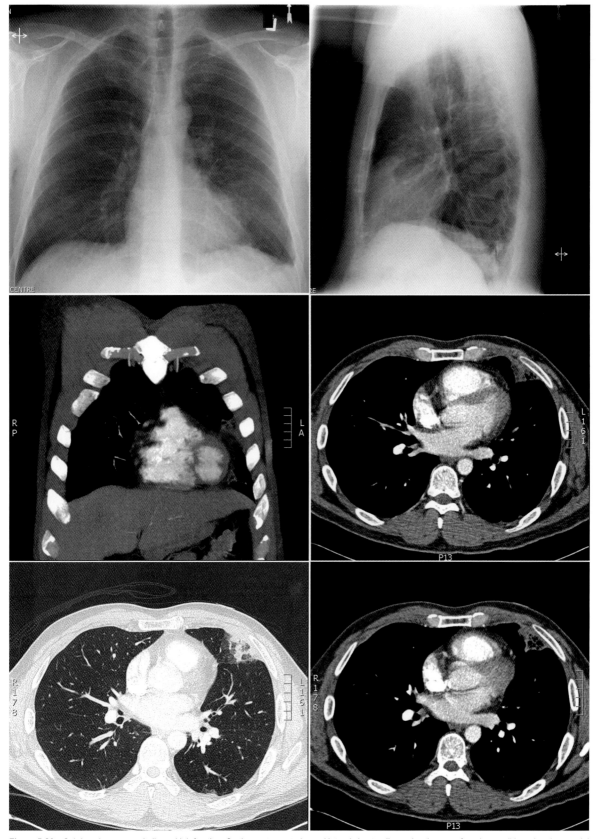

Figure 5-26. Subtle pulmonary embolism with infarction. On the posteroanterior and lateral chest radiographs, there are few abnormalities other than partial silhouetting of the mid-left heart border. The contrast-enhanced computed tomography scans reveal an area of consolidation extending from the left heart border anteriorly and superiorly and with a wedge shape that is pleural based.

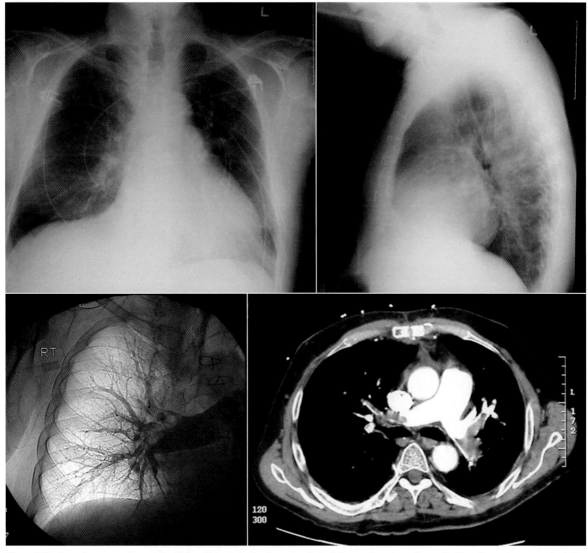

Figure 5-27. Upper images: posteroanterior (PA) and lateral chest radiographs. On both images there is cardiomegaly. Sternotomy wires are present. The patient had undergone aortocoronary bypass grafting 3 weeks previously. There is enlargement of the main pulmonary artery and of the interlobar pulmonary artery seen on the PA chest radiograph. There is the appearance of but not the definite sign of oligemia in the right upper lobe and in the left upper lobe. No pleural effusions are present. Lower images: contrast pulmonary angiogram (*left*) and contrast-enhanced computed tomography pulmonary angiogram (*right*). A large bulk of thrombus is present at the bifurcations of both the right main and left main pulmonary arteries.

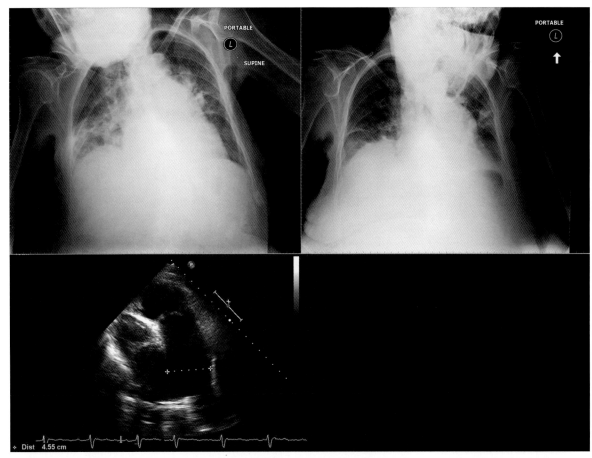

Figure 5-28. Anteroposterior radiographs demonstrating interstitial pulmonary edema and cardiomegaly. The contours of the cardiopericardial silhouette are for the most part difficult to resolve given the rotation of the heart. However, there is prominent dilation of the main pulmonary artery, which measures 4.6 cm in diameter, as is seen on the transthoracic echocardiography view on the lower image; this was idiopathic.

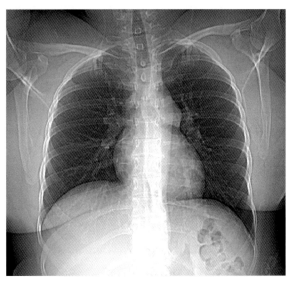

Figure 5-29. Dilation of the main pulmonary artery trunk, without pulmonic stenosis or pulmonary hypertension ("idiopathic dilation of the main pulmonary artery").

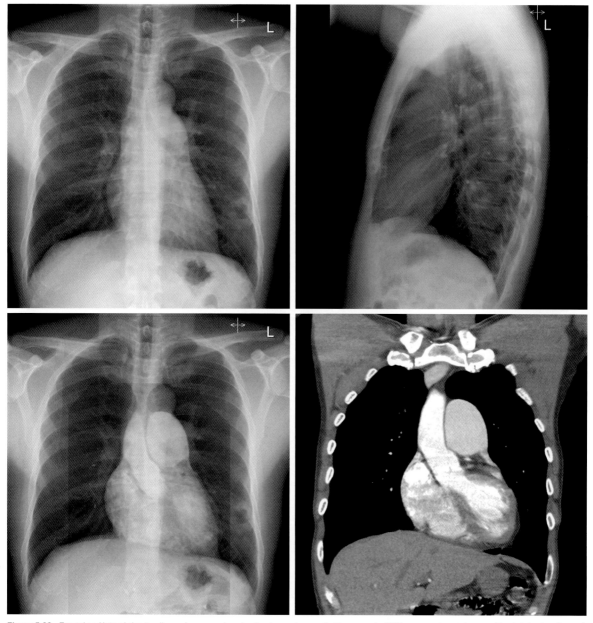

Figure 5-32. Frontal and lateral chest radiographs, coronal contrast-enhanced computed tomography (CT) scan, and superimposed frontal chest radiograph and coronal contrast-enhanced CT scan of a patient with valvar pulmonic stenosis and poststenotic dilation of the main pulmonary artery. The shape of the main pulmonary artery on the CT scan is consistent with the main pulmonary artery dilation not being associated with severely elevated pulmonary artery pressures, because the cross-sectional shape is not circular.

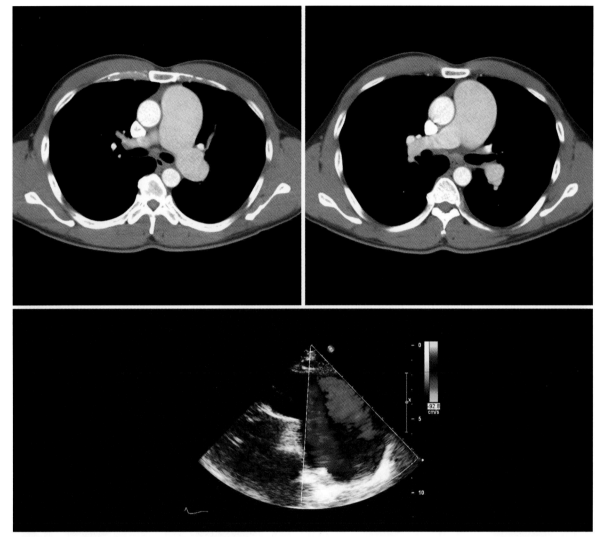

Figure 5-33. Axial contrast-enhanced computed tomography scans of the patient in Figure 5-32, with poststenotic dilation of the main pulmonary artery. The left images reveal that the associated dilation of the left pulmonary artery exceeds that of the right pulmonary artery, shown in the right image. The lower transthoracic echocardiogram shows again the plump poststenotic dilation of the main pulmonary artery.

bronchial walls [peribronchial "cuffing"], and between fissures) (Figs. 6-2 to 6-4)

☐ Hazy hila (Fig. 6-5). Embryologically, the lung parenchyma grew out from the hila. The pulmonary septa therefore radiate away from the hilum and are closest together at the hila and farthest apart at the pleural surface. Accumulation of septal edema therefore is most apparent at the hila, where the septa converge.

☐ Interstitial edema/infiltrates that render the right lower pulmonary artery indistinct

☐ Common Kerley B lines (see later discussion)

☐ Thickened interstitial spaces with pulmonary edema that are indistinct (whereas those due to lymphangitic cancer and to pulmonary fibrosis may be better defined)

Stage 3: (Intra-)alveolar Edema

This stage is characterized by alveolar or intra-alveolar edema, which appears as puffy 2 to 3 mm round or confluent opacities.

Stage 4: Hemosiderosis plus Ossification of Lung

This stage is characterized by the following:

☐ Hemosiderosis and ossification of the lung that occur as an airspace pattern with a "stippled" appearance due to multiple nodules. This is an uncommon finding of very severe mitral stenosis with repeated episodes or pulmonary edema and hemorrhage.

☐ Differential diagnosis: prior granulomatous disease, calcified metastases (e.g., osteosarcoma)

KERLEY LINES

Kerley A lines are thin, straight, or oblique lines in the upper lobes, due to fluid in the interlobular septa. Kerley A lines are uncommon and therefore are not often cited.

Kerley B lines are costophrenic septal lines:

☐ Due to visible interlobular lymphatics and their surrounding connective tissue

☐ 1 to 3 cm long and nonbranching

☐ Less than 1 mm thick

☐ Extending from and perpendicular to the pleural surface

☐ Best seen in the costophrenic angles

☐ The most cited of these three signs

Kerley C lines are a "spider web" appearance of the lower lobes. These lines probably result from the overlap of Kerley B lines. They are also uncommon, and are therefore uncommonly cited.

DIFFERENTIAL DIAGNOSIS

Differential diagnoses are discussed in the following sections.

Peribronchial "Cuffing:" Differential
(Figs. 6-6 to 6-9)

☐ Asthma (mucosal and wall edema)
☐ Chronic bronchitis (mucosal and wall edema)
☐ Bronchiectasis (mucosal and wall edema)

Vascular Redistribution: Differential
☐ Pulmonary embolus to the lower lobes
☐ Chronic obstructive pulmonary disease
☐ Severe precapillary pulmonary hypertension

Kerley B Lines: Differential
☐ Lymphatic obstruction
☐ Fibrosis from lymphangitic cancer, pneumoconioses, or sarcoidosis

Unilateral Pulmonary Edema: Differential
☐ Prolonged lateral decubitus position ("gravitational")
☐ Unilateral aspiration
☐ Reexpansion pulmonary edema: rapid thoracentesis of air or fluid from the ipsilateral side
☐ Bronchial obstruction
☐ Systemic artery to pulmonary artery shunts
  • Waterston shunt on the right side
  • Potts shunt on the left side
  • Blalock-Taussig on the left or right side
☐ Pulmonary venous obstruction (unilateral)
☐ Left atrial tumor, mediastinal tumor, fibrosing mediastinitis
☐ Pulmonary artery obstruction (unilateral)
☐ Intraluminal: thromboembolus
☐ Extraluminal: tumor, fibrosing mediastinitis, aortic aneurysm
☐ Congenital absence/hypoplasia of a pulmonary artery
☐ Unilateral emphysema or lobectomy

Lag Phase in Radiographic Signs of Pulmonary Edema

It is important to recall that there is a "lag phase" (time difference) between the radiographic signs of pulmonary edema and left atrial pressures. The lag phase occurs because it takes time for fluid to be mobilized from the interstitial and alveolar compartments and removed by venous and lymphatic channels. Thus, there is often discordance between radiographic and clinical impressions of the degree of pulmonary edema.

Causes of Pulmonary Edema with a Normal Cardiopericardial Silhouette

Causes include the following:

☐ Acute myocardial infarction in a previously normal heart (Figs. 6-10 to 6-19)

☐ Acute severe mitral or aortic insufficiency (Figs. 6-20 and 6-21)

☐ Noncardiogenic pulmonary edema

☐ Other types of pulmonary disease (e.g., pneumonia, carcinomatosis)

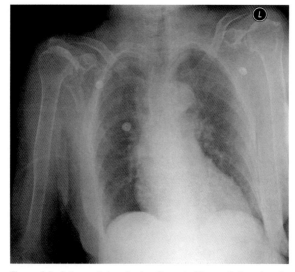

Causes of Noncardiogenic Pulmonary Edema

Causes include the following:

- ❒ Drowning/asphyxia
- ❒ Upper airway obstruction
- ❒ Negative pressure pulmonary edema
- ❒ High-altitude pulmonary edema
- ❒ Elevated intracranial pressure
- ❒ Reexpansion pulmonary edema
- ❒ Noxious gas inhalation
- ❒ Drug-related conditions
- ❒ Poisons
- ❒ Recreational drug–related conditions
- ❒ Blood transfusion–related conditions
- ❒ Contrast media–related conditions
- ❒ Pancreatitis, sepsis

Figure 6-1. Cardiomegaly with interstitial edema, vascular redistribution, Kerley B lines, indistinct and mildly fluffy hilar definition, and bilateral small pleural effusions.

Figure 6-2. The cardiothoracic ratio and contours of the cardiopericardial silhouette are difficult to assess due to obscuring of the borders of the heart by interstitial and airspace pulmonary edema and also superimposition of breast shadow. There is acute pulmonary edema due to hypertensive crisis in a patient with left ventricular hypertrophy and normal systolic function. Note the severe calcification of the abdominal aorta apparent best on the lateral view, a contributor to the systolic hypertension by rendering of the aorta extremely noncompliant.

Figure 6-3. Anteroposterior chest radiograph. The cardiothoracic ratio is increased without particular contour abnormality. There is rotation of the chest. There are both interstitial and airspace pulmonary edema with obscuring of the hilar structures resulting in the "bat wing" pattern. The aorta is heavily calcified at the arch level. There is acute pulmonary edema due to hypertensive crisis in a patient with systolic hypertension, left ventricular hypertrophy, and normal systolic function.

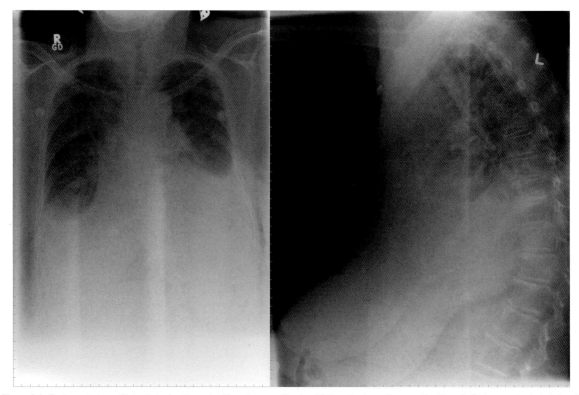

Figure 6-4. Posteroanterior and lateral chest radiographs. There is congestive heart failure due to cardiomyopathy. Pleural effusions are typical of chronic biventricular heart failure. Due to the presence of significant size bilateral pleural effusions, the cardiothoracic ratio and the cardiopericardial contours cannot be assessed. There is extensive interstitial pulmonary edema and increased pulmonary venous prominence.

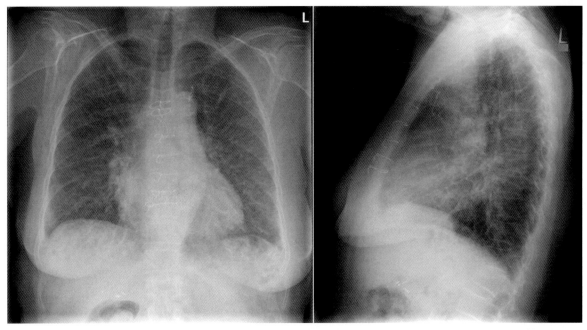

Figure 6-5. Severe bilateral airspace and interstitial pulmonary edema, most apparent over the hila. The cardiac silhouette is nearly impossible to interpret due to rotation, poor inspiration, and silhouetting of the heart by the pulmonary edema.

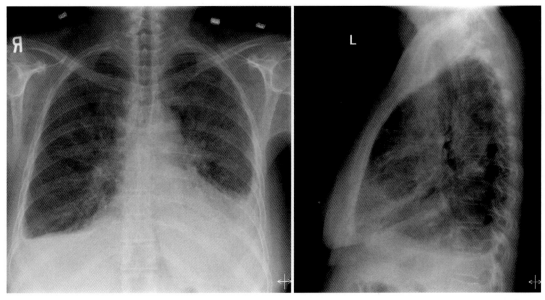

Figure 6-6. Bilateral pleural effusions, apparent cardiomegaly, and widely accentuated interstitial markings are found in this patient with widely disseminated carcinoma and pleural fluid–proven–positive carcinomatosis. The left heart function was normal/supranormal, and all of the pulmonary findings were attributed to lymphangitic carcinamatosis and pleural carcinamatosis. The overall appearance is readily confused with left-sided heart failure.

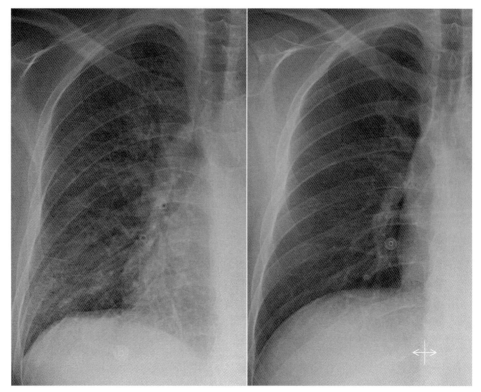

Figure 6-7. Congestive heart failure (*left*) versus normal condition (*right*). On the image of congestive heart failure, note the prominent pulmonary vasculature and markings, the less than distinct hilar silhouettes, and the obvious peribronchial cuffing. By way of comparison, the image of the normal chest shows clear hilar silhouettes, normal subtle pulmonary vasculature, and no peribronchial cuffing.

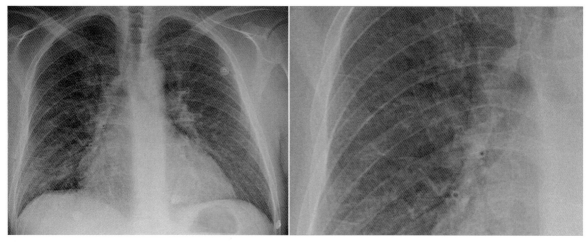

Figure 6-8. Interstitial pulmonary edema with prominent peribronchial edema (cuffing).

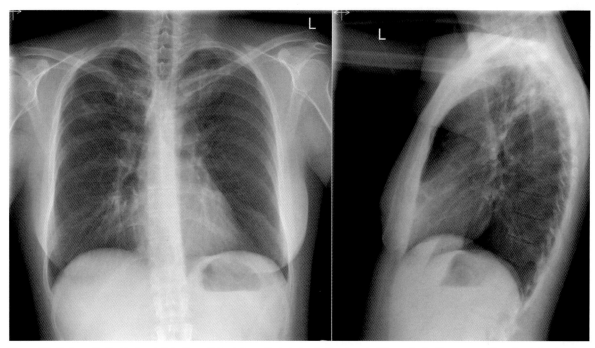

Figure 6-9. Peribronchial "cuffing" and dilated bronchi due to bronchiectasis (cystic fibrosis variant) in a patient with a coronary dissection, but no heart failure.

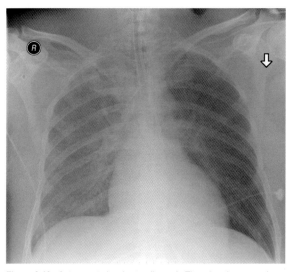

Figure 6-10. Anteroposterior chest radiograph. There is pulmonary edema secondary to myocardial infarction of a previously normal heart. The cardiothoracic ratio is normal, as is the cardiopericardial silhouette. There is airspace and interstitial pulmonary edema with ill distinction of the hila and a slight "bat wing" pattern. The endotracheal tube is within 2 cm of the carina.

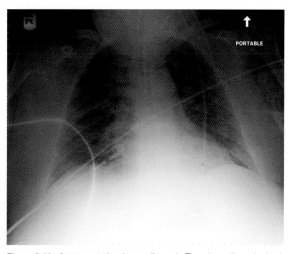

Figure 6-11. Anteroposterior chest radiograph. There is cardiogenic shock with acute pulmonary edema due to a third myocardial infarction. The cardiothoracic ratio is increased. There is no specific abnormality apparent of the cardiopericardial silhouette. There is bilateral interstitial pulmonary edema rendering the hilar vessels indistinct. The position of the endotracheal tube is difficult to establish with respect to the carina.

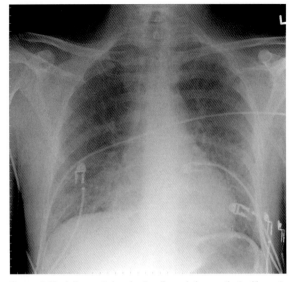

Figure 6-12. Anteroposterior chest radiograph in a patient with acute pulmonary edema due to acute myocardial infarction. The cardiothoracic ratio is increased. There is no specific abnormality of the cardiopericardial silhouette. There is both airspace and interstitial pulmonary edema and pulmonary venous engorgement.

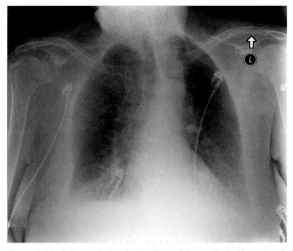

Figure 6-13. Anteroposterior chest radiograph in a patient with acute pulmonary edema due to acute myocardial infarction. The cardiopericardial silhouette is at most mildly increased. The aorta at the arch level is mildly enlarged. The pulmonary vasculature is engorged. There is interstitial pulmonary edema, rendering the hilar area indistinct.

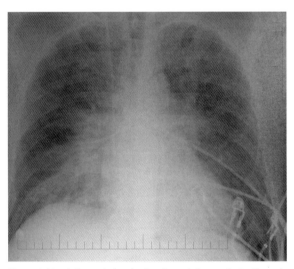

Figure 6-14. Anteroposterior chest radiograph in a patient with acute pulmonary edema due to acute myocardial infarction. Note the multiple electrocardiogram leads and the pulmonary artery catheter. The patient is not intubated. There is confluent perihilar opacification due to pulmonary edema, which is both interstitial and air-space.

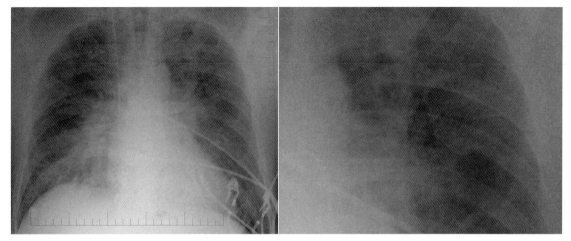

Figure 6-15. Interstitial and air-space pulmonary edema post–myocardial infarction. The hilar silhouettes are completely indistinct due to the presence of interstitial pulmonary edema.

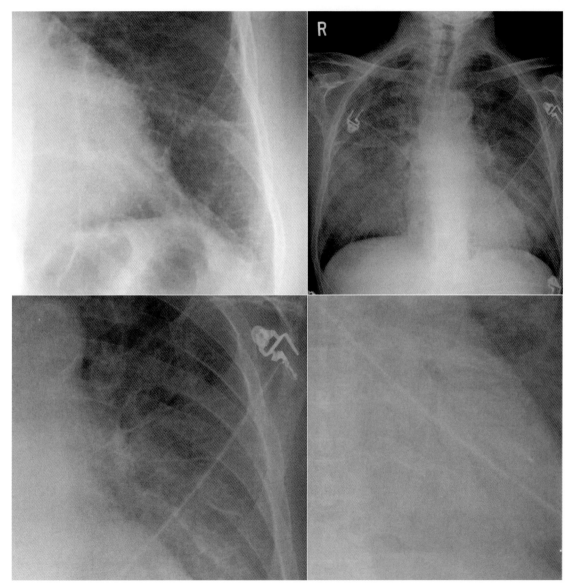

Figure 6-16. Severe pulmonary edema, post–myocardial infarction. Note the indistinct hilar and cardiac silhouettes and the bronchial silhouettes from the air-space pulmonary edema.

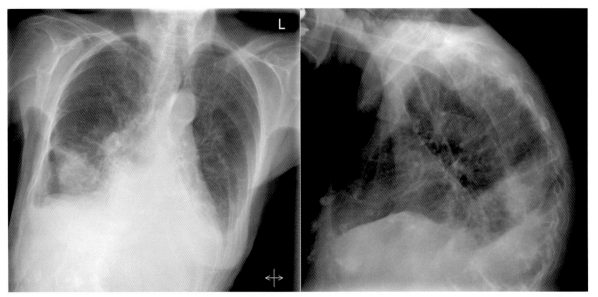

Figure 6-17. Congestive heart failure in an elderly patient with severe aortic stenosis and mitral regurgitation. There are prominently increased interstitial vascular markings, and small pleural effusions. The right pleural effusion is eccentrically located.

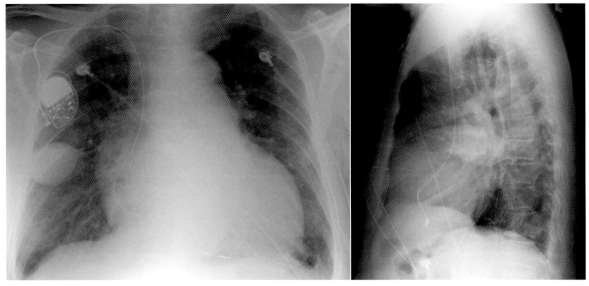

Figure 6-18. Fluid in the minor fissure (right middle lobe to right upper lobe interface) due to congestive heart failure (pseudotumor). Note the cardiomegaly, signs of multichamber enlargement, and pulmonary vascular markings.

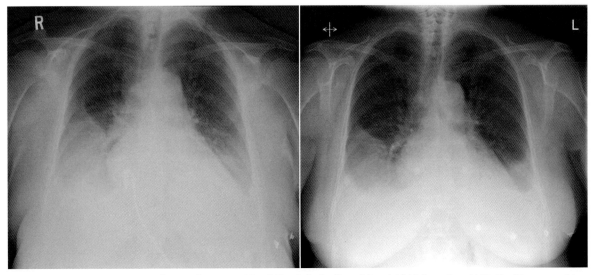

Figure 6-19. A patient with ischemic cardiomyopathy at presentation (*left*) and after two liters of diuresis (*right*); the peribronchial "cuffing," the venous distention, and the perihilar haze have all improved. As is usual, the pleural effusions are persisting longer.

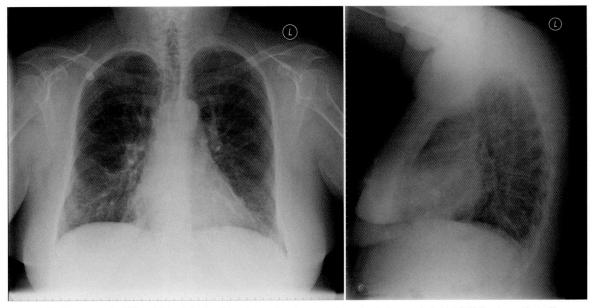

Figure 6-20. Posteroanterior (PA) and lateral chest radiographs; acute pulmonary edema due to the onset of atrial fibrillation in a patient with severe mitral stenosis. On the PA chest radiograph, there is no definite increase of the cardiothoracic ratio. The cardiopericardial silhouette is only abnormal in the straightening of the upper left heart border consistent with left atrial appendage enlargement. The pulmonary vasculature is prominent, and there is interstitial pulmonary edema marked over the hilar areas. On the lateral chest radiograph, there is left atrial posterior enlargement and probably increased apposition of the right ventricle into the sternum. Pulmonary edema is apparent.

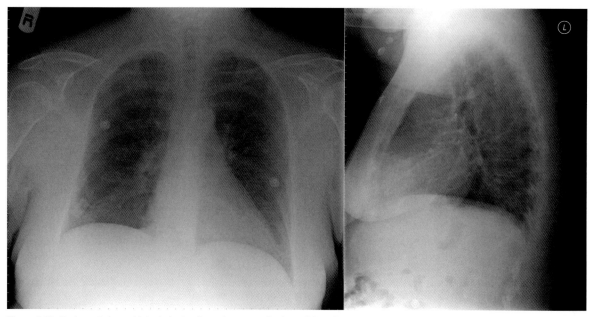

Figure 6-21. Posteroanterior and lateral chest radiographs; congestive heart failure due to the onset of atrial fibrillation in a patient with severe mitral stenosis. The cardiothoracic ratio is mildly increased. There is straightening of the upper left heart border consistent with the left atrial appendage enlargement. There is moderate interstitial pulmonary edema rendering the hilar vessels indistinct. On the lateral radiograph, left atrial enlargement is apparent as posterior displacement. There is increased apposition of the right ventricle against the sternum.

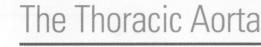

7 The Thoracic Aorta

ISSUES CONCERNING CHEST RADIOGRAPHIC IMAGING OF THE THORACIC AORTA

It is important to remember that (1) the chest radiograph does not image the aorta comprehensively and (2) abnormalities of the aorta evident on the chest radiograph represent substantial pathology that is often clinically important and sometimes life-threatening. Therefore, to not overlook major aortic pathology when reading a chest radiograph, it is imperative to scrutinize aortic contours and appearance (Fig. 7-1). The aorta is evident on the chest radiograph wherever the air-filled lung is in contact with it and there is a silhouette to evaluate.

It is critical to recall that major aortic pathologies, such as dissection, may occur with a normal or near-normal chest radiograph. A final diagnosis for aortic pathology requires a more advanced and comprehensive test such as CT, MRI, TEE, or aortography.

Review of Silhouettes of the Aorta

The aortic root begins behind the pulmonary artery at the level of the aortic valve and lies within the pericardium. The root is surrounded by soft tissue (the pulmonary artery in front, the left atrium inferiorly, the pericardium, and pericardial and mediastinal fat) and the aortic valve is usually not evident unless it is either heavily calcified or prosthetic; therefore, the aortic root cannot be localized accurately on the chest radiograph on either the frontal or lateral radiographs. Marked dilation (Graphic 7-1) of the root, which usually occurs

concurrently with dilation of at least the ascending aorta, is evident on the chest radiograph. The ascending aorta, the continuation of the aorta after the root, is better depicted on the lateral chest radiograph, and when enlarged, the ascending aorta may also be seen on the frontal chest radiograph. The aortic arch is fairly well depicted on the lateral radiograph, but the images are foreshortened and the orientation of the arch in the chest renders considerable variability in its appearance. The superior and lateral aspects of the distal portion of the arch are generally well depicted on the frontal radiograph in the region egregiously referred to as the "knuckle." The lateral aspect of the proximal descending thoracic aorta is again well depicted as it abuts (normally) air-filled lung, but the medial portion lies against the thoracic vertebrae; therefore, the medial border of the proximal descending aorta is very difficult to identify on the chest radiograph. The middle and lower portions of the thoracic aorta, which run downward with the lateral portion abutted by lung, are well visualized. The medial portion, which lies generally against the vertebral column, is poorly seen. The middle and lower portions of the thoracic aorta are frequently rendered tortuous by disease, especially aneurysmal and hypertensive disease. The cardiopericardial silhouette (CPS) may obscure the middle and lower thoracic aorta on the frontal radiograph.

ACQUIRED PATHOLOGIES OF THE AORTA

Atherosclerosis

Advanced atherosclerosis of the aorta is radiographically evident as associated intimal calcification (Fig. 7-2). Aortic calcification is usually caused by atherosclerosis, although syphilitic and noninfectious aortitis may result in calcification. Calcification due to atherosclerosis is best appreciated on the frontal chest radiograph and is seen in the distal aortic arch/proximal descending aorta. Perhaps the most commonly calcified site of the thoracic aorta is the floor and lateral wall of the distal arch, which happens to project edge-on and quite cleanly and clearly on the frontal projection.

Calcification due to atherosclerosis resides in intimal plaques and therefore serves as a marker of the inner surface of the aorta such that aortic wall thickness can

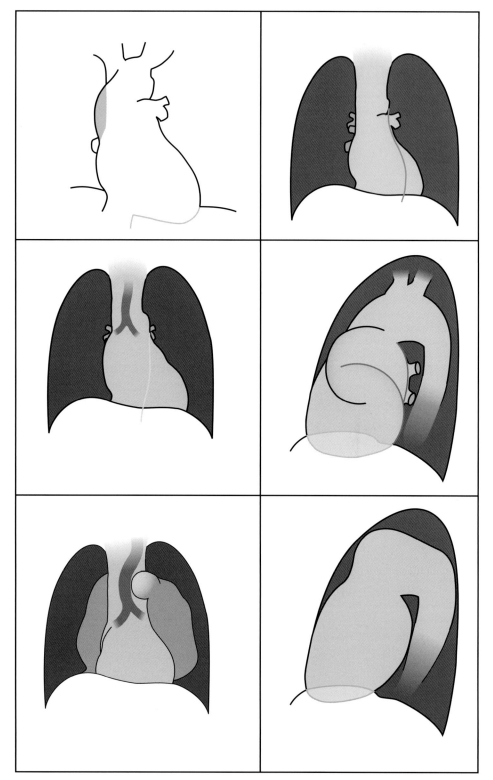

Graphic 7-1. Schematic renderings of enlargement of different portions of the aorta. *Left upper graphic*: Dilation of the ascending aorta may be evident on the frontal radiograph as a curvilinear shadow overlying the right hilum ("hilar overlay"). *Right upper graphic*: Dilation of the descending aorta may be apparent on the frontal radiograph as a leftwardly displaced curvilinear structure posterior to the heart or right hilum. Distinguishing dilation of the descending aorta from marked tortuoisity is a potential challenge. *Middle left graphic*: Aneurysmal dilation of the aortic root, if prominent, may be apparent on the frontal radiograph as a curvilinear structure projecting to the right side of the heart, rather than over the more superior right hilum. *Middle right graphic*: Aneurysmal dilation of the aortic root may be apparent on the lateral radiograph as a rounded central structure. *Lower graphics*: Enormous aneurysmal dilation of the thoracic aorta may generate complex, mass-like silhouettes.

be estimated when the diagnosis of aortic dissection is sought. Aortic intimal calcification is most visible on the lateral wall of the aortic "knuckle." Calcification of the ascending aorta is most commonly due to atherosclerosis but may also be caused by syphilis or aortic vasculitis. Gross calcification of the ascending aorta visible on the chest radiograph is worrisome to the cardiovascular surgeon because it engenders difficulty in cross-clamping the aorta and increased stroke risk with bypass. Other consequences of atherosclerosis that may be evident on the chest radiograph are elongation and tortuosity of the aorta, which result in greater prominence of the aorta and a higher aorta in the chest (Fig. 7-3).

Arterial Hypertension

Long-standing hypertension results in elongation, tortuosity, and atherosclerosis of the aorta, as well as occasionally mild dilation, dissection, or aneurysmal formation of the aorta. As with atherosclerosis, the aorta is more evident in patients with hypertension because of its unfolding.

Aneurysms and False Aneurysms of the Aorta

Aneurysmal disease of the aorta may occur without antecedent disease (hypertension, aortitis, or associated aortic valvulopathy), particularly when the aortic syndrome is heritable/familial. Most aneurysms of the thoracic aorta are apparent on the PA chest radiograph, although aneurysms at the root and ascending level, and also ones posterior to the heart, may be difficult to appreciate with any confidence (Figs. 7-4 to 7-9) unless they are very large (Fig. 7-10). The impossibility of having both sides of the aorta silhouetted against air makes it impossible to establish maximal transverse diameter of an aneurysm accurately, except for a few arch-only aneurysms. Furthermore, there are insufficient signs available in the chest radiograph to ascertain the development of a dissection of an aneurysm. The lateral radiograph contributes to the perception of thoracic aneurysms, and as well, the lateral chest radiograph may inadvertently capture the finding of a calcified anterior wall of an abdominal aortic aneurysm—if the field of view and penetration are optimal. (See Figures 7-11 to 7-24; see also Graphic 7-1).

False aneurysms of the aorta distort the aortic contours if they become large enough (Fig. 7-25). False aneurysms at the arch level are the most readily detected (Fig. 7-26; see also Fig. 7-24). Contrast-enhanced CT scanning, MRI, and TEE are far more robust modalities to assess aneurysmal and false aneurysmal disease of the aorta, as well as their complications. Distinction of true from false aneurysms of the aorta, and identification of most of their complications, requires use of more advanced imaging modalities.

Aortic Dissection

The chest radiograph is somewhat useful for the evaluation of suspected aortic dissection but should not be considered of sufficient diagnostic reliability to yield a final diagnosis for this major disorder. By far the most common test in the current era to evaluate the clinically suspected diagnosis of aortic dissection is CT. The chest radiograph is usually abnormal with several of the features listed subsequently, but a minority of patients (approximately 20%) with proven dissections have normal chest radiographs. Therefore, a normal chest radiograph is never sufficient evidence against aortic dissection.

It should be recalled that there are several types of dissections: type A is where some or all of the intimal flap is within the ascending aorta and type B is where no intimal flap is available within the ascending aorta. The radiographic appearance therefore depends on the location of the involved area and the complications that have occurred.

The main radiographic findings of aortic dissection are as follows:
- ❏ Widening of the aortic contour caused by the false lumen
- ❏ Signs of leaking or bleeding externally to the aorta
- ❏ Intimal displacement or signs of a thickened aortic wall (see later discussion)

Chest Radiographic Findings of Aortic Dissection

On chest radiography, several findings point to aortic dissection.

SIGNS OF ABNORMAL AORTIC CONTOURS (Graphic 7-2; Fig. 7-27)
- ❏ Widened superior mediastinum (seen in only 70% of cases) on the frontal chest radiograph. A widened mediastinum is generally defined as a mediastinal width on an anteroposterior radiograph of greater than 8 cm at the T4 vertebrae level or at the carinal level.
- ❏ Displacement to the right of the trachea or esophagus (best appreciated as rightward displacement of a nasogastric tube)
- ❏ Prominent ascending aorta
- ❏ Enlargement of the aortic "knuckle"

SIGNS OF THICKENED AORTIC WALL. Thickening of the wall of the aorta of greater than 1 cm is reasonably specific for dissection or intramural hematoma involving the arch, at the tradeoff of some sensitivity (Graphic 7-3). Thickening is used as a sign of presence of a false lumen (hematoma within the wall thickening the wall) (Figs. 7-28 and 7-29). The thickness of the wall is measured at the "knuckle" level looking at the superolateral portion of the aorta. When there is intimal calcification, the inside surface of the aorta can be well appreciated because calcification is usually intimal (a complication of intimal atherosclerosis). When there is no intimal calcification, determination of the internal side of the aortic wall is more difficult (Fig. 7-30). The outside of the wall is taken to be the most superolateral shadow of the aortic "knuckle" silhouette. Given the limitations of chest radiography, it is not possible to measure wall thickness accurately elsewhere in the aorta. Therefore, if the dissection involves

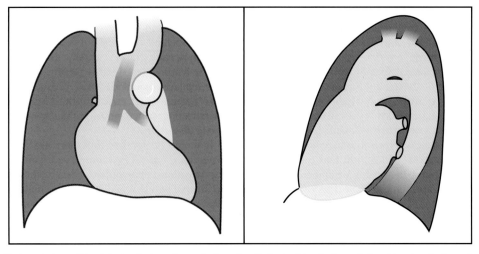

Graphic 7-2. Posteroanterior and lateral chest projections of an aortic dissection. On the frontal projection, note the widened mediastinum, the dilated aorta, the displaced tracheal air column, and mild cardiomegaly. There is also inward intimal displacement denoted by intimal calcium at the distal aortic arch level. On the lateral projection, note the general enlargement of the aorta.

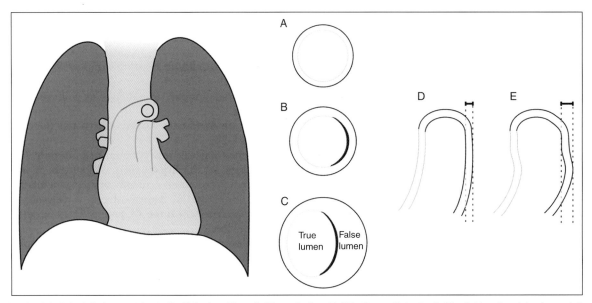

Graphic 7-3. Intimal displacement denoted by thickening of the wall of the aortic "knuckle." The floor and lateral wall of the distal aortic arch is a frequent site of atherosclerotic calcification, which may lead to a useful sign of aortic dissection or intramural hematoma. The lateral wall of the aortic knuckle is normally 2 to 3 mm thick but its thickness is difficult to discern (**A**) without the presence of intimal calcification (**B**) to denote the inside margin of the lateral wall. The outside margin of the wall is denoted by the silhouette. The presence of a false lumen from dissection or intramural hemaotoma along the lateral aspect of the aortic arch will displace the intima inwards, which may be apparent on the frontal radiograph as inward "intimal displacement" if there is calcified plaque on the intima (**C**). Thickening of the wall is only a fair sign for an aortic dissection because the presence of intimal calcification is variable, and a tortuous aorta may project a thick-appearing wall shadow (**D**) versus normal (**E**).

other regions of the aorta, this sign may be falsely negative. Conversely, if the arch is tortuous, the sign may be falsely positive.

SIGNS OF EXTERNAL BLEEDING FROM THE AORTA

❏ Displacement to the right of the trachea/esophagus (best appreciated as rightward displacement of a nasogastric tube) (Fig. 7-31)

❏ Enlargement of/haziness of the descending aorta (caused by hematoma)

❏ Enlargement of/haziness of the ascending aorta (caused by hematoma)

❏ Loss or haziness of the aortic "knuckle"

❏ Left (or right) pleural effusion/cap (caused by external bleeding)

❏ Para-aortic mass (hematoma)

❏ Haziness of the ascending aorta (caused by adventitial hematoma)

SIGNS OF CARDIAC COMPLICATIONS

❏ Signs of acute pulmonary edema (secondary to acute aortic insufficiency due to prolapse of a valve leaflet or acute myocardial infarction due to coronary occlusion by the intimal flap)

❏ A large azygous vein. This suggests elevated central venous pressure, which in the context of aortic dissection suggests tamponade due to intrapericardial rupture or right heart failure from torrential aortic insufficiency.

Aortographic Signs of Aortic Dissection

DIRECT SIGNS
☐ Double channel
☐ True lumen plus false lumen
☐ Linear radiolucency (equals intimal flap)
☐ Entry of contrast into a false lumen
☐ Reentry of contrast into a true lumen

INDIRECT SIGNS
☐ Narrowed true lumen
☐ Thickening of the aortic wall: greater than 5 to 6 mm (normal, 2–3 mm)
☐ Abnormal catheter position (assumed to be displaced by the intimal flap)
☐ Aortic insufficiency
☐ Branch artery involvement

Intramural Hematoma/Penetrating Ulcer of the Aorta

The chest radiograph is insensitive to the difficult diagnoses of intramural hematoma and penetrating ulcer of the aorta (Fig. 7-32). More sophisticated imaging modalities are required to establish these diagnoses.

Thoracic Aortic Aneurysms

Aneurysms of the thoracic aorta are evident on the chest radiograph as widening of the aorta in the affected portion. Aneurysms may involve any combination of the root, the ascending aorta, the arch, the descending aorta, or the entire aorta. Aneurysms involving the arch may result in displacement of the mediastinum and occasionally of compression of the right bronchus.

Other Arch Lesions

These include the following:
☐ Post-traumatic pseudoaneurysms of the arch and proximal descending aorta. There is focal outpouching, often with double density overlying or beneath the aortic knuckle, which may calcify, if long-standing.
☐ Penetrating ulcers with associated pseudoaneurysms of the arch and proximal descending aorta.
☐ Arch anomalies. Aberrant subclavian arteries can be seen on the lateral chest radiograph as soft tissue density posteriorly, indenting the esophageal shadow.

Traumatic Rupture of the Aorta

Blunt chest trauma or more commonly deceleration injury (usually a motor vehicle accident with rapid deceleration) may result in partial or complete disruption or trans-section of the aorta (Fig. 7-33). This most frequently occurs at the proximal portion of the descending aorta. There, a shear injury may occur at the site where the well-tethered aortic arch (by ligaments to other mediastinal structures and to the chest wall) joins the poorly tethered descending aorta, which

is joined to other structures only through its intercostal and spinal branches (Figs. 7-34 and 7-35). Many cases of aortic trauma are frank disruptions of the aorta and immediately fatal due to internal hemorrhage; however, many cases are partial, and therefore life-threatening, but potentially surgically correctable. Thus, rapid detection is necessary.

Traumatic disruption of the aorta results in a tear into the wall of the aorta with false aneurysm lesion type formation or complete tearing of the aorta and internal hemorrhage (Figs. 7-36 and 7-37). True dissection may occur but is much less common and tends to be localized versus the extensive nature of most typical primary dissection lesions.

The radiographic signs include widening of the distal aorta or aortic arch and possibly left pleural effusion (which is nonspecific in a trauma situation but suggests aortic injury and rupture, especially in the context of an abnormal-appearing aorta). The widening is the result of the bulk of the false aneurysm or of the bulk of associated mediastinal hematoma. Mediastinal hematoma may occur due to vascular or bone injury without disruption of the aorta, and disruption of the aorta may occur without mediastinal hematoma. Any abnormal aortic contours in the context of severe deceleration injury require further evaluation of the aorta with a more definitive test such as CT, angiography, or TEE.

Important ancillary findings in the setting of trauma include pneumothorax, pneumomediastinum, pneumopericardium, lung contusion, and rib fractures.

CONGENITAL ABNORMALITIES OF THE AORTA

Coarctation of the Aorta

The chest radiograph is strongly suggestive of coarctation of the aorta in more than 90% of cases. The diagnosis of coarctation may be often made from the frontal chest radiograph and essentially confirmed with more advanced modalities. See Chapter 19 (Graphic 19-2) for the radiographic appearance of coarctation of the aorta.

Cardiac Findings on Chest Radiography

Coarctation of the aorta is often associated with an enlargement of the CPS (increased left ventricular dimensions) because of the pressure load on the left ventricle from the hypertension arising from the coarctation or the volume or pressure load imparted on the left ventricle by dysfunction of an associated bicuspid aortic valve.

Vascular Findings of Coarctation on Chest Radiography (Figs. 7-38 to 7-40)

Findings include the following:
☐ Aorta and "knuckle" with a rather constant abnormal contour—the "figure 3"

□ Upper bulge: aortic knuckle plus dilated subclavian artery with or without dilated proximal aorta. The upper bulge may be less apparent if the shadow of the left subclavian artery is obscuring it.

□ Indentation: coarctation itself

□ Lower bulge: dilated distal aorta (poststenotic dilatation)

As a historical note: in coarctation of the aorta, a barium esophagram yielded mirror image curves, the "reverse figure 3," because the esophagus is immediately adjacent to (posterior to) the aorta.

A bicuspid aortic valve is present in approximately 50% of cases of coarctation of the aorta. Signs of dysfunction of an associated bicuspid valve should be sought in coartation cases: aortic insufficiency (left ventricular elongation, dilation, and generalized enlargement of the aorta) and aortic stenosis (left ventricular enlargement). As well, signs of dilation or aneurysm of the ascending aorta, which may reflect associated aortopathy or poststenotic dilation, should be sought.

Rib notching is usually seen along the third to the ninth ribs. It requires more than 5 years to become radiographically apparent. Unilateral right-sided versus bilateral rib notching points to the site of the obstruction; the coarctation with unilateral right notching is at or before the left subclavian artery. Rib notching is usually present in significant coarctation but may be absent in one fourth of adult patients with this diagnosis. Rib notching may result from enlargement of any of the three elements of the arterial-venous-nervous bundle that runs under a rib (see later discussion).

RIB NOTCHING: DIFFERENTIAL

Causes of Pseudo–Rib Notching (Fig. 7-41)
Causes include the following:
□ Congenital (nonsclerotic margins of adjacent bone)
□ Hyperparathyroidism

Causes of True Rib Notching
Causes include the following:
□ Aortic obstruction
□ Coarctation (enlarged intercostal artery)
□ Interrupted aorta (enlarged intercostal artery)
□ Subclavian artery obstruction
□ Markedly reduced pulmonary blood flow
□ Tetralogy of Fallot
□ Pulmonary atresia
□ Tricuspid atresia
□ Absence of a pulmonary artery
□ Superior vena cava syndrome (enlarged intercostal vein)
□ Neurofibromatosis enlarged intercostal nerve

Causes of Unilateral Rib Notching
Causes include the following:
□ Ipsilateral Blalock-Taussig shunt (upper two ribs)
□ Coarctation presubclavian artery (subclavian artery may or may not be aberrant)

Causes of Bilateral Rib Notching
Causes include the following:
□ Bilateral Blalock-Taussig shunt
□ Coarctation distal to both subclavian arteries

Postrepair Coarctation Complications
Complications include the following:
□ Recoarctation (which is difficult to identify by chest radiography)
□ Postintervention aneurysm/pseudoaneurysm formation. Usually seen with a patch–flap repair or a tube–graft repair. Radiographically, postcoarctation aneurysm/pseudoaneurysm formation may be apparent as a focal area of enlargement in the proximal descending aorta, generally best seen on the frontal radiograph. It may be associated with dysplastic ribs in the left upper thoracic cage from prior thoracotomy.

Causes of Isolated Right-Sided Aortic Arch (Figs. 7-42 to 7-46)
The incidence of an isolated right-sided aortic arch is 1:2500. A right-sided aortic arch is apparent when no aortic "knuckle" is seen on the left side, displacement of the trachea is to the left, and an aortic "knuckle" is on the right. With an isolated right-sided aortic arch, there is a high incidence of associated congenital heart disease (10 to 100 times that of the general population). Associations include truncus arteriosus, pulmonary atresia with ventricular septal defect, tetralogy of Fallot, tricuspid atresia, and transposition of the great arteries.

THE ABDOMINAL AORTA

It must be stated that the chest radiograph is not a suitable means to evaluate the abdominal aorta. However, on occasion, on the lateral chest radiograph of an individual with an abdominal aortic aneurysm, the calcified anterior wall of the aneurysm may be seen. In the majority of individuals (approximately 70%) with an abdominal aortic aneurysm, an abdominal lateral "shoot through" radiograph depicts calcification in the anterior wall of the aneurysm. The lateral chest radiograph may serendipitously achieve this depiction.

Causes of a Small Thoracic Aorta
Causes include the following:
□ Intracardiac left-to-right shunt, especially atrial septal defects. The heart is rotated to the left and

the arch folds on itself, looking smaller, and the main pulmonary trunk is rotated and appears to be more prominent and often is as well.

❐ Coarctation (with a long hypoplastic arch)
❐ Transposition of the great arteries: rotation of the aorta, which appears to be small but actually is not

Causes of a Large Thoracic Aorta

Causes include the following:

❐ Proximal: valvular aortic stenosis proximal to the right innominate artery, coarctation, patent ductus arteriosus, annuloaortic ectasia or ascending aorta, syphilis (usually just the ascending aorta), aortitis, dissection

❐ Generalized: hypertension, "unfolded" (atherosclerotic) aorta, aortic insufficiency, dissection

Inheritable Disorders of the Aorta

(Figs. 7-47 to 7-54)

Marfan syndrome and related disorders, such as Loeys-Dietz syndrome, are complex syndromes that involve the aorta and musculoskeletal systems (among others). Chest radiography is frequently notable for the following:

❐ Pectus deformities
❐ Kyphosis and scoliosis
❐ Aneurysmal dilation of the aorta, especially the aortic root and ascending aorta

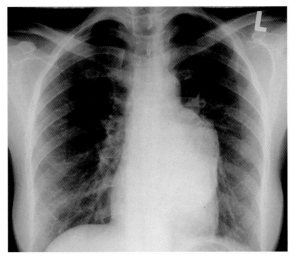

Figure 7-1. There is a markedly abnormal contour to the left of the heart, which is actually of the descending aorta from which a very large sarcoma of the aorta is growing into the left chest cavity.

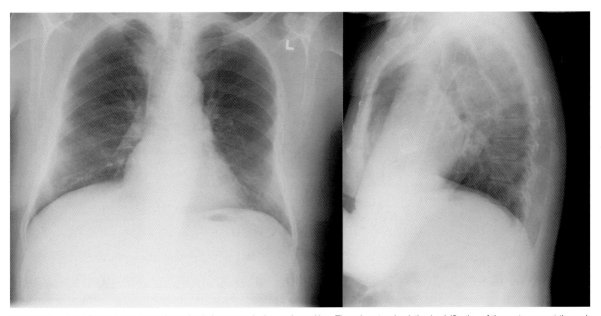

Figure 7-2. A Starr-Edwards mechanical prosthesis is present in the aortic position. There is extensive intimal calcification of the aorta seen at the arch level on the posteroanterior radiograph and at the descending thoracic aorta seen on the lateral radiograph, which is consistent with the advanced age of the patient and the type of prothesis.

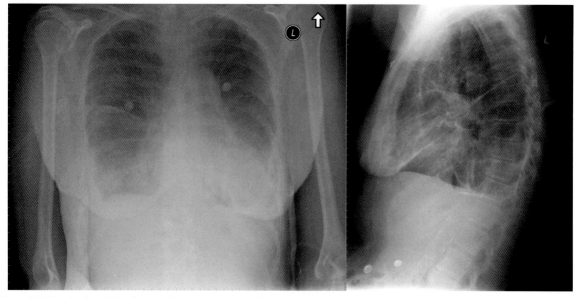

Figure 7-3. Hypertensive crisis and acute pulmonary edema in an elderly patient. Note the extensive calcification of the aorta, best seen on the abdominal aorta on the lateral radiograph.

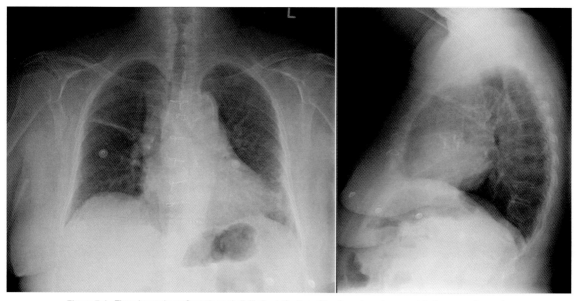

Figure 7-4. There is nearly confluent "egg shell–like" calcification of the thoracic aorta, especially the ascending aorta.

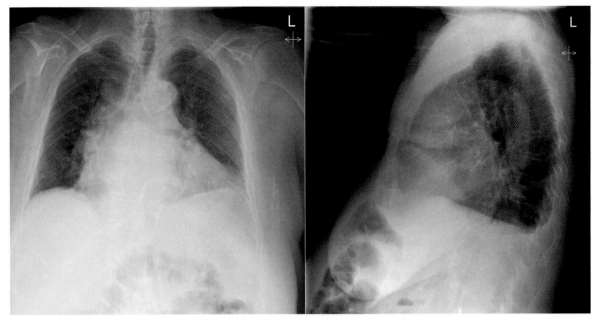

Figure 7-5. Cardiomegaly due to left heart chamber enlargement. The thoracic aorta is prominently calcified.

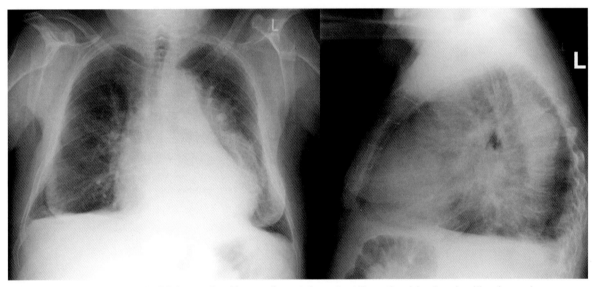

Figure 7-6. The cardiothoracic ratio is mildly increased, and the ascending aorta is prominent. The aortic arch is enlarged, and there is a very large aneurysm of the entire descending thoracic aorta visible lateral to the heart shadow and posterior to it.

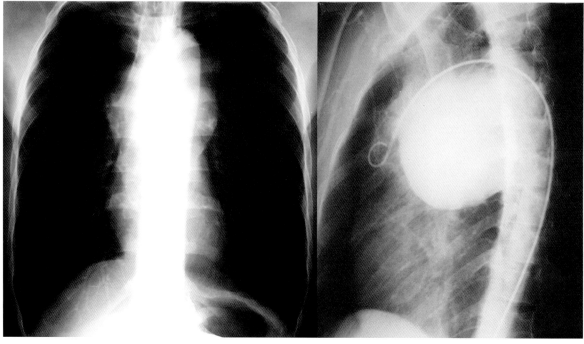

Figure 7-7. Posteroanterior radiograph and contrast aortogram of a luetic aneurysm of the ascending aorta.

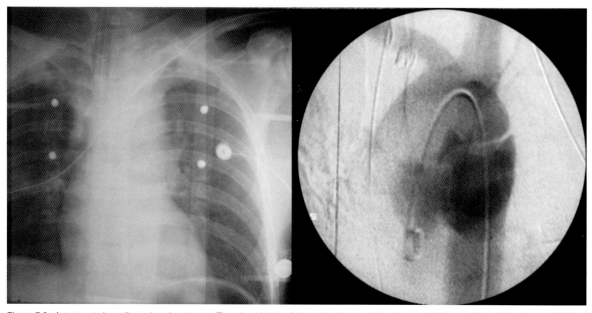

Figure 7-8. Anteroposterior radiograph and aortogram. There is widening of the mediastinum and displacement of the endotracheal tube from mediastinal hematoma associated with the traumatic disruption of the proximal descending ("isthmus") portion of the aorta and from a false aneurysm produced by the disruption. The margins of the aortic arch and proximal descending aorta are hazy due to associated mediastinal hematoma.

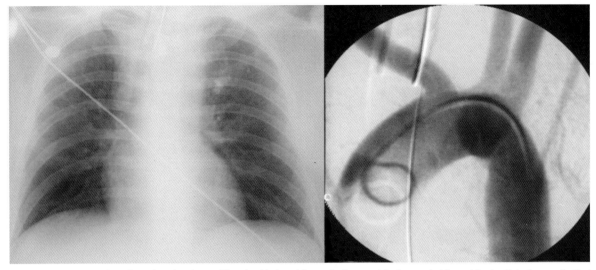

Figure 7-9. Anteroposterior radiograph and aortogram. There is widening of the mediastinum and displacement of the endotracheal tube from mediastinal hematoma associated with the traumatic disruption of the proximal descending ("isthmus") portion of the aorta.

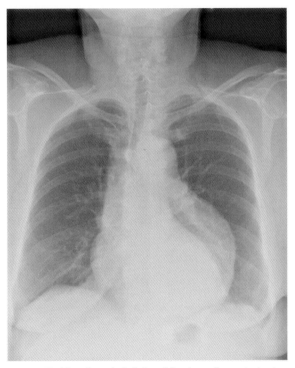

Figure 7-10. There is marked dilation of the descending aorta due to a 10-cm aneurysm. Intimal calcification follows and denotes the left lateral margin of the wall of the aneurysmal aorta.

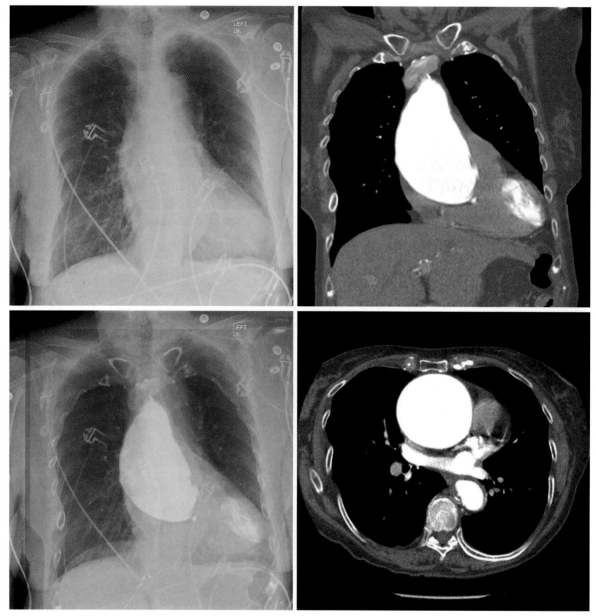

Figure 7-11. Chest radiographs, coronal and axial contrast computed tomography (CT) scans, and superimposed coronal CT scan on the frontal chest radiograph, which reveal the hilar overlay sign of dilation of the ascending aorta overlying and obscuring the right hilum.

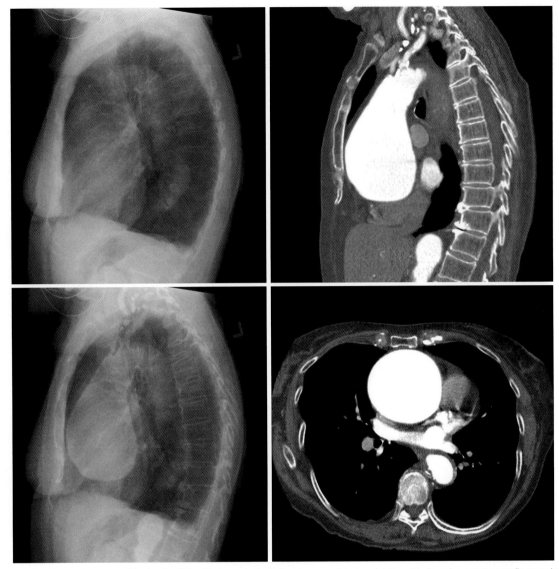

Figure 7-12. The anterior aspect of the heart, which achieves contact with the sternum, a fair sign of right ventricular enlargement generally, may also be formed by enlargement and dilation of the ascending aorta, as in this case.

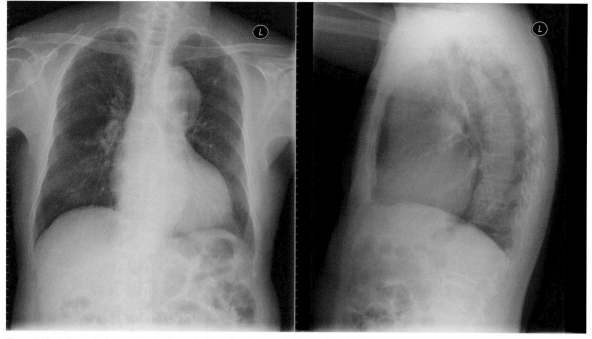

Figure 7-13. Anteroposterior and lateral radiographs. There is enlargement of the aortic arch, depressing the left mainstem bronchus. The descending aorta is tortuous. The intimal calcification is difficult to localize. The cardiothoracic ratio is increased, and on the lateral radiograph left ventricular posterior displacement is apparent (due to aortic insufficiency complicating dilation of the aorta).

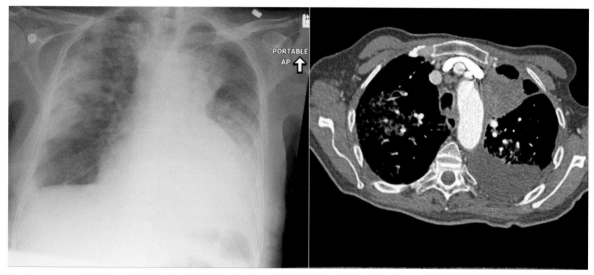

Figure 7-14. What appears to be a prominent aneurysmal aortic arch is seen on a contrast-enhanced axial CT scan to be due to a lung cancer mass arising beside and against the aortic arch.

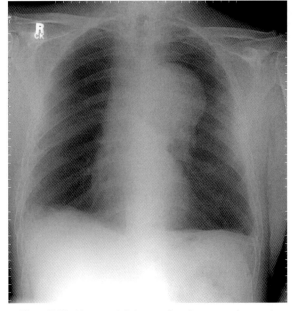

Figure 7-15. A large, and obvious, aortic arch aneurysm is present.

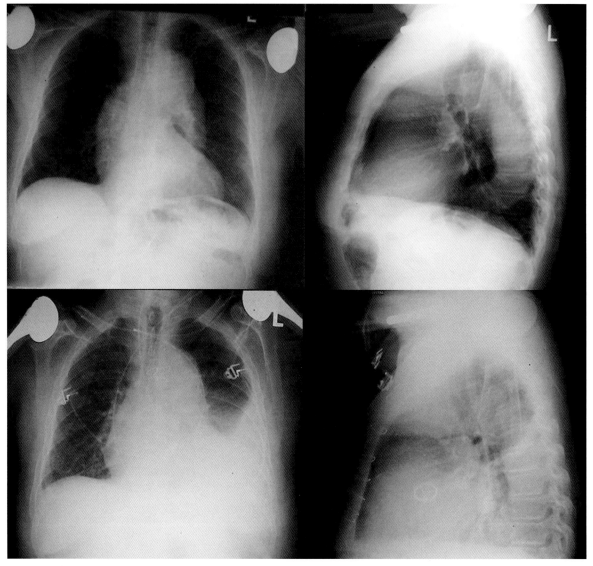

Figure 7-16. Pre–Bentall procedure (*top*); post–Bentall procedure (*bottom*). Preoperatively, there is enlargement of the ascending aorta denoted by right hilar overlay, enlargement of the arch apparent as dilation and left mainstem bronchus depression, and unfolding/tortuosity of the descending aorta. Post-operatively, only the aortic root and ascending aorta have been replaced, and only their shadow has (partially) normalized—the appearance of the arch and descending aorta have not changed.

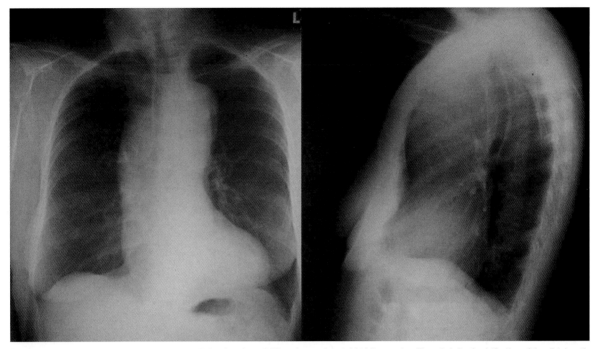

Figure 7-17. The ascending aorta and arch are obviously enlarged. There is prominent right hilar overlay. There is intimal calcification of the distal aortic arch/proximal descending aorta. A pectus excavatum is apparent on the lateral radiograph.

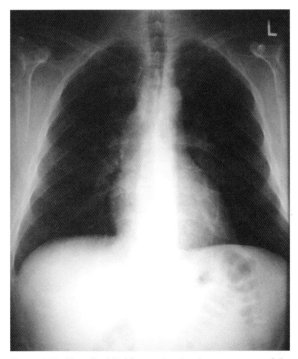

Figure 7-18. There is right hilar overlay due to an aneurysm of the ascending aorta.

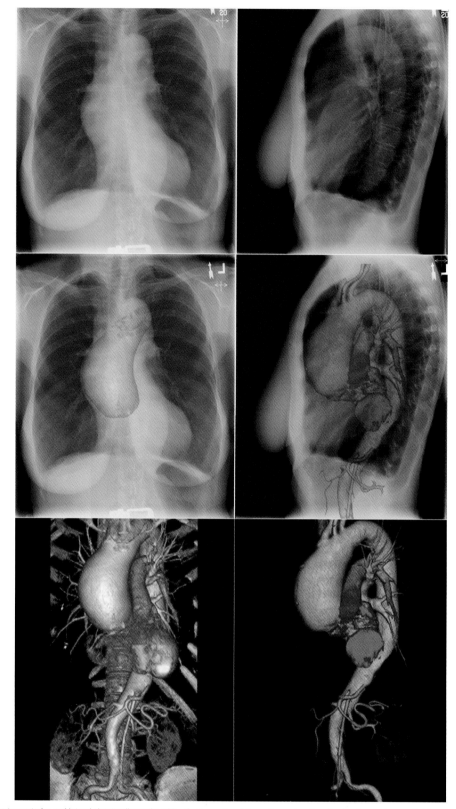

Figure 7-22. Posteroanterior and lateral chest radiographs with volume-rendered three-dimensional contrast-enhanced computed tomography images. The hilar overlay sign is revealed to be due to aneurysmal dilation of the ascending aorta that extends into the arch. The aneurysm abutts the sternum, as seen on the lateral projection images.

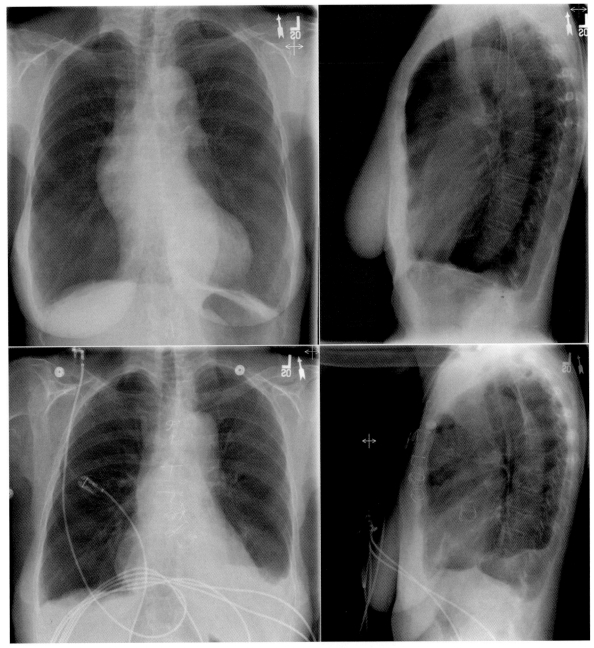

Figure 7-23. Images before and after replacement of the ascending aorta and arch and aortic valve (with a bioprosthesis that is best seen on the lateral radiograph, where it cannot be confused with sternal wires). The size of the ascending aorta has diminished.

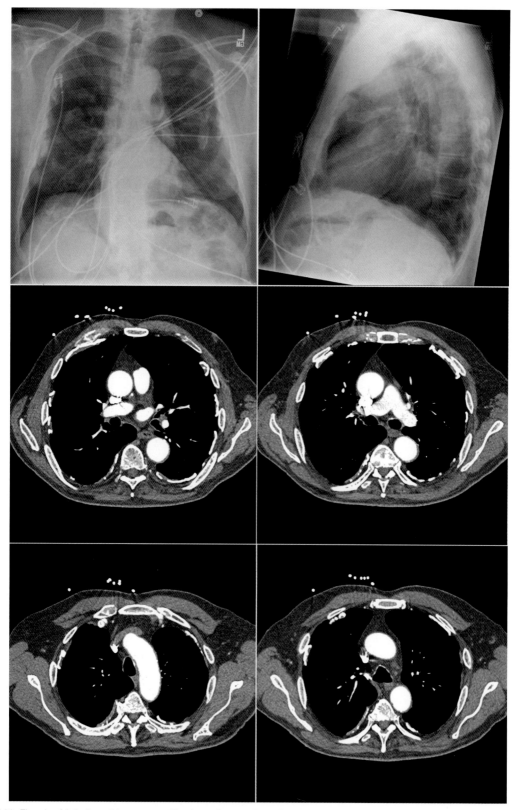

Figure 7-24. There is a faintly discernible aneurysm of the descending aorta located, as depicted on the contrast computed tomography scans, retrocardiac at the level of the diaphragm. What are considerably more obvious on the computed tomography scans are the numerous calcified pleural plaques due to prior asbestos exposure, although some of them are certainly appreciable on the chest radiographs.

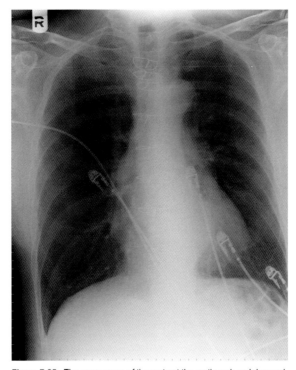

Figure 7-25. The appearance of the aorta at the aortic arch and descending levels is normal and without dilation, displacement, or calcification. There is a questionable slight prominence of the silhouette of the ascending aorta. A false aneurysm of several centimeters in diameter was present arising off the ascending aorta (due to prior surgical manipulation at the time of bypass surgery) but is radiographically scarcely apparent.

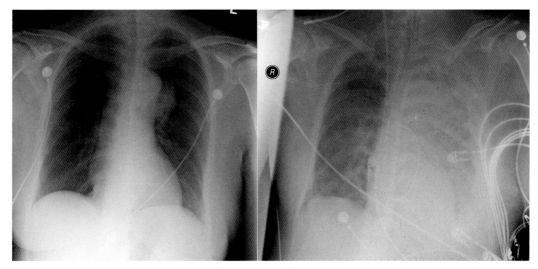

Figure 7-26. Anteroposterior radiographs at admission and after rupture. In the left radiograph, the cardiothoracic ratio is normal. The ascending aorta is dilated/displaced. To the left lateral aspect of the arch there is an abnormal shadow, which is a false aneurysm due to aortitis. No intimal calcium or calcium displacement is present. In the right radiograph, rupture into the left pleural cavity has occurred. An intra-aortic balloon pump and pulmonary artery line have been inserted to manage an acute coronary syndrome. Either the anticoagulents/antiplatelet agents and/or the intra-aortic balloon pump contributed to the bleeding from the aneurysm.

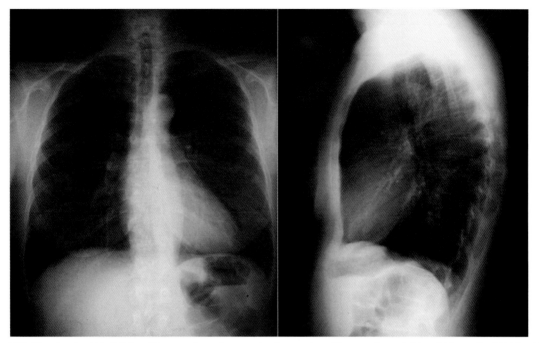

Figure 7-27. There is only a hint of dilation of the ascending aorta apparent as the curvature of the ascending aorta lying slightly over the right hilum. There is hyperinflation of the lungs from chronic obstructive pulmonary disease.

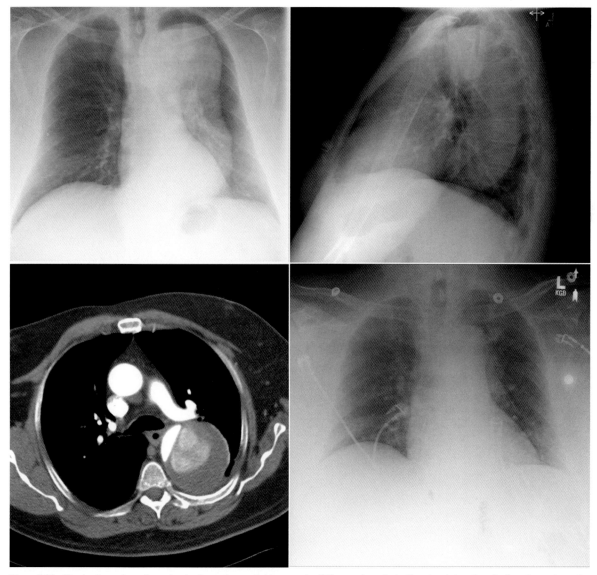

Figure 7-28. Chest radiographs and a contrast-enhanced computed tomography (CT) scan of a patient with a chronic type B aortic dissection and massive enlargement of the false lumen. The right lower image is from 2 years previously at the time of presentation with an acute type B aortic dissection. At that time, the aortic arch and descending aorta were enlarged. The amount of further dilation of the false lumen within 2 years was striking.

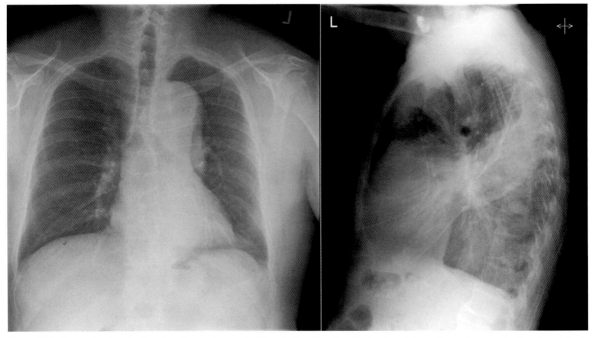

Figure 7-29. Chronic distal aortic dissection after surgical repair of Type A dissection. The distal arch and descending aorta are markedly enlarged due to expansion of the false lumen.

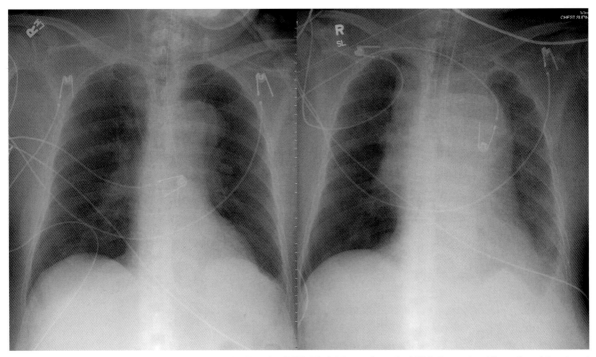

Figure 7-30. Anteroposterior radiographs, type A acute aortic dissection (AAD). The left image shows the AAD before rupture. The aortic arch is enlarged and there is a double contour, with no haziness to the contour. No intimal calcification or intimal displacement is apparent. There is no left pleural effusion. The right image shows the AAD after rupture. The mediastinum has widened due to mediastinal hematoma, the aortic contour is hazy due to periaortic hematoma, and there is a new left pleural effusion due to tracking of the hematoma.

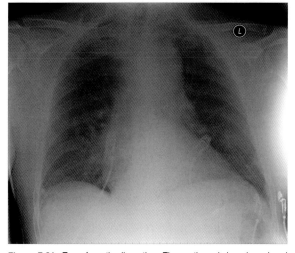

Figure 7-31. Type A aortic dissection. The aortic arch is enlarged and displacing the trachea. There is no intimal displacement, double contour, or haziness of the aorta present. The cardiothoracic ratio is normal. There is no pulmonary congestion and no pleural effusion.

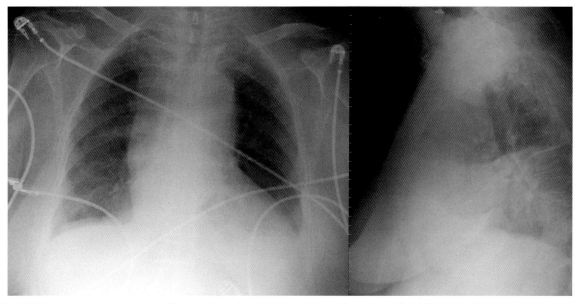

Figure 7-32. Type A intramural hematoma. The ascending aorta, aortic arch, and descending aorta are dilated. The contour of the descending aorta may have a double appearance. A small left pleural effusion is present.

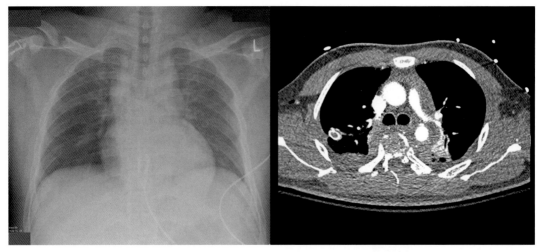

Figure 7-33. A 25-year-old male, post–motor vehicle accident—an ejected, non–seat-belted driver. The mediastinum is widened and can be seen to be due to a mediastinal hematoma on the contrast-enhanced computed tomography scan. The degree of aortic injury was actually only a minor traumatic disruption. Note the fractured clavicle, one of eleven bone fractures.

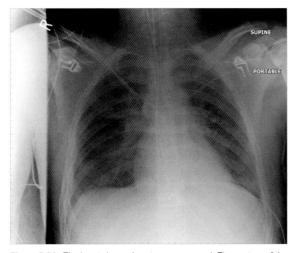

Figure 7-34. The heart size and contours are normal. The contour of the aorta is normal. The mediastinum is not prominently widened, and the nasogastric tube is not displaced. However, the patient had a very extensive traumatic disruption of the "isthmus" portion of the aorta, but without an associated hematoma to displace mediastinal structures.

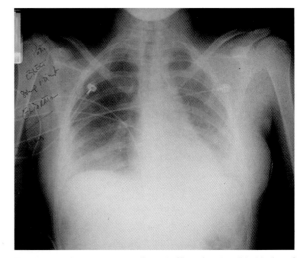

Figure 7-35. Anteroposterior radiograph. There is only mild widening of the mediastinum and displacement of the tracheal air column from mediastinal hematoma associated with a traumatic disruption of the proximal descending aorta.

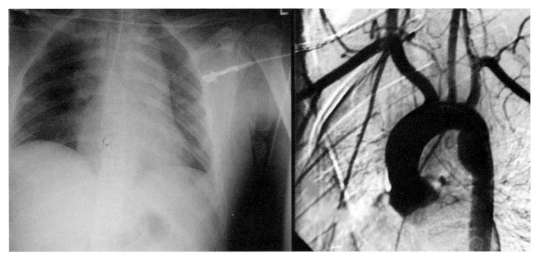

Figure 7-36. Anteroposterior radiograph and aortogram. There is widening of the mediastinum and displacement of the nasogastric tube, from mediastinal hematoma associated with traumatic disruption of the proximal descending ("isthmus") portion of the aorta and from a false aneurysm produced by the disruption.

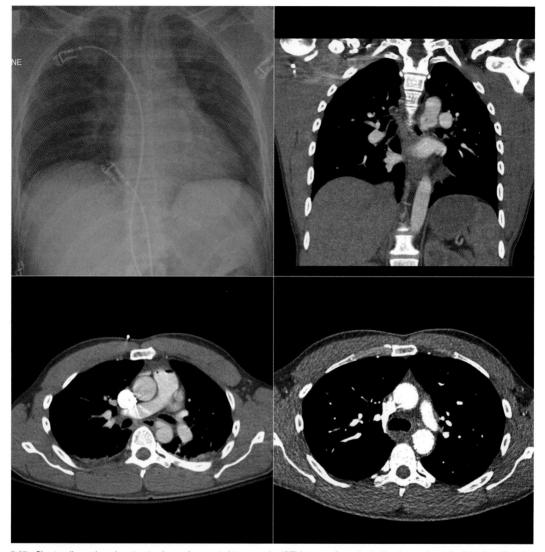

Figure 7-37. Chest radiograph and contrast-enhanced computed tomography (CT) images of a patient with a traumatic aortic disruption. The chest radiograph does not reveal significant mediastinal widening, but there is rotation. The right upper and left lower CT images demonstrate the intimal disruption and false lumen of the traumatic disruption and the "isthmus" portion of the aorta. There is little, if any, mediastinal hematoma, despite the injury to the aorta. The right lower image follows endograft deployment to the disrupted area, with exclusion of the false aneurysm.

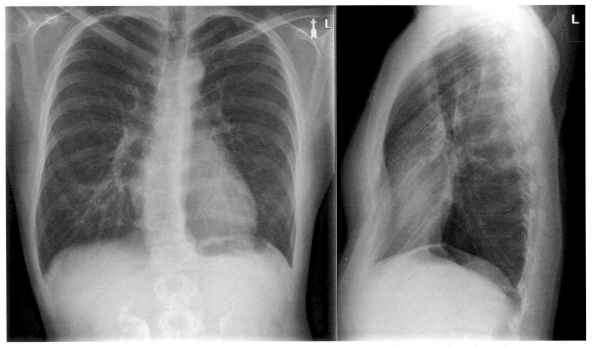

Figure 7-51. Marfan syndrome. Patient with a tall body habitus and little subcutaneous fat. There is scoliosis of the spine and a small pectus excavatum of the sternum. The heart and pulmonary vasculature appear normal.

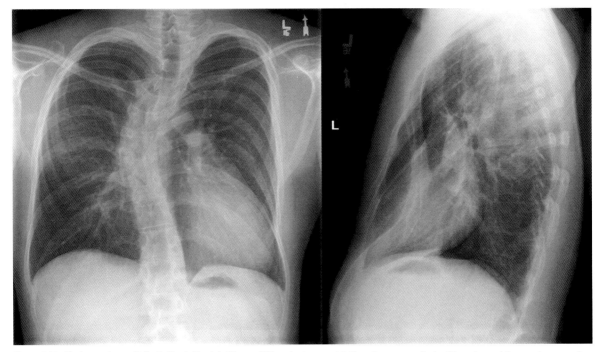

Figure 7-52. Marfan syndrome. Patient with a tall body habitus and little subcutaneous fat. There is severe scoliosis of the spine and deep pectus excavatum of the sternum.

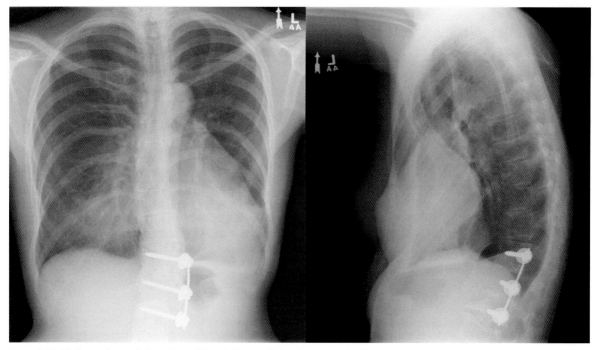

Figure 7-53. Marfan syndrome. Patient with a tall body habitus and little subcutaneous fat. There is scoliosis of the spine and in dwelling reconstructive hardware to align the spine. There is a deep pectus excavatum of the sternum.

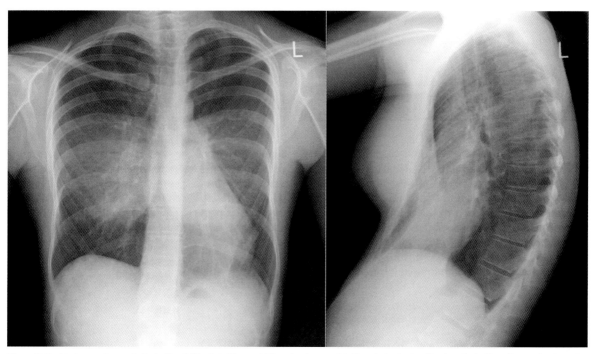

Figure 7-54. Marfan syndrome. Patient with a tall body habitus and little subcutaneous fat. There is kyphosis without scoliosis. There is a moderate pectus excavatum of the sternum.

Localizing Prosthetic Valves

Key Points

- Radiographically apparent aortic, mitral, tricuspid, and pulmonic valve prostheses can all be identified and localized by chest radiography. Older mechanical and biological valves were easy to identify because they generally had obvious metallic components. Contemporary mechanical and biological valves have far less or no ferrometallic or other metallic components; therefore, they are more difficult to recognize, especially if the heart shadow is dense. Furthermore, the momentum of prosthetic valve insertion has shifted toward bioprostheses (4:1 ratio), several of which have no radiographically evident components at all.
- The frontal radiograph alone is often adequate to identify and to localize a prosthesis, but superimposition of the shadow of a prosthesis onto that of the spine and obscuring of a prosthesis shadow by that of a large heart reduce the sensitivity of the frontal radiograph somewhat.
- The lateral radiograph is invaluable to allow projection of the prosthesis shadow off that of the spine.
- Both the position of the prosthesis shadow and its orientation are used to establish its location.

The chest radiograph can localize the great majority of valve prostheses to the aortic, mitral, or tricuspid positions, and it can usually determine whether the prosthesis is mechanical or bioprosthetic. In addition, the chest radiograph can offer radiographic evidence of the presence or absence of congestive heart failure. Both the posteroanterior and lateral radiographs are required (Graphic 8-1).

AORTIC VALVE PROSTHESIS

On the frontal radiograph, an aortic prosthesis overlies part of, or the whole, vertebral column and may not be apparent due to superimposition of the aortic valve prosthesis shadows onto that of the spine, especially if the heart shadow is also dense. The lateral radiograph is particularly important to identify and to localize a prosthesis to the aortic position, because it projects the prosthesis away from the spine such that it can be clearly seen and its orientation understood. An aortic prosthesis lies above an imaginary line from the left mainstem bronchus to the sternodiaphragmatic angle, on an oblique/horizontal plane (Fig. 8-1).

MITRAL VALVE PROSTHESIS

On the frontal radiograph, a mitral prosthesis partially or completely lies to the left of the vertebral column and is usually visually obvious. A large and radiopaque heart, particularly on a poorly exposed radiograph, may obscure a mitral prosthesis. The lateral radiograph is important to project the prosthesis away from the spine and to localize a prosthesis to the mitral position. A mitral prosthesis lies below an imaginary line from the left mainstem bronchus to the sternodiaphragmatic angle, on a vertical plane facing the frontal projection.

TRICUSPID VALVE PROSTHESIS

On the frontal radiograph, a tricuspid prosthesis lies on or to the right of the vertebral column and is usually visually obvious. Again, a large and radiopaque heart, particularly on a poorly exposed radiograph, may obscure a tricuspid prosthesis. The tricuspid position is on a similar plane to the mitral position, but lies on the diaphragm, on the right side of the cardiopericardial silhouette (Fig. 8-2).

PULMONIC VALVE PROSTHESIS

On the frontal radiograph, a pulmonic valve prosthesis overlies the vertebral column and may not be apparent. The lateral radiograph is particularly important to identify and to localize a prosthesis to the pulmonic position. As with an aortic prosthesis, a pulmonic prosthesis lies above an imaginary line from the left mainstem bronchus to the sternodiaphragmatic angle. It lies on an oblique or horizontal plane more anteriorly than, and against, the anterior border of the heart.

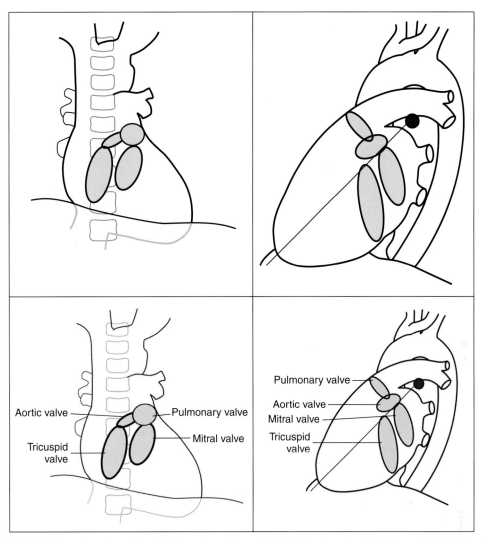

Graphic 8-1. Projection of the cardiac valves and annuli on the posteroanterior and lateral chest radiographs. A line between the left mainstem bronchus and the apex of the heart on the lateral radiograph separates the pulmonic and aortic valves (*above*) and the mitral and tricuspid valves (*below*).

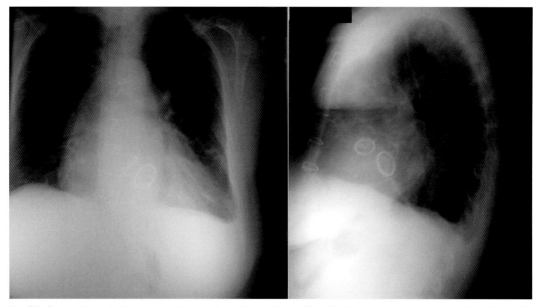

Figure 8-1. Bileaflet occluder mechanical valve prostheses in the aortic and mitral positions. On the posteroanterior radiograph, the occluders of the aortic prosthesis are seen in systole edge-on and in the open position.

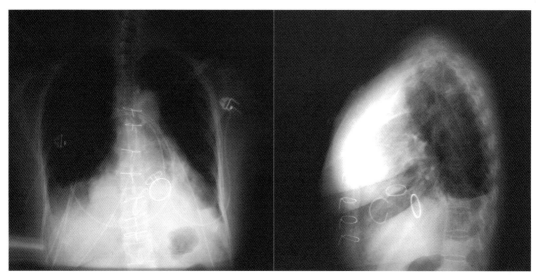

Figure 8-2. Bileaflet occluder mechanical valve prostheses are present in the aortic and mitral positions, and there is a tricuspid annuloplasty ring in the tricuspid position.

9 Mechanical Prosthetic Valves

MECHANICAL PROSTHESES

Most often, mechanical valve prostheses (Table 9-1) are inserted into the aortic and the mitral positions. Many different models have been made over the 40 years of valve replacement surgery, but currently the great majority that are inserted are bileaflet hemidisk models. However, there are many older types and models still in situ, and therefore it is necessary to have an appreciation of the different types. Mechanical prostheses are evident principally because of their radiopaque sewing rings, and for some models, radiographically evident struts, cages, or occluders. The more ferrous or other metallic material within the prosthesis, the more radiographically evident the prosthesis; current mechanical prostheses contain little ferrous or metallic material and are much less radiographically evident by comparison.

A chest radiograph may reveal if a mechanical prosthesis is in the open or closed position, depending on (by chance occurrence) which phase of the cardiac cycle occurred when the exposure was taken. A chest radiograph is not a sufficient means to determine whether the occluder elements of a prosthesis are moving correctly or whether the sewing ring is stable. To determine occluder motion, fluoroscopy, gated cardiac computed tomography, or transesophageal echocardiography is required.

Bileaflet Occluder

Because of excellent hemodynamics, reliability, and longevity, bileaflet occluder prostheses are the current mechanical valve prostheses of choice (Graphic 9-1).

There are more than a dozen designs of bileaflet occluder valves, with small differences between them. Most are of St. Jude or CarboMedics designs.

The ring of the older St. Jude model was barely visible on the chest radiograph because it contained little radiopaque alloy. More recent models contain more radiopaque alloy, and hence the sewing ring is radiographically more readily apparent. CarboMedics valves have a more radiopaque sewing ring than do St. Jude prostheses. The sewing ring may not be seen when it overlies the spine on an underpenetrated frontal radiograph. The ring is circular, with two small curve bulges opposite each other that support the hinges of the occluder elements (Figs. 9-1 and 9-2).

The occluder elements (two hemidisks) are made of carbolite (pyrolitic carbon/graphite) and are faintly radiographically visible, again, especially when viewed edge-on. Occluder hemidisks of older prostheses contain less alloy than do current models and are therefore less obvious. When viewed en-face, or obliquely, the occluders are often not sufficiently radiopaque to be visible. The occluders do not open fully to 90°, but rather to 78° or 85°. Bileaflet occluder prosthesis hemidisks do not close flat but rather to an oblique angle of 35°. The hemidisk occluders pivot on small hinges on their inside margin. Generally, the two occluders should be seen as symmetric. However, visualization of one occluder and not the other may occur despite normal occluder motion if the angle of incidence of the x-ray beam is adequate for one occluder but not the other.

Because the sewing rings are relatively thin and because the occluder elements open nearly to 90°, bileaflet occluder valves (particularly the larger diameter ones) are only mildly obstructive to blood flow.

Fluoroscopy has been the most reliable means of determining normal or abnormal occluder motion and normal or rocking sewing ring motion. However, electrocardiography-gated cardiac computed tomography is increasingly able to assess occluder motion although is heart rate–dependent in doing so.

Single Tilting Disk

The Björk-Shiley prosthesis (Graphic 9-2) is an example of a single tilting disk type of mechanical prosthesis and has an obviously distinct radiographic appearance. Single tilting disk prostheses represent older

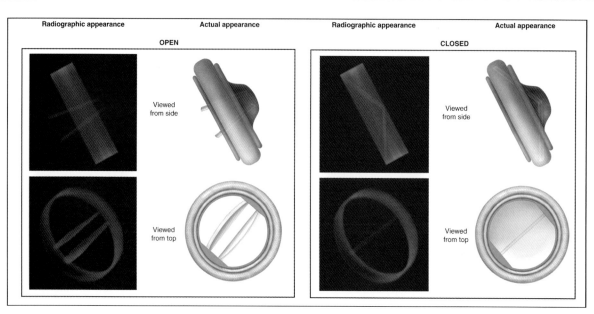

| Radiographic appearance | Actual appearance | | Radiographic appearance | Actual appearance |

OPEN **CLOSED**

Viewed from side

Viewed from top

Graphic 9-1. Mechanical prosthesis Bileaflet occluder (St. Jude and CarboMedics).

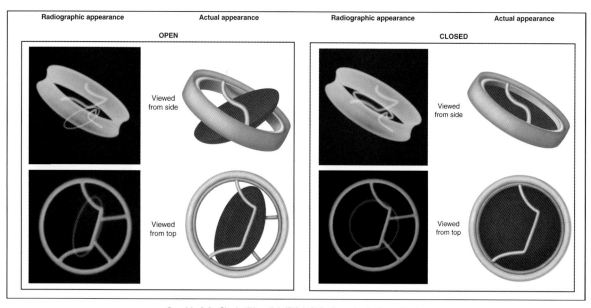

| Radiographic appearance | Actual appearance | | Radiographic appearance | Actual appearance |

OPEN **CLOSED**

Viewed from side

Viewed from top

Graphic 9-2. Single tilting disk (Björk-Shiley) mechanical prosthesis.

technology and currently are rarely inserted, but many are still in existence and functioning well. They are quite easily visualized and identified (Fig. 9-3). Some early production Björk-Shiley prostheses of the convexoconcave 60-degree model were mechanically unreliable because of minor strut failure, resulting in embolization of the tilting disk occluder.

The valve sewing ring is easily visualized as a metal containing ring that yields a dense shadow. There are two radiographically apparent struts (a major and a minor) that retain the tilting disk within the sewing

ring, and this limits the angle to which the disk can open (60°) and close (0°).

The tilting disk is not radiopaque, but a circular wire rim toward the center of the disk is easily seen and is very useful for following the motion of the otherwise radiographically invisible tilting disk (Figs. 9-4 to 9-6). The tilting disk is usually well imaged on any plane. The disk is not attached by hinges but moves passively according to blood flow and pressure, and it is restrained by the two struts. The Björk-Shiley 60° convexoconcave single tilting disk closes at 0° and opens to 60°; the Björk-Shiley 70° model, not inserted in North America, closes at 0° and opens to 70°.

The Medtronic-Hall prosthesis is another single tilting disk type of prosthesis that also contains radiographically obvious struts and has a unique appearance (Graphic 9-3). With its unique design, a bent finger–like major strut penetrates the center of the tilting disk, which slides over the curved strut to from a closed position of 0° to an open position of 60°. As the major strut penetrates the center of the disk, there is, among single tilting disk prostheses, a unique central jet of mild insufficiency. A minor strut controls the extent of occluder disk motion (Fig. 9-7).

The Omniscience valve (Graphic 9-4) is an example of a single tilting disk occluder valve prosthesis that does not contain struts. Strutless valves were designed in response to strut failure. The tilting disk motion is restrained by small flanges within the sewing ring (Figs. 9-8 and 9-9).

There were considerable numbers of designs of single tilting disk valves—by different manufacturers and even by the same manufacturers. Therefore, there are many types of struts that range from C- or U-shaped to curved lines or straight bars. Because the occluder element generally only opened to 60°, single tilting disk prostheses were moderately obstructive to

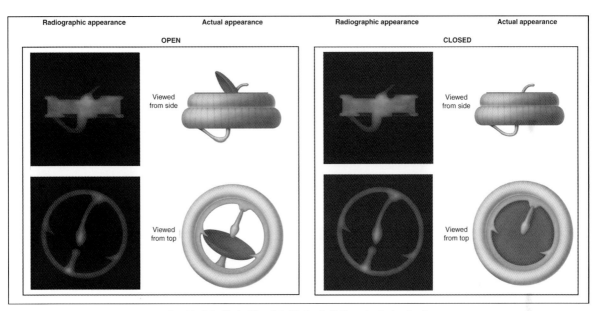

Graphic 9-3. Single tilting disk (Medtronic-Hall) mechanical prothesis.

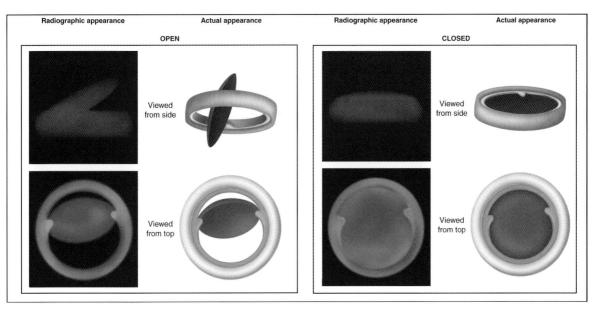

Graphic 9-4. Single tilting disk (Omniscience) mechanical prothesis.

transvalvar blood flow and partitioned the flow through a major and a minor orifice.

Single (Nontilting) Disk

Single (nontilting) disk valve prostheses represent old technology. However, there are still single nontilting disk prostheses in use. Fundamental to their design is an inherent obstructiveness to blood flow and a susceptibility of the occluder to wear.

The Beall model (Graphic 9-5) was most common. Several other designs and manufacturers were also available.

The sewing ring is dense and easily visualized. There are two struts that restrain the motion of the plastic occluder when the valve is in the open position. The struts are easily seen. The single disk is not visible, and therefore radiographically the motion of the occluder cannot be reliably determined.

Ball-in-Cage

The ball-in-cage design is the oldest design of valve prosthesis that was widely inserted. The Starr-Edwards (Graphic 9-6) was the most common (Figs. 9-10 to 9-14). Other models included the

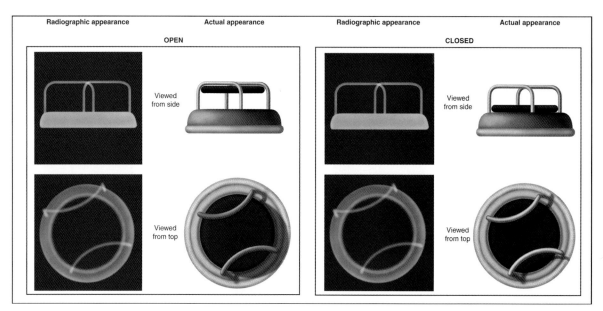

Graphic 9-5. Single nontilting disk (Beall) mechanical prosthesis.

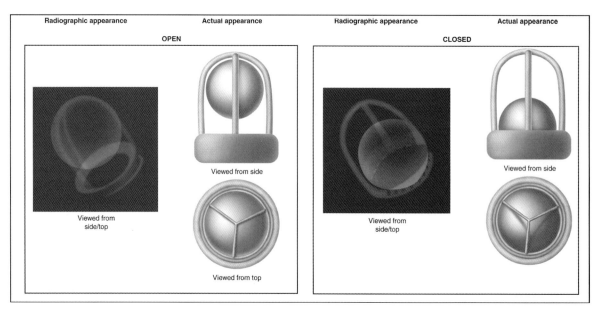

Graphic 9-6. Ball-in-cage (Starr-Edwards) mechanical prosthesis.

DeBakey-Surgitool, the Magovern-Cromie, and the Smeloff-Cutter (Graphic 9-7). Ball-in-cage valves were inherently very obstructive, and the balls were prone to wear and tear.

The sewing rings were radiographically dense, and the struts (i.e., the "cage") that retained the ball when the prosthesis was in the open position were radiographically obvious. The design of the struts was variable. The stents of the Starr-Edwards and Smeloff-Cutter designs came close to joining at the apex but did not. The stents of the DeBakey-Surgitool and Magovern-Cromie valves did join at the apex.

The ball of the Starr-Edwards valve and most other types was made of plastic and was not radiographically visible. Therefore, radiographically, it was not possible to determine the occluder position or movement. The DeBakey-Surgitool valve had a metal ball that was radiographically glaringly obvious.

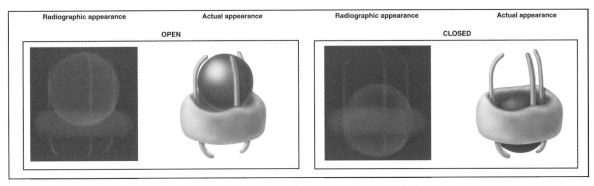

Graphic 9-7. Ball-in-cage (Smeloff-Cutter) mechanical prosthesis.

TABLE 9-1 Mechanical Prosthetic Heart Valves

VALVES	OCCLUDERS	HOUSING/SEWING RING
Bileaflet Occluders		
Sorin		
CarboMedics Standard	Bileaflet, radiopaque tungsten-impregnated pyrolytic carbon over graphite. Opening: 78°; Closing: 35°	Radiopaque titanium pyrolytic carbon over graphite ring/thick sewing ring
CarboMedics Aortic "R" series	Bileaflet, radiopaque tungsten-impregnated pyrolytic carbon over graphite. Opening: 78°; Closing: 35°	Radiopaque titanium pyrolytic carbon over graphite ring
CarboMedics Top Hat	Bileaflet, radiopaque tungsten-impregnated pyrolytic carbon over graphite. Opening: 78°; Closing: 35°	Supra-annular/radiopaque titanium pyrolytic carbon over graphite ring
CarboMedics Mitral mechanical	Bileaflet, radiopaque tungsten-impregnated pyrolytic carbon over graphite. Opening: 78°; Closing: 35°	Radiopaque titanium pyrolytic carbon over graphite ring/very thick sewing ring
CarboMedics Optiform Mitral	Bileaflet, radiopaque tungsten-impregnated pyrolytic carbon over graphite. Opening: 78°; Closing: 35°	Radiopaque titanium pyrolytic carbon over graphite ring
Monoleaflet Allcarbon	Bileaflet, radiopaque tungsten-impregnated pyrolytic carbon over graphite. Opening: 60°; Closing: 0°	Radiopaque titanium pyrolytic carbon over graphite ring
Bicarbon	Bileaflet, radiopaque tungsten-impregnated pyrolytic carbon over graphite. Opening: 80°	Radiopaque titanium pyrolytic carbon over graphite ring
Bicarbon Slimline	Bileaflet, radiopaque tungsten-impregnated pyrolytic carbon over graphite. Opening: 80°	Radiopaque titanium pyrolytic carbon over graphite ring
Bicarbon Overline	Bileaflet, radiopaque tungsten-impregnated pyrolytic carbon over graphite. Opening: 80°	Supra-annular/radiopaque titanium pyrolytic carbon over graphite ring

Table continues on following page.

TABLE 9-1   Mechanical Prosthetic Heart Valves—Cont.

VALVES	OCCLUDERS	HOUSING/SEWING RING
Medtronic		
Medtronic-Hall (mechanical prosthesis)	Radiopaque tungsten-containing single tilting disk with a central hole. Central curved radiopaque titanium guidepost. Opening: 70-75°	Radiopaque titanium-containing housing ring
Medtronic-Hall Easy-Fit	Radiopaque tungsten-containing single tilting disk with a central hole. Central curved radiopaque titanium guidepost. Opening: 70-75°	Supra-annular/radiopaque titanium-containing housing ring
Advantage	Bileaflet, radiopaque occluders. Opening: 86°	NA
Advantage Supra	Bileaflet, radiopaque occluders. Opening: 86°	Supra-annular
(Carpentier) Edwards		
Edwards Mira (mechanical prosthesis)	Bileaflet occluders Opacity not known. Opening: 80°	Radiopaque tungsten-titanium
St. Jude Medical Biocor		
Standard	Bileaflet, radiopaque tungsten-impregnated pyrolytic carbon over graphite. Opening: 85°; closing: 35°	Nonradiopaque pyrolytic carbon over graphite ring/thick sewing ring
Masters	Radiopaque tungsten-impregnated pyrolytic carbon over graphite. Opening: 85°; closing: 35°	Nonradiopaque pyrolytic carbon over graphite ring/thick sewing ring
Masters HP (Hemodynamic Plus)	Radiopaque tungsten-impregnated pyrolytic carbon over graphite. Opening: 85°; closing: 35°	Supra-annular, nonradiopaque pyrolytic carbon over graphite ring/thick sewing ring
Regent	Radiopaque tungsten-impregnated pyrolytic carbon over graphite. Opening: 85°; closing: 35°	Supra-annular, nonradiopaque pyrolytic carbon over graphite ring/thick sewing ring
Bileaflet (Other)		
Triflo (mecahnical prosthesis)	Bileaflet	NA
CarboMedics Orbis Universal	NA	NA
St. Jude Medical Masters	NA	NA
St. Jude Medical HP	NA	NA
CarboMedics "R" Series Aortic	NA	NA
Sorin Bicarbon	NA	NA
ATS Open Pivot (mechanical bileaflet)	Bileaflet, nonradiopaque pyrolytic carbon. Opening: 85°	Nonradiopaque pyrolytic carbon
On-X	Bileaflet, nonradiopaque pyrolytic carbon. Opening: 85°	Nonradiopaque pyrolytic carbon
Single (Nontilting) Disk		
Beall-Surgitool	Nonopaque flat plastic occluders	NA
Cooley-Cutter	Radiopaque single faceted domed disk	Densely radiopaque housing with four densely radiopaque pronglike struts that do not close at the top

TABLE 9-1   Mechanical Prosthetic Heart Valves—Cont.

Single Tilting Disk

Björk-Shiley	Single tilting disk with a central radiopaque rim. Opening: 60°; closing: 0°	Densely radiopaque housing with two densely radiopaque bridgelike struts
Björk-Shiley Convexoconcave (BCC60)	Single tilting disk with a central radiopaque rim. Opening: 60°; closing: 0°	Densely radiopaque housing with two densely radiopaque bridgelike struts
Björk-Shiley Convexoconcave (BCC70)	Single tilting disk with a central radiopaque rim. Opening: 70°; closing: 0°	Densely radiopaque housing with two densely radiopaque bridgelike struts
Björk-Shiley Monostrut	Single tilting disk with a central radiopaque rim. Opening: 60°; closing: 0°	Densely radiopaque housing with two densely radiopaque struts; one bridge shaped and the other a post
Omnicarbon	Single tiling disk; pyrolytic carbon/graphite. Opening: 80°; closing: 0°	Radiopaque titanium, includes small struts/flanges that hold the occluder and are visible
Koehler Ultracor	Radiopaque single tilting disks. Aortic with opening of 73° and mitral with opening of 68°; closing angle unknown	NA
Lillehei-Kaster	Radiopaque single tilting disk	Radiopaque housing with two radiopaque fanglike struts
Omniscience	Radiopaque single tilting disk	Radiopaque housing and flanges
Aortech UltraCor	Radiopaque single tilting disk	Radiopaque housing and wire struts
Bicer	Single tilting disk	Radiopaque housing and wire struts
Sorin Monocast	Single tilting disk	Radiopaque housing and wire struts

Ball-in-Cage

Starr-Edwards	Radiopaque (barium-containing) silastic ball; radiopaque alloy cage	Radiopaque post; cage domed at the top
Smeloff-Cutter	Silastic ball	Radiopaque post; cage (open at the top)
McGovern-Crombie	Silastic ball	Radiopaque post; cage (open at the top)
Debakey-Surgitool	Radiopaque steel ball	Radiopaque post; cage domed at the top

NA, not available.
Data from Surgical Technology International Online: http//www.surgicaltechnology.com/15-149-CS-Page2-.html#Top.

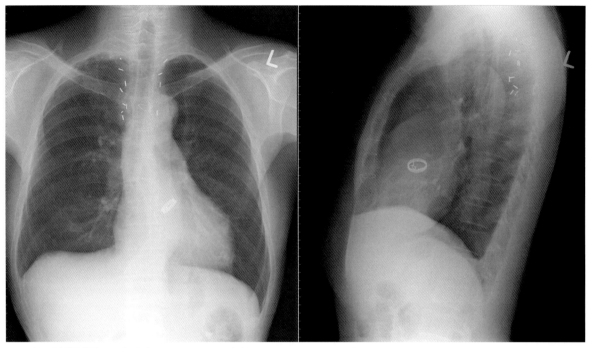

Figure 9-3. A Björk-Shiley mechanical prosthesis is present in the aortic position. Because of optimal penetration, it is appreciated on both the posteroanterior and lateral films. The cardiothoracic ratio is not increased. The cardiopericardial silhouette suggests left ventricular hypertrophy.

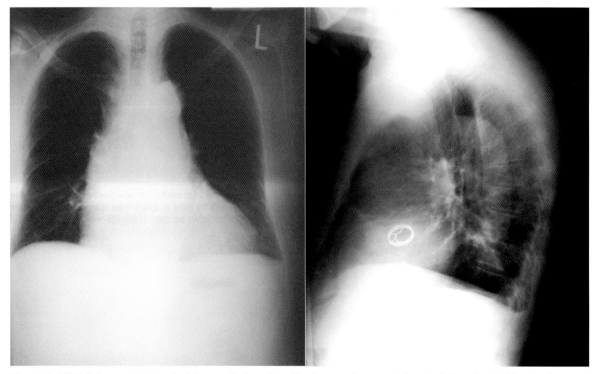

Figure 9-4. A Björk-Shiley mechanical prosthesis is present in the aortic position. Because of poor penetration, despite its radiopacity, it is not easily appreciated on the posteroanterior film.

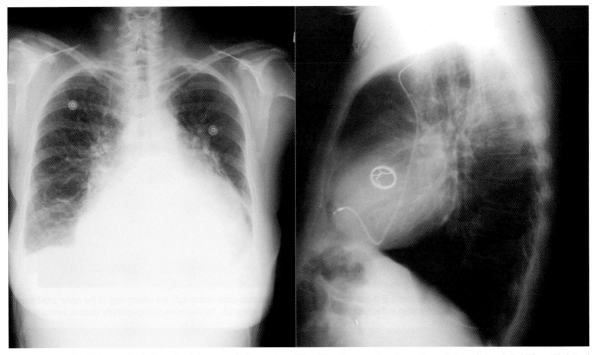

Figure 9-5. A Björk-Shiley mechanical prosthesis is present in the aortic position. It is not apparent on the posteroanterior radiograph, but it is on the lateral radiograph.

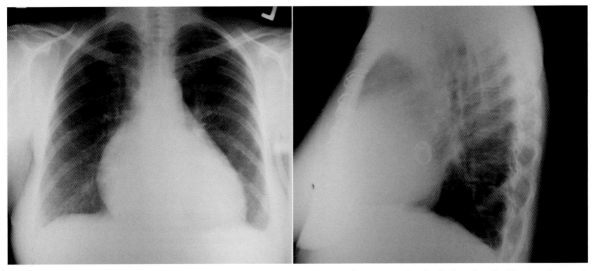

Figure 9-6. A Björk-Shiley mechanical prosthesis is present in the mitral position. Because of poor penetration, despite its radiopacity, it is not easily appreciated on the posteroanterior (PA) film. On the PA film, the left heart border is straightened and lengthened due to left atrial appendage enlargement and left ventricular lengthening. On the lateral film, there is posterior displacement of the left ventricle, consistent with enlargement. There is also increased right ventricular apposition to the sternum on the lateral film, consistent with right ventricular chamber enlargement. The right atrial curvature is increased on the PA film as well.

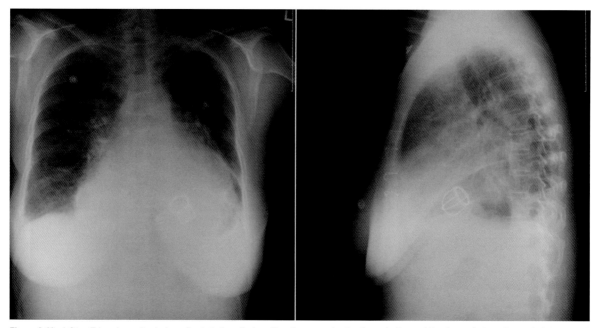

Figure 9-11. A Starr-Edwards mechanical prosthesis in the mitral position. Because of optimal penetration and despite marked cardiomegaly, it is appreciated on both the posteroanterior (PA) and lateral radiographs. On the PA radiograph, the carina is splayed and on the lateral radiograph, the marked posterior displacement of the left atrium is appreciated. The PA radiograph also suggests right atrial enlargement, and the lateral radiograph suggests right ventricular enlargement.

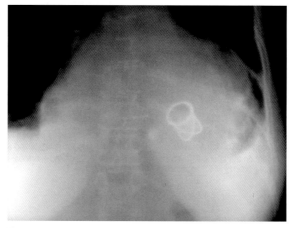

Figure 9-12. The shadow of a Starr-Edwards mechanical prosthesis is apparent on this zoom view of a posteroanterior radiograph.

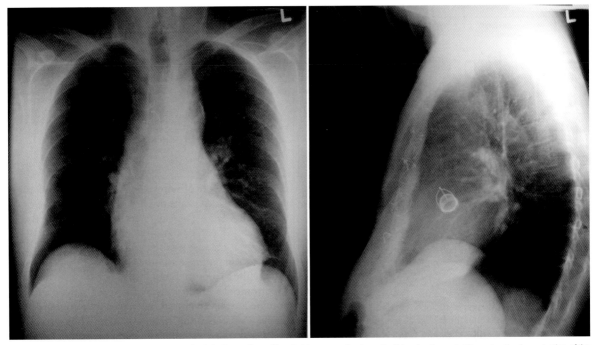

Figure 9-13. A Starr-Edwards mechanical prosthesis in the aortic position that is apparent only on the lateral radiograph. The suboptimal penetration of the posteroanterior (PA) radiograph and the projection of the shadow over that of the spine obscure it on the PA image.

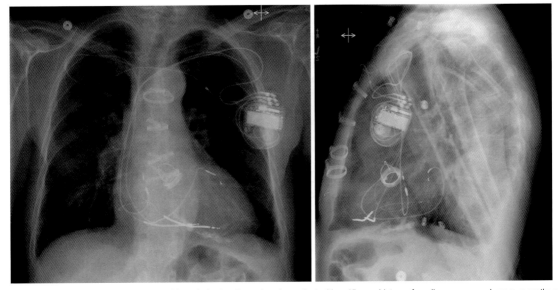

Figure 9-14. A set of 2011 posteroanterior and lateral chest radiographs of a patient with a 45-year history of cardiac surgery and, more recently, electrophysiological interventions. There are right atrial endocardial pacemaker, left lateral cardiac vein, cardiac resynchronization, and two right ventricular endocardial/implantable cardioverter defibrillator leads. As well, there are sternal bands and the characteristic appearance of a Starr-Edwards ball-in-cage aortic valve.

TABLE 10-1   Bioprosthetic Heart Valves

VALVE	LEAFLET MATERIAL	STENTS	RING/SEWING RING
Sorin			
MORE	Pericardial tissue	Polymer stents; low profile; radiopaque wire marker	Nonradiopaque polyester sewing ring/supra-annular
Pericarbon Freedom (stentless)	Pericardial tissue	Stentless	No sewing ring or mesh
Freedom Solo (stentless)	Pericardial tissue	Stentless	NA
Soprano	Pericardial tissue	Nonradiopaque polymer stents	Sewing cloth; no ring
Mitroflow	Pericardial tissue	Radiopaque polymer stents	Radiopaque (tungsten-impregnated silicone ring)
Medtronic			
Mosaic	Porcine aortic valve	Nonradiopaque polymer stent; low profile	Nonradiopaque sewing ring/supra-annular
Mosaic Ultra	Porcine aortic valve	Nonradiopaque polymer stent; low profile	Nonradiopaque sewing ring/supra-annular
Freestyle Stentless	Porcine aortic valve and root	Stentless	Nonradiopaque/sewing cuff, not sewing ring
Hancock II	Porcine aortic valve	Nonradiopaque polymer stent; low profile	Nonradiopaque sewing ring/supra-annular
Advantage			
Melody	Bovine jugular stented, percutaneous pulmonic valve replacement, "Bonnhoeffer"	Stented	NA
	Supported and non-supported	NA	NA
VenPro Contegra (unsupported)	Bovine jugular vein valve conduit	Stentless	NA
VenPro Contegra (supported)	Bovine jugular vein valve conduit	Stentless	With two plastic rings—sometimes seen on fluoroscopy; seldom seen on chest radiography
Carpentier-Edwards			
Perimount (aortic and mitral bioprostheses)	Bovine pericardial tissue	Radiopaque wire (Elgiloy) stent frame	Sewing ring is not radiopaque; partially supra-annular position slightly increases available orifice
Perimount Magna (aortic bioprosthesis)	Bovine pericardial tissue; different fixation/preservation technique	Radiopaque wire (Elgiloy) stent frame	Redesigned Perimount valve, fully supra-annular/sewing ring is not radiopaque
Perimount Magna (mitral bioprosthesis)	Bovine pericardial tissue; different fixation/preservation technique	Radiopaque wire (Elgiloy) stent frame	Redesigned Perimount valve; saddle-shaped ring/sewing ring is not radiopaque
Perimount Plus (mitral bioprosthesis)	Different fixation/preservation technique	Radiopaque wire (Elgiloy) stent frame	Redesigned Perimount valve/sewing ring is not radiopaque
Perimount Theon (mitral replacement)	Different fixation/preservation technique	Radiopaque wire (Elgiloy) stent frame	Redesigned Perimount valve/sewing ring is not radiopaque

TABLE 10-1   Bioprosthetic Heart Valves—Cont.

Carpentier-Edwards—Cont.

S.A.V.	Porcine aortic valve	Radiopaque wire (Elgiloy) stent frame; low profile	Sewing ring is not radiopaque; supra-annular position increases available orifice
Duraflex Low-Pressure	Porcine aortic valve; asymmetric orifice (includes muscle shelf); low-pressure fixation to lessen stiffening of leaflets	Radiopaque wire (Elgiloy) stent frame	Larger sewing ring to fit the mitral orifice
Prima Plus (stentless porcine prosthesis)	Porcine aortic valve and root	No stent frame	No separate sewing ring
BioPhysio (pericardial aortic bioprosthesis)	Bovine pericardial tissue	Radiopaque wire (Nitinol) stent frame	Supra-annular position; nonradiopaque silicone sewing ring

St. Jude Medical Biocor

Porcine (bioprosthesis)	Porcine aortic valve	Nonradiopaque plastic stents	Nonradiopaque (polyester) sewing ring
Supra Porcine (bioprosthesis)	Porcine aortic valve	Nonradiopaque plastic stents	Nonradiopaque (polyester) sewing ring; supra-annular position
Epic Porcine (bioprosthesis)	Porcine aortic valve	Nonradiopaque plastic stents; low profile	Nonradiopaque (polyester) sewing ring
Epic Supra Porcine (bioprosthesis)	Porcine aortic valve	Nonradiopaque plastic stents; low profile	Nonradiopaque (polyester) sewing ring; supra-annular position
Toronto (stentless porcine bioprosthesis)	Porcine aortic valve and root	NA	Nonradiopaque sewing mesh, not sewing ring; subcoronary
Toronto (stentless root porcine bioprosthesis)	Porcine aortic valve and root	NA	Nonradiopaque sewing mesh, not sewing ring
Biocor	Bovine pericardial tissue	Nonradiopaque plastic stents	Nonradiopaque (polyester) sewing ring; supra-annular position
Biocor Stentless	Composite porcine aortic valve/pericardial conduit mount	Stentless	NA
Trifecta	Pericardial tissue	Stents	Sewing ring; supra-annular position

Others

CryoValve aortic valve/conduit	Human cadaveric	Stentless	No sewing ring or mesh
CryoValve pulmonary valve/conduit	Human cadaveric	Stentless	No sewing ring or mesh
CryoValve mitral valve	Human cadaveric	Stentless	No sewing ring or mesh
Cryolife-O'Brien (stentless)	Porcine aortic valve	Stentless	No sewing ring or mesh
Shelhigh Skeletonized Super-Stentless	Porcine aortic valve	Stentless	NA
Shelhigh Skeletonized Super-Stentless	Porcine aortic valve	Stentless	NA

Table continues on following page.

TABLE 10-1 Bioprosthetic Heart Valves—Cont.

VALVE	LEAFLET MATERIAL	STENTS	RING/SEWING RING
Others—Cont.			
Shelhigh BioMitral	Porcine mitral valve	NA	NA
Shelhigh porcine pulmonic valve conduit	Porcine pulmonic valve and conduit	NA	NA
Koehler Aspire porcine bioprosthesis	Porcine aortic valve	NA	NA
Koehler Elan stentless porcine aortic valve	Porcine aortic valve	Stentless	No sewing ring or mesh
Koehler Elan stentless porcine root prosthesis	Porcine aortic valve and root	Stentless	Sewing mesh

NA, not available.
Data from Surgical Technology International Online: http://www.surgicaltechnology.com/15-149-CS-Page2-.html#Top.

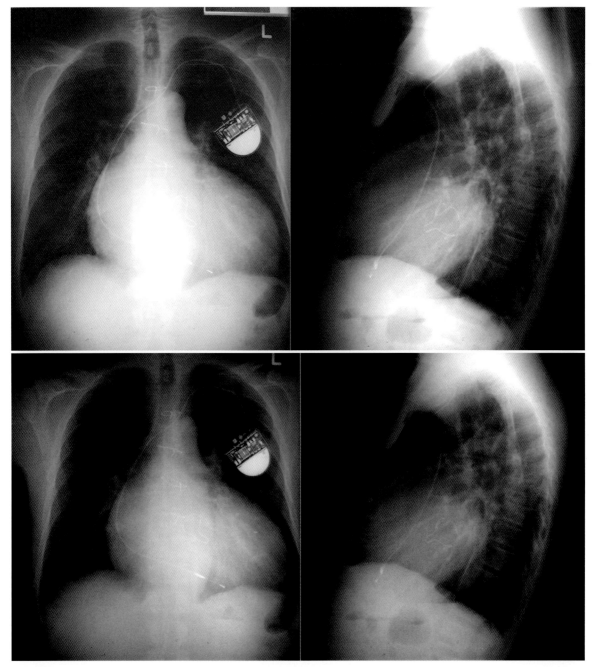

Figure 10-1. Upper and lower radiographs from the same patient, but with different "windowing." There is prominent cardiomegaly with enlargement signs of all cardiac chambers. The ventricular pacer lead is obvious on all images. The effect of the large heart is to increase attenuation, and to add this to the attenuation of the spine, thereby tending to obscure findings within the heart. On the upper frontal radiograph, detail within the heart is poor. On the lower frontal radiograph (with the windowing changed—less brightness and more contrast), a stented mitral bioprosthesis is readily seen. On the lateral radiographs, because the projection is free of the spine, there is less tendency for cardiomegaly to obscure intracardiac findings and the stented bioprosthesis is just as obvious, regardless of windowing.

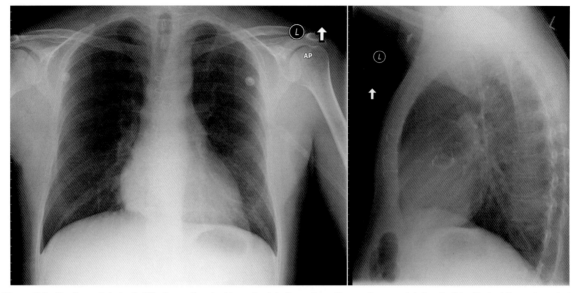

Figure 10-2. The ring and struts of a Mitroflow aortic valve bioprosthesis in the aortic position can be appreciated on the lateral but not the posteroanterior (PA) radiograph, where the valve shadow falls over the spine on the PA radiograph. The superior orientation of the prosthesis is compatible with the aortic valve position.

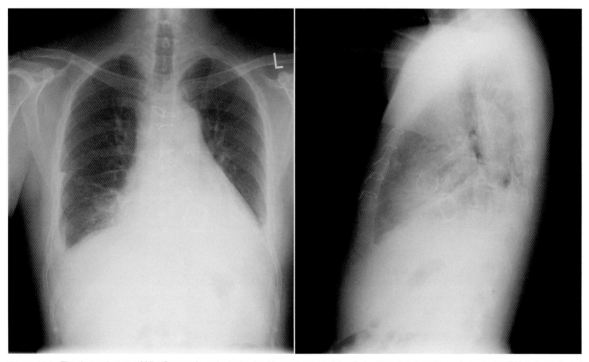

Figure 10-3. The ring and struts of Mitroflow aortic and mitral valve bioprostheses can be dimly appreciated on the posteroanterior (PA) radiograph and much better appreciated on the lateral radiograph. The valve shadow falls over the spine on the PA radiograph. The different positions and orientations of the aortic and mitral prosthesis are demonstrated.

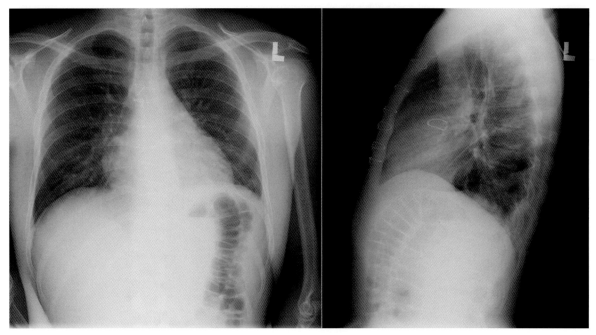

Figure 10-4. The sewing ring of a Mitroflow aortic valve bioprosthesis in the aortic position can be appreciated on the lateral radiograph better than on the posteroanterior radiograph (PA). The ring shadow falls over the spine on the PA radiograph.

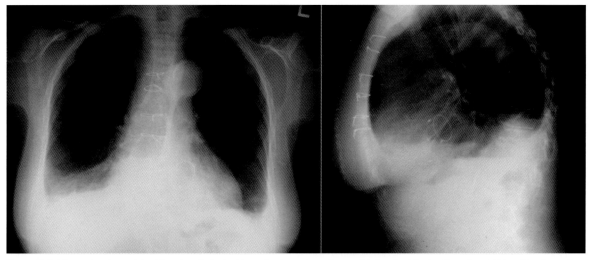

Figure 10-5. The sewing ring and stent tips of a mitral valve bioprosthesis can be well appreciated on the lateral radiograph and fairly well on the posteroanterior (PA) radiograph. The shadow of the prosthesis falls to the side of the spine on the PA radiograph.

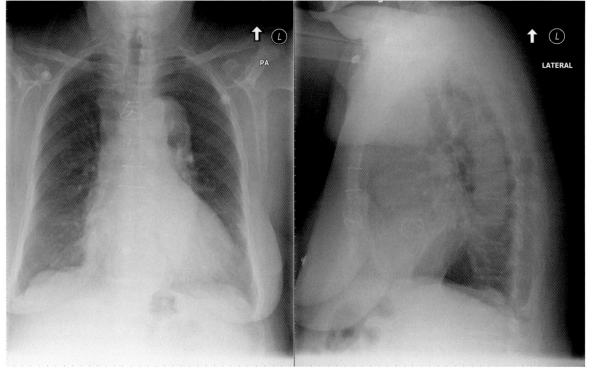

Figure 10-6. Bioprosthetic stented aortic valve replacement (Mitroflow). There is cardiomegaly, extensive calcification of the aorta, and sternal wires. Lying on the left border of the spine seen on the posteroanterior view is the shadow of the wire stents of the prosthesis. The orientation is consistent with that of the aortic valve. The stents of the valve prosthesis are more clearly depicted on the lateral chest radiograph.

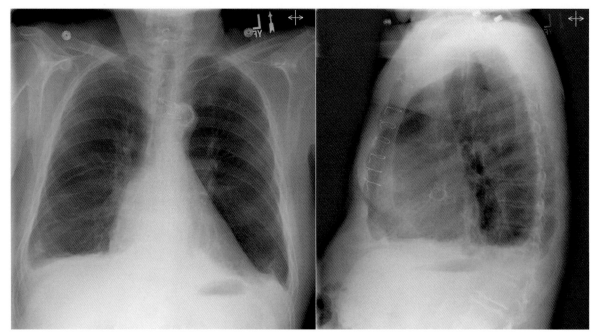

Figure 10-7. There is cardiomegaly, a calcified aortic arch, sternal wires, and a left pleural effusion. On the posteroanterior radiograph, it is possible to barely discern that inferior to the lowest sternal wire is the shadow of the struts of a bioprosthesis lying on the left border of the spine. On the lateral chest radiograph, the stented bioprosthesis (Mitroflow) is much more clearly depicted.

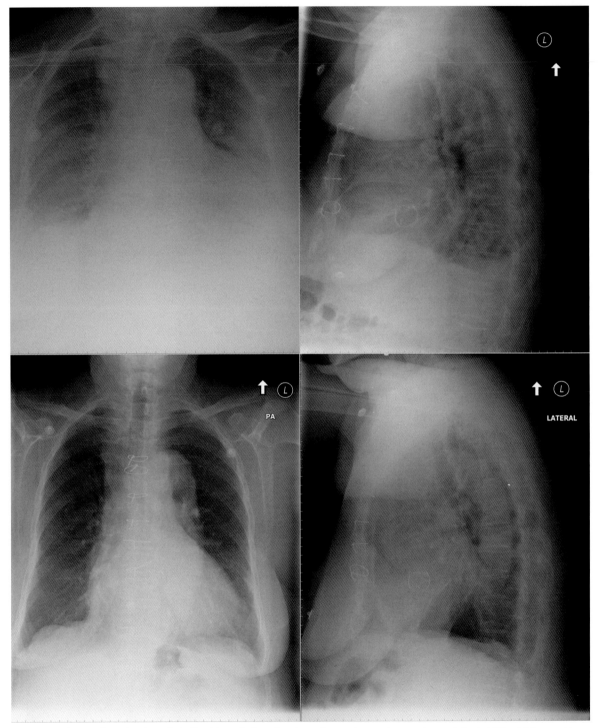

Figure 10-8. Chest radiographs of a patient with a bioprosthetic aortic valve replacement: upper images at presentation in left heart failure, and lower images, with treatment and resolution of heart failure. There is cardiomegaly, sternal wires, and the radiopaque struts of a bioprosthetic aortic valve prosthesis. On the posteroanterior chest radiographs, the radiopaque struts can only barely be seen along the left margin of the spine. In the presence of sternal wires, the radiopaque struts of aortic valve bioprosthesis are commonly overlooked. The bioprosthesis is far more apparent on the lateral chest radiographs. The heart failure in this case was not due to prosthesis dysfunction but to progressive left ventricular failure.

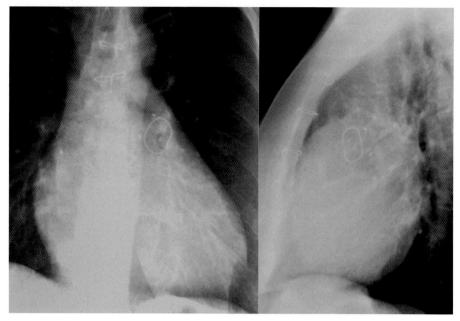

Figure 10-9. Bioprosthetic pulmonary valve replacements.

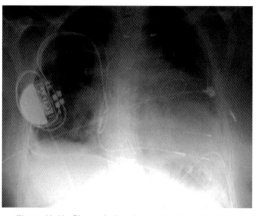

Figure 10-10. Bioprosthetic pulmonary valve replacement.

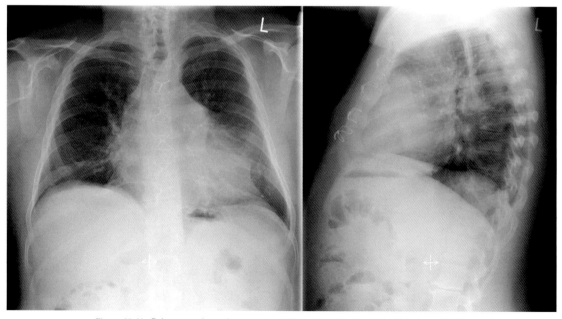

Figure 10-11. Pulmonary valve replacement in a patient with previously repaired tetralogy of Fallot.

Annuloplasty Rings

Key Points

- Annuloplasty rings may be inserted to support mitral or tricuspid valve repairs.
- The radiographic appearance of annuloplasty rings varies according to the design and includes partial (C-shaped) and complete (O-shaped and kidney-shaped) rings, and two-dimensional and three-dimensional round and kidney-shaped rings.
- Most annuloplasty rings can be identified on and localized by chest radiography. The lateral chest radiograph often assists with obviating the projection of a mitral annuloplasty ring onto the spine, particularly in large hearts that otherwise may diminish the depiction of annuloplasty rings on the frontal radiograph.

A nnuloplasty rings may be inserted onto either the mitral or tricuspid valve annulus to correct annular dilation as a contributing cause of mitral or tricuspid insufficiency (Graphic 11-1 and Table 11-1). Novel percutaneously inserted devices that crimp the coronary sinus, and thus the nearby mitral annulus, are increasingly inserted (Fig. 11-1). Mitral annular rings may be inserted within the context of pure mitral valve surgery, usually, but not always, in conjunction with a mitral repair procedure. Alternatively, they may be placed as a secondary indication for ischemic or myxomatous mitral regurgitation in the context of primary indication of coronary bypass surgery (Figs. 11-2 to 11-9). Conversely, tricuspid annular rings are almost always inserted in the context of a primary indication of mitral valve surgery (repair/replacement of commissurotomy) when there is a problematic degree of associated tricuspid insufficiency due to right heart dilation. Only in rare and highly selected patients is tricuspid valve repair/annuloplasty a primary and sole intervention.

Annuloplasty rings are considerably less radiographically conspicuous than prosthetic valves. Distinction between tricuspid and mitral annular rings is readily accomplished using a frontal chest radiograph and noting the position of the ring.

There are numerous designs of annuloplasty rings with different radiographic appearances (Graphic 11-2):
- ❐ Complete (kidney-shaped or round) versus partial (C-shaped)
- ❐ Flat (two-dimensional) versus three-dimensional
- ❐ Smooth and curved versus smooth and angulated
- ❐ Smooth versus "crinkled"

For example, annuloplasty rings are kidney-shaped, C-shaped (e.g., the Cosgrove-Edwards and Carpentier-Edwards models), or O-shaped. The Duran annuloplasty ring, which is O-shaped, often appears "crinkled" because of distortion of the soft ring by sutures.

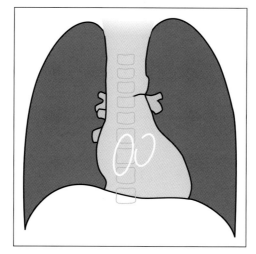

Graphic 11-1. Posteroanterior projection: Tricuspid and mitral annuloplasty rings.

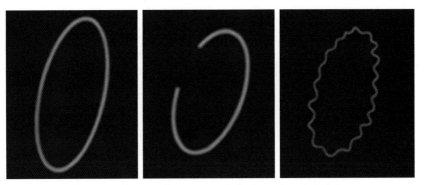

Graphic 11-2. Radiographic appearance of a few types of annuloplasty rings.

TABLE 11-1 Annuloplasty Rings

	SHAPE	RADIOPACITY
Mitral Rings		
Complete Rings		
Carpentier-Edwards Classic	Kidney-shaped	Radiopaque (titanium-containing)
Carpentier-Edwards Physio	Flatter on top, rounder on bottom	Radiopaque (Elgiloy)
Carpentier-McCarthy-Adams IMR ETlogix	Asymmetrically shaped to obviate the effect of asymmetric annular dilation	NA
Edwards GeoForm	Complex shape to obviate the effect of left ventricular dilation on the annulus	NA
Medtronic Duran flexible ring	Round	Radiopaque
St. Jude Medical Séguin	Round or kidney-shaped	NA
St. Jude Medical Tailor	Kidney-shaped Can be trimmed anteriorly to be open	NA
Sorin-CarboMedics Annulo Flex	Complete or partial ring — can be cut	Radiopaque (barium-containing)
Sorin Sovering	Includes round	Radiopaque (barium-containing)
Genesee Sculptor	NA	NA
Jostra fully flexible	NA	NA
Jostra La Pitié	NA	NA
Shelhigh BioRing	Polyester and pericardium	Nonradiopaque?
ATS Simulus FLX-O	NA	NA
Partial Rings		
Cosgrove-Edwards	Widely open C shape	Radiopaque (barium-containing)
Medtronic Duran Flexible band	Widely open C shape, for posterior annular repair	NA
Medtronic Colvin-Galloway Future Band	Widely open C shape with wider ends	Radiopaque
St. Jude Medical Tailor	Kidney-shaped Complete ring but can be trimmed anteriorly to be open	NA
St. Jude Medical Tailor (band)	Kidney-shaped	NA
St. Jude Medical Rigid Saddle	Kidney-shaped	NA
Sorin-CarboMedics Annulo Flo	Kidney-shaped	Radiopaque (titanium-containing)
Sorin-CarboMedics Annulo Flex	Complete or partial ring (can be cut)	Radiopaque (barium-containing)
Sorin Sovering	Includes partially open C-shaped ring	Radiopaque (barium-containing)
Sorin Memo 3D		Radiopaque
Koehler Mitral Repair System (MRS)		Radiopaque (barium-containing)
ATS Simulus Annuloplasty FLX-O (band)		NA
Tricuspid Rings		
Complete Rings		
Medtronic Duran Flexible	Round	Radiopaque
Jostra Fully Flexible	NA	NA
Jostra La Pitié	NA	NA
Partial Rings		
Carpentier-Edwards Classic	Oval-shaped	Radiopaque (titanium-containing)
Edwards MC3	NA	NA
Sorin Sovering	Include widely open C-shaped ring and more than half open C-shaped rings	Radiopaque (barium-containing)

NA, not applicable.
Data from Surgical Technology International Online: http://www.surgicaltechnology.com/15-149-CS-Page2-.html#Top.

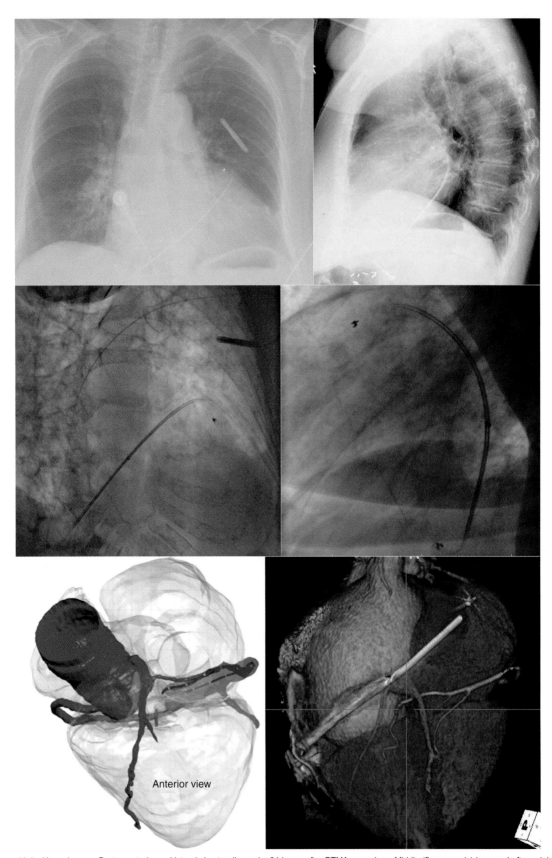

Figure 11-1. *Upper images:* Posteroanterior and lateral chest radiographs 24 hours after PTMA procedure. *Middle (fluoroscopic) images:* Left cranial (*left*) and lateral (*right*) views showing the PTMA device with two rods. Observe the proximal marker at the ostium of the coronary sinus and the distal marker in the anterior interventricular vein. *Lower images:* CT scan with three-dimensional reconstruction and colorization of native coronary arteries, coronary sinus, and mitral annulus (*left*). In this case, maximum distance between coronary sinus and mitral annulus was measured at 20 mm. Thirtieth-day CT scan showing the PTMA catheter in the coronary sinus, which is located above the mitral apparatus (*right*). (From Bertrand OF, Philippon F, St. Pierre A, et al: Percutaneous mitral valve annuloplasty for functional mitral valve regurgitation: acute results of the first patient treated with the Viacor permanent device and future perspectives. *Cardiovasc Revasc Med* 11[4]:e1–e265, 2010. Used with permission.)

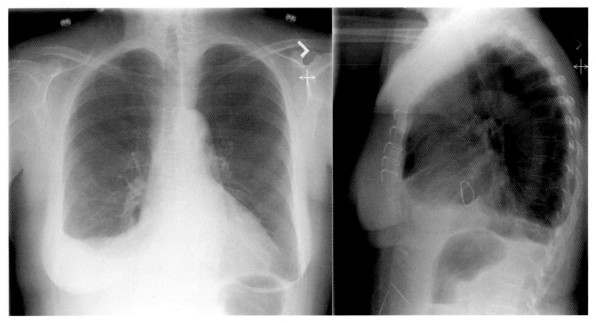

Figure 11-2. Posteroanterior and lateral views early post–cardiac surgery (sternal wires and pacing leads on the skin and pleural effusions). There is cardiomegaly with left ventricular, left atrial, and right ventricular enlargement due to prior severe mitral regurgitation. A mitral annuloplasty ring is evident.

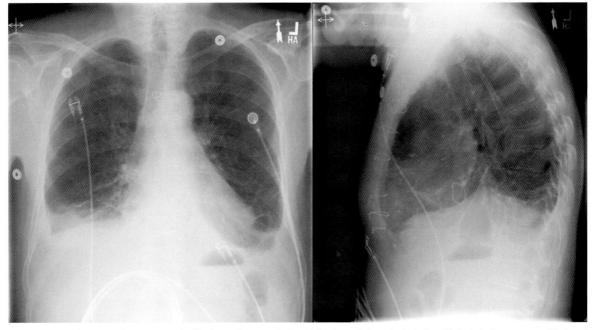

Figure 11-3. Barely seen on the posteroanterior film, but well seen on the lateral film, is a mitral annuloplasty ring with the typical appearance of that used to repair type IIB mitral regurgitation (due to ischemic dilation of the ventricle). There are bilateral pleural effusions, many surgical clips for the aortocoronary bypasses, and sternal wires.

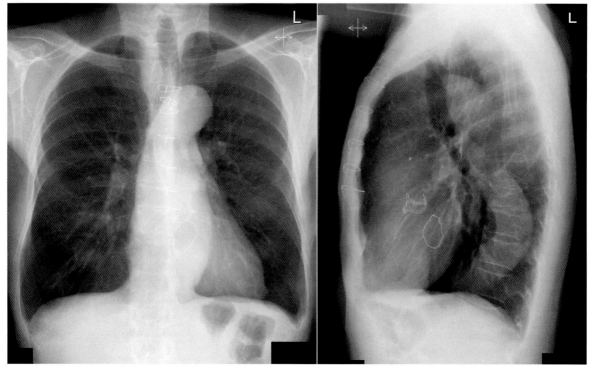

Figure 11-4. A mitral annuloplasty ring and an aortic bioprosthesis. Note the aortic elongation and also tortuosity in this patient.

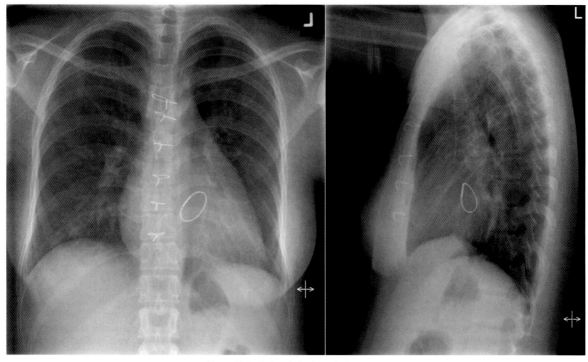

Figure 11-5. A closed mitral annuloplasty ring.

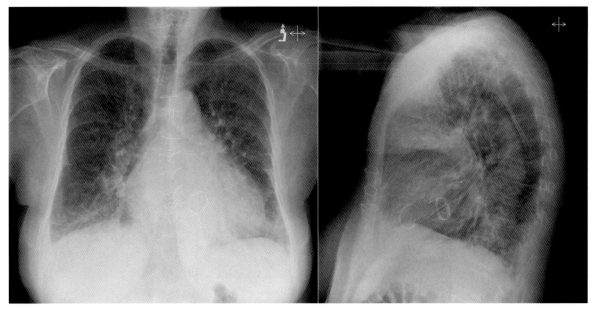

Figure 11-6. An open tricuspid annuloplasty ring and a bioprosthetic mitral valve replacement in a patient in heart failure. There are "double contours" on the right heart border, as may be expected in a patient with mitral and tricuspid valve disease.

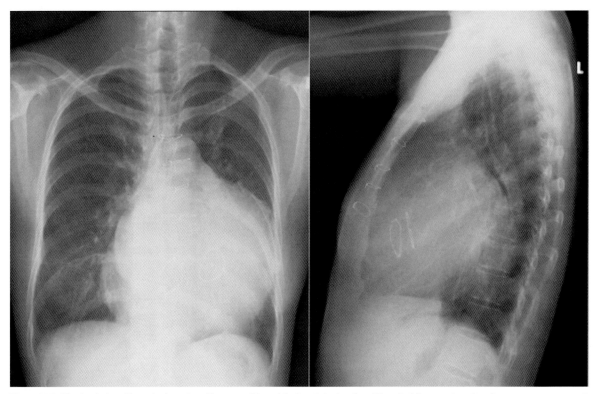

Figure 11-7. Mitral and tricuspid annuloplasty rings. Note as well the relatively anterior location of the mitral ring, as yet another sign, among many present, of left atrial dilation. Note as well the double heart contours from left (upper contour) and right (lower contour) rightward dilation.

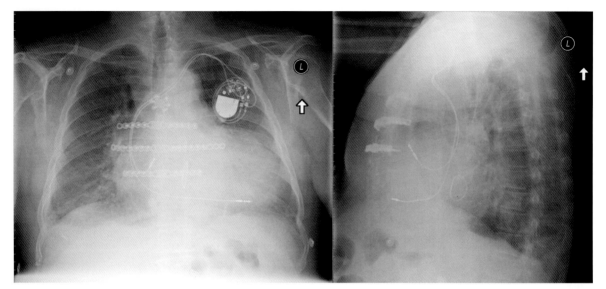

Figure 11-8. Sternal reconstruction hardware is prominently seen on both the posteroanterior and lateral chest radiographs. There are also a dual chamber pacemaker and a mitral annuloplasty ring.

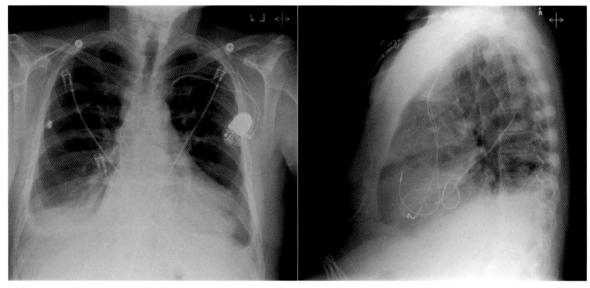

Figure 11-9. A (closed) mitral annuloplasty ring, an (open) tricuspid annuloplasty ring, and dual chamber pacer leads.

12 Prosthetic Valve Dysfunction

Key Points

- Bioprostheses may develop transvalvar or perivalvar insufficiency, and mechanical prostheses may develop thrombotic or pannus-mediated obstruction or paravalvar insufficiency.
- The consequences of valve prosthesis dysfunction may be evident on the chest radiograph; left-sided prosthesis insufficiency or obstruction may result in radiographically evident heart failure.
- In the absence of another apparent reason, when a patient with a valvular prosthesis develops hemodynamic duress, the prosthesis should be suspected of dysfunction, until disproven.

PROSTHESIS DYSFUNCTION

The presence of heart failure in a patient with a valve prosthesis warrants due consideration of prosthesis dysfunction.

Bioprostheses are susceptible to transvalvar insufficiency due to wear-and-tear degeneration or infection and to perivalvar insufficiency, which is usually caused by infection (Fig 12-1). Bioprostheses may develop obstruction, likewise due either to wear-and-tear degeneration or infection.

Mechanical prostheses rarely develop significant transvalvar insufficiency but often develop paravalvar insufficiency, which may be sterile, but usually is due to infection, and often includes dehiscence (Figs. 12-2 and 12-3). Obstruction of a mechanical prosthesis may occur because of thrombosis, pannus (fibrous scar tissue) ingrowth, both conditions, or, rarely, to infection with large vegetations (Figs. 12-4 to 12-7).

All mechanical prostheses are apparent on chest radiograph. Most, but not all, bioprostheses are radiographically apparent. Prior sternotomy wires may be the only sign of prior stentless bioprosthesis insertion. For now, all percutaneously or transapically inserted aortic valve bioprostheses are radiographically apparent.

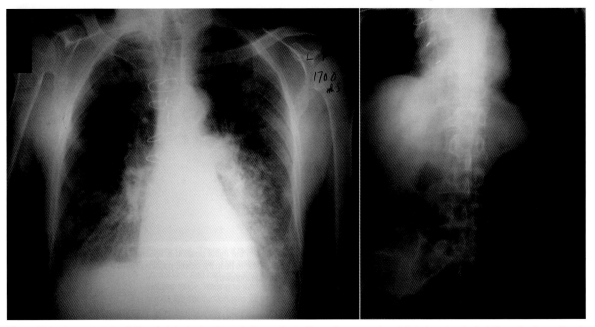

Figure 12-1. Anteroposterior (AP) and abdominal radiographs in a patient with emphysema and an infected, ruptured mitral bioprosthesis resulting in pulmonary edema. At the time of presentation, the bioprosthesis was fortuitously apparent on the abdominal film. The AP radiograph demonstrates a normal cardiothoracic ratio. Sternotomy wires are evident. There are extensive infiltrates, predominantly in the inferior lobes and around the hila. The lungs are overinflated. The abdominal film reveals a stented mitral bioprosthesis at its very top.

Interventional Material

❑ Coiling embolization material, into
  • Aortic false aneurysm (see Fig. 13-8)
  • Coronary fistulae (Fig. 13-29)
  • Vacular lesions (see Fig. 13-29)
❑ The Evalve mitral clip (Figs. 13-30 and 13-31)

Surgical Material

❑ The Heartmesh/CorCap Cardiac Support Device (Acorn Cardiovascular) (Graphic 13-3)

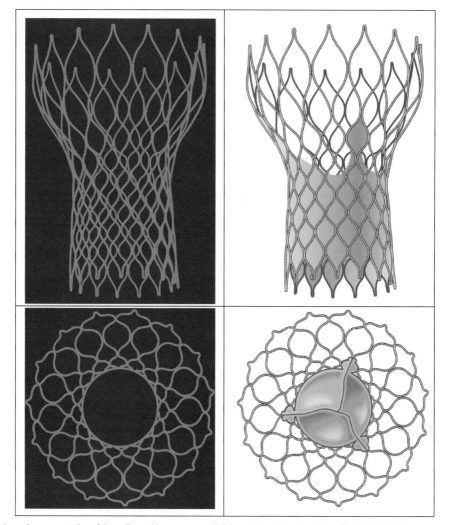

Graphic 13-1. Schematic representation of the radiographic appearance (*left images*) and drawings of the CoreValve (*right images*), seen side-on (*upper images*), and from top down (*lower images*).

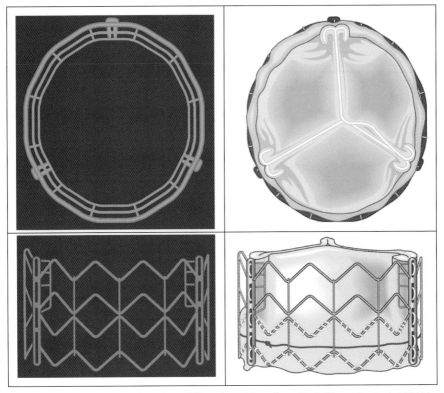

Graphic 13-2. "En-face" (*upper images*) and side-on (*lower images*) illustrations of the radiographic (*left images*) and actual (*right images*) appearance of the Edwards Sapien percutaneous aortic valve.

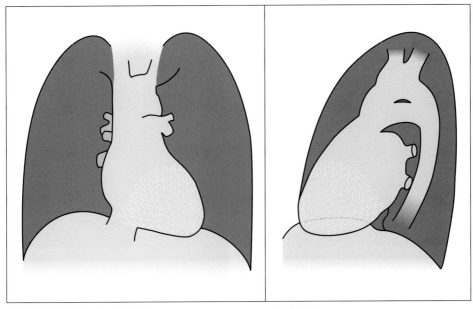

Graphic 13-3. HeartNet mesh "girdle."

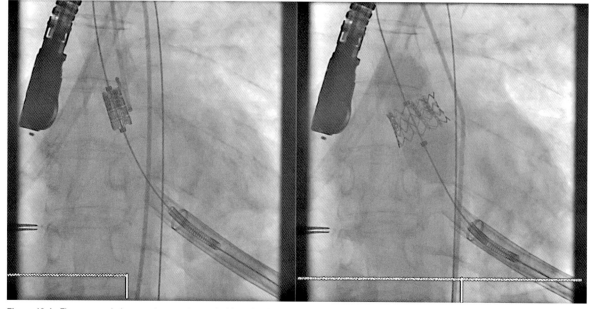

Figure 13-4. Fluoroscopy during percutaneous transapical insertion (*left image*) and deployment of Edwards Sapien valve (*right image*). Note the fluoroscopic appearance of transesophageal echocardiography probe.

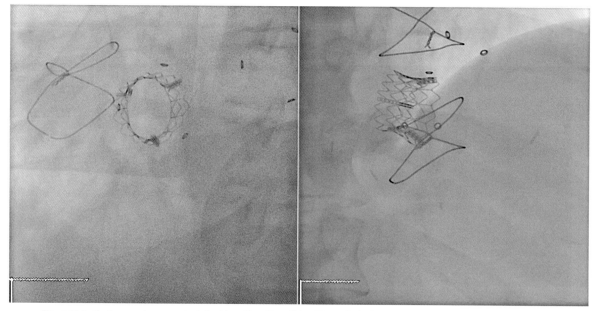

Figure 13-5. Sapien percutaneous valve in the tricuspid position within a bioprosthetic tricuspid valve. Note the bioprosthetic mitral valve.

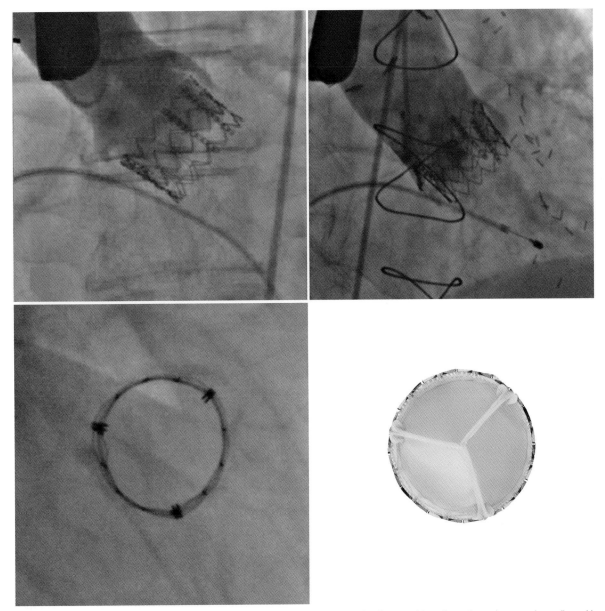

Figure 13-6. Fluoroscopic images and photograph of the Edwards Sapien percutaneous aortic valve seen side-on (*upper images*), seen end-on radiographically (*lower left image*), and seen top-down in actuality (*lower right image*).

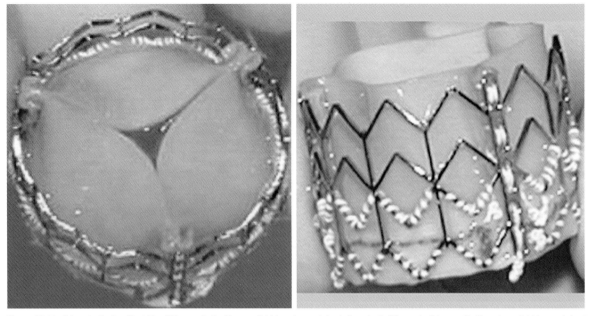

Figure 13-11. Edwards Sapien Stent-Fixed Transcatheter Xenograft. Valve size and stent diameter is 23 mm. *Left image*: Outflow view; *right image*: lateral view. (From Walther T, Falk V, Dewey T, et al: Valve-in-a-valve concept for transcatheter minimally invasive repeat Xenograft implantation. *J Am Coll Cardiol* 50:56–60, 2007. Used with permission.)

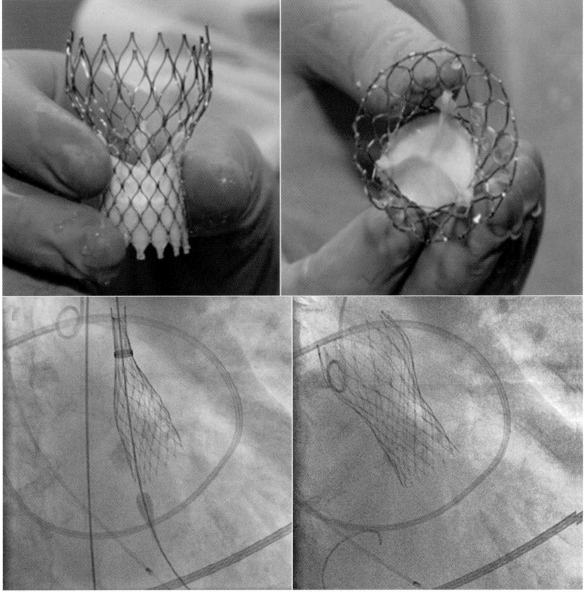

Figure 13-12. *Upper images*: Third generation of the CoreValve prosthesis (18-F) before loading into the delivery catheter. *Lower images*: Implantation of the CoreValve Prosthesis. Prosthesis partially released (still possible to retrieve the valve) (*lower left image*); prosthesis completely released (*lower right image*). (From Grube E, Schuler G, Buellesfeld L, et al: Percutaneous aortic valve replacement for severe aortic stenosis in high-risk patients using the second-generation and current third-generation self-expanding CoreValve prothesis device: success and 30-day clinical outcome. *J Am Coll Cardiol* 50:69–76, 2007. Used with permission.)

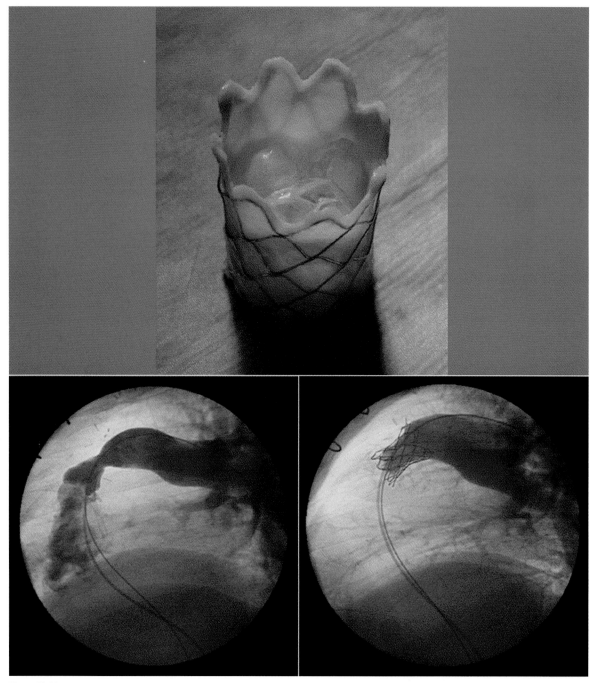

Figure 13-13. *Upper image*: The percutaneous bovine jugular venous valve mounted within an expandable platinum-iridium stent (Numed, Hopkinton, USA). *Lower images*: Percutaneous pulmonary valve stent insertion. Severe pulmonary regurgitation (*lower left image*) is absent following the deployment of the valve (*lower right image*). (Upper image from Coats L, Tsang V, Khambadkone S, et al: The potential impact of percutaneous pulmonary valve stent implantation on right ventricular outflow tract re-intervention. *Eur J Cardiothorac Surg* 27:536–543, 2005. Used with permission.)

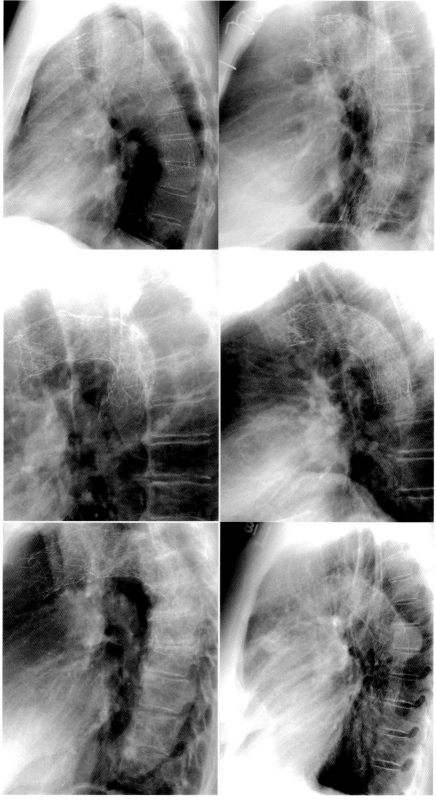

Figure 13-14. Chest radiographic views of six patients with a Gore thoracic aortic endograft.

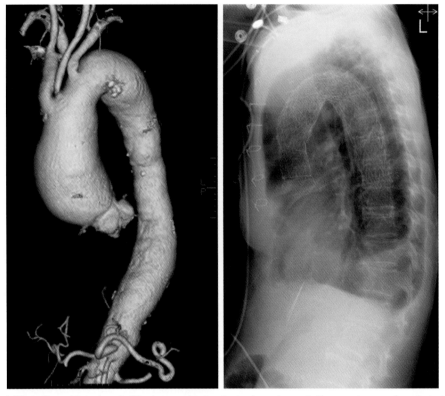

Figure 13-15. The left image is an oblique view of a 3D volume-rendered contrast-enhanced computed tomography scan of a patient prior to endovascular repair. There are atherosclerotic plaques evident by their calcification at the arch level at origin of the innominate artery. The ascending aorta is dilated above the sinotubular junction. The lateral chest radiograph (*right*) of the same patient after debranching of the aortic arch and stenting the ascending aorta, the arch, and half of the descending thoracic aorta.

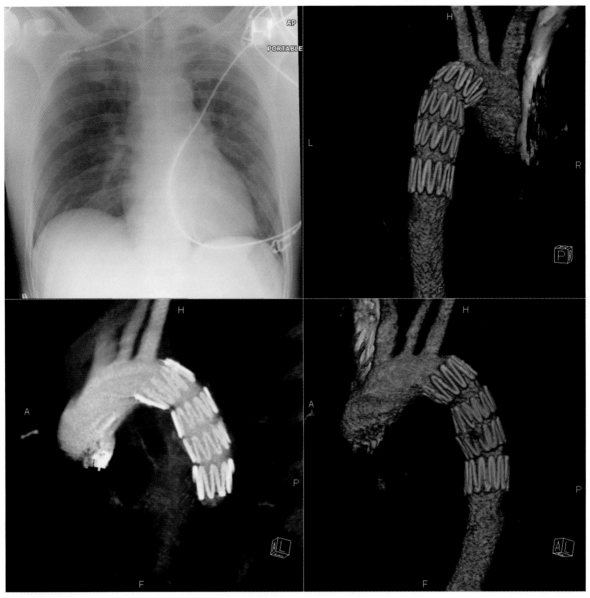

Figure 13-16. Chest radiographic and volume-rendered 3D and MIP contrast-enhanced computed tomography scans of a patient with a Medtronic thoracic aortic endograft.

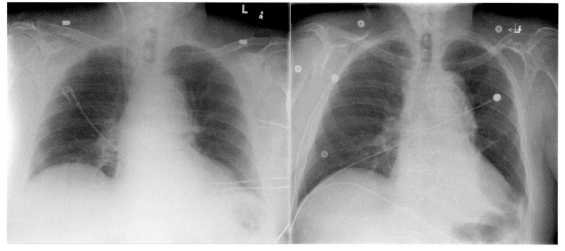

Figure 13-17. In the left image, the descending aorta has been stented to address malperfusion complications of a type B acute aortic dissection. Note how the margins of the stent are inwardly displaced due to the intimal flap/false lumen. This is a reiteration of the conventional intimal displacement sign. In the right image, 2 weeks later, the patient has experienced a type A dissection and underwent median sternotomy and surgical repair.

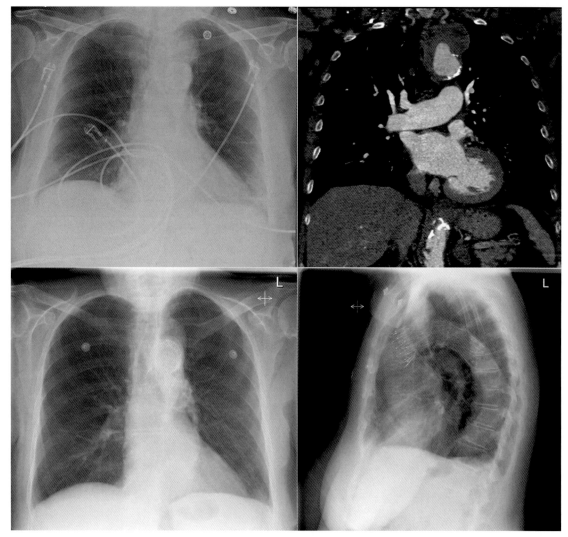

Figure 13-18. The upper images are a chest radiograph and coronal contrast-enhanced computed tomography (CT) scan of a patient with a large penetrating ulcer of the distal arch, which prominently protrudes superiorly on the frontal radiograph and the CT scan. The lower images are following endovascular repair to exclude the penetrating ulcer.

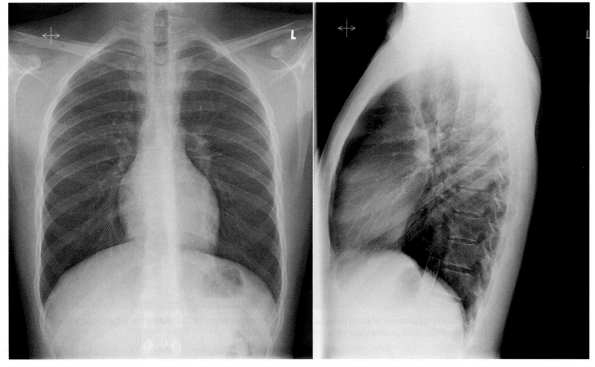

Figure 13-19. On the posteroanterior and lateral radiographs, an aortic stent is apparent straddling the level of the diaphragm. The heart size is within normal parameters, and there is no heart failure or pulmonary vascular prominence, although there is evidence of rib notching. Aortic stenting had been performed at the level of coarctation of the isthmus of the aorta; however, the stent has embolized further distally in the aorta.

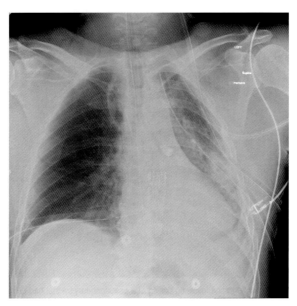

Figure 13-20. Anteroposterior radiograph of a patient recently postoperative from aortic endografting of an aneurysm of the lower thoracic aorta.

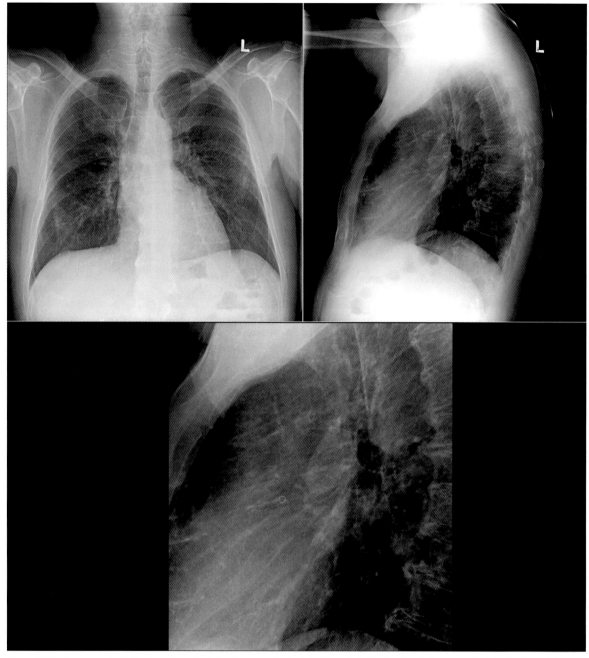

Figure 13-24. A coronary stent in the circumflex artery is barely seen on the frontal radiograph, but is almost perfectly seen on the lateral radiograph because the perspective is end-on.

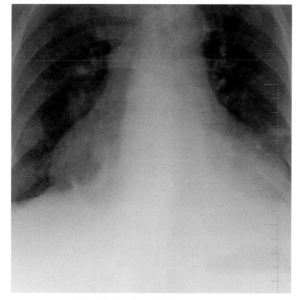

Figure 13-25. A stented innominate vein.

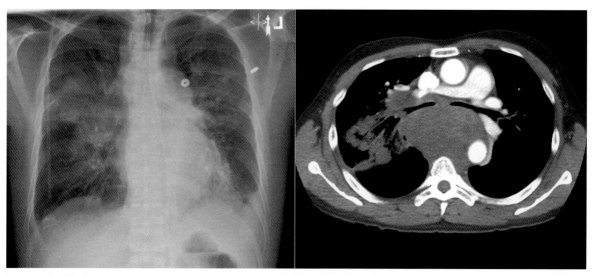

Figure 13-26. Massive hilar and mediastinal adenopathy due to non–small cell lung cancer (*left image*). Note the stenting of the left and right mainstem bronchi to alleviate compression, as is demonstrated by the axial contrast-enhanced computed tomography scan on presentation (*right image*).

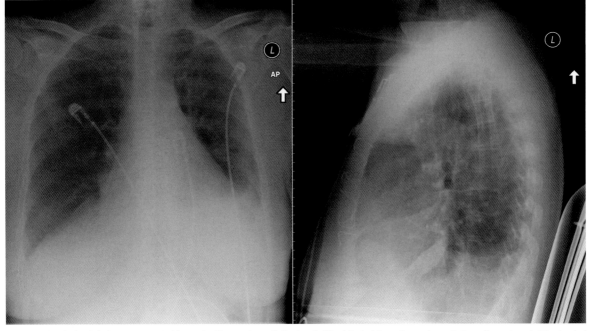

Figure 13-27. Left subclavian artery stent. A large stent is seen beneath the head of the left clavicle on the posteroanterior radiograph and at the level of the manubrium on the lateral radiograph. A tight ostial left subclavian stenosis had been stented before the patient underwent aortocoronary bypass grafting, including use of the left internal thoracic artery as a bypass conduit.

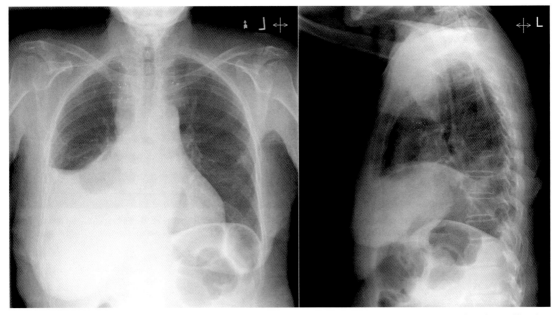

Figure 13-28. There is a large right-sided pleural effusion and a widened mediastinum in this patient with widely disseminated carcinoma. Note the radiographic appearance of the superior vena cava (SVC) and innominate vein stents, deployed to alleviate SVC syndrome.

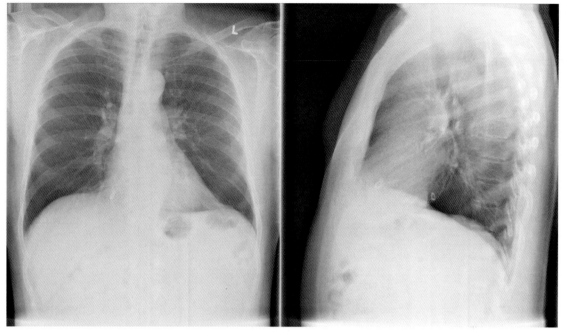

Figure 13-29. Posteroanterior and lateral chest radiographs of a patient who had undergone percutaneous coiling of the proximal and distal ends of a right coronary artery to coronary sinus fistula.

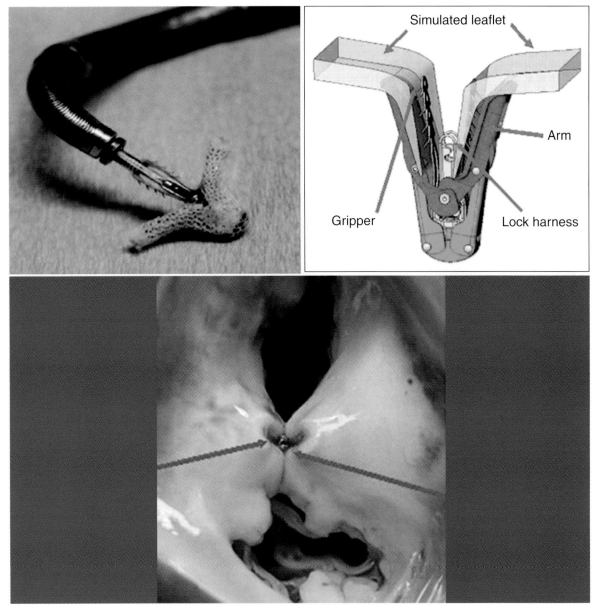

Figure 13-30. The Evalve Mitraclip (Evalve, Inc.). *Upper left image*: Clip device on distal tip of triaxial catheter delivery system. *Upper right image*: Illustrated components of clip device grasping mitral valve leaflet. *Lower image*: Animal pathology specimen of the mitral valve with clip resulting in a double-orifice mitral valve. (Courtesy of Evalve, Inc., Abbott Park, IL. Used with permission.)

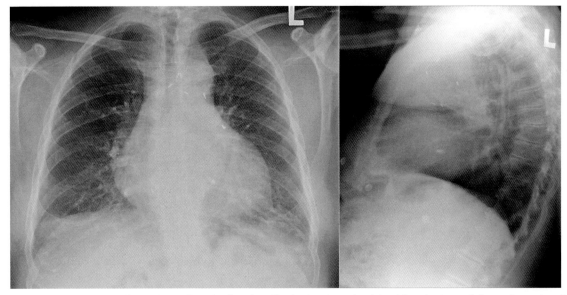

Figure 13-31. Posteroanterior and lateral chest radiographs of a patient with prior sternotomy wires, internal thoracic artery graft clips, cardiomegaly and left heart failure, and an Evalve mitral valve percutaneous clip.

Radiographic Findings by Diagnosis: Cardiomyopathies

Key Points

- Chest radiography in the context of cardiomyopathies is an important means by which to incrementally increase the sensitivity and specificity of determination of the presence of, particularly, cardiomegaly associated left-sided heart failure.
- The chest radiographic appearance of the different forms of cardiomyopathy is established by the expected enlargement of specific chambers (dilated cardiomyopathy: all chambers; hypertrophic cardiomyopathy: left atrium; and restrictive cardiomyopathy: both atria), and the relative amounts of expected left (hypertrophic cardiomyopathy) versus biventricular failure (dilated cardiomyopathy, restrictive cardiomyopathy).

ACQUIRED MYOPATHIES

Hypertrophic Cardiomyopathy

Enlargement of the left atrium is present in the majority of cases of hypertrophic cardiomyopathy (Figs 14-1 to 14-4). Left atrial enlargement is greater in patients with hypertrophic cardiomyopathy when there is con-current mitral insufficiency. The degree of left ventricular enlargement is variable but is usually mild and consistent with left ventricular hypertrophy. About 50% of cases have cardiomegaly, usually mild to moderate. Mitral annular calcification is common.

Dilated Cardiomyopathy (Figs. 14-5 and 14-6)

With four-chamber enlargement, the cardiopericardial silhouette usually assumes a globular shape, which also occurs with pericardial effusions. Some evidence of pulmonary venous hypertension is common, and frank pulmonary edema may be seen.

Restrictive Cardiomyopathy (Figs. 14-7 to 14-9)

Biatrial enlargement is seen in the majority of cases. In the late stages of the disease, there is enlargement of all cardiac chambers. Evidence of pulmonary venous congestion is very common. The azygous vein may be enlarged, consistent with elevated central venous pressure. An important negative finding is absence of calcification of the pericardium; constrictive pericarditis is the principal differential diagnosis.

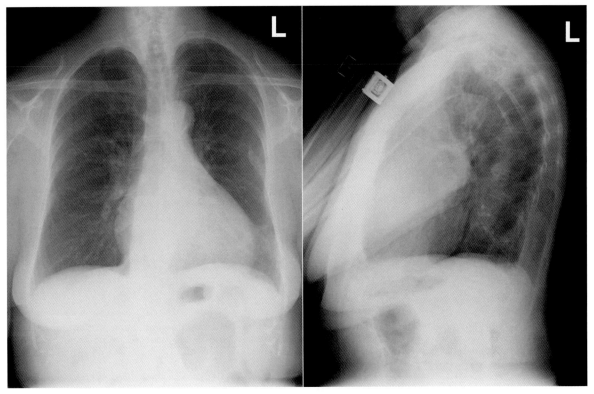

Figure 14-1. Hypertrophic cardiomyopathy. On the posteroanterior radiograph, the cardiothoracic ratio is mildly increased, and the upper left heart border is more prominent due to left atrial appendage enlargement. The lateral radiograph reveals posterior left ventricular displacement behind the supradiaphragmatic inferior vena cava.

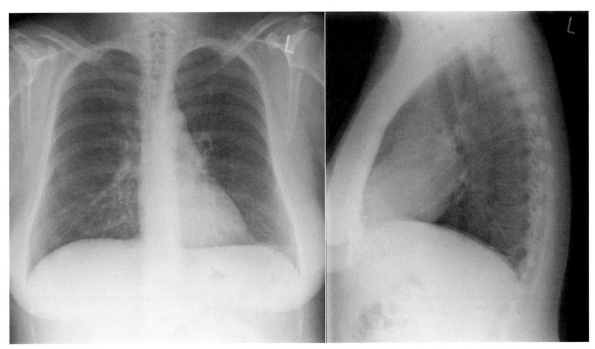

Figure 14-2. Anteroposterior and lateral chest radiographs of a patient with hypertrophic cardiomyopathy of a mild form. The left atrial appendage is likely enlarged, depicted by a straightening of the left superior heart border on the anteroposterior chest radiograph. There is no frank cardiomegaly. There is borderline posterior displacement of the left ventricular silhouette and probable enlargement of the left atrial silhouette on the lateral chest radiograph.

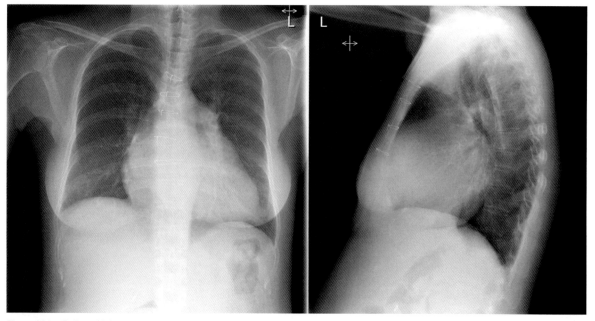

Figure 14-3. Patient with long-standing hypertrophic cardiomyopathy years after a myotomy/myectomy. The sternal wires attest to the previous cardiac surgery. There is gross cardiomegaly with signs of enlargement of all four cardiac chambers. Although myotomy and myectomy had afforded relief from the left ventricular tract obstruction, eventually severe right-sided heart failure and enlargement have developed.

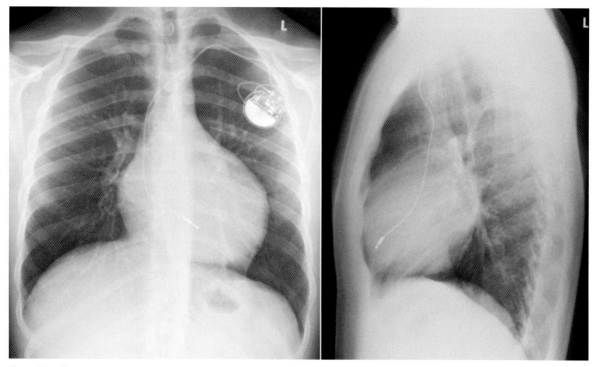

Figure 14-4. Hypertrophic obstructive cardiomyopathy, with a ventricular pacemaker lead. The left upper heart border is straightened by left atrial appendage enlargement, and the left heart border (elevated apex) reflects the severe left ventricular hypertrophy.

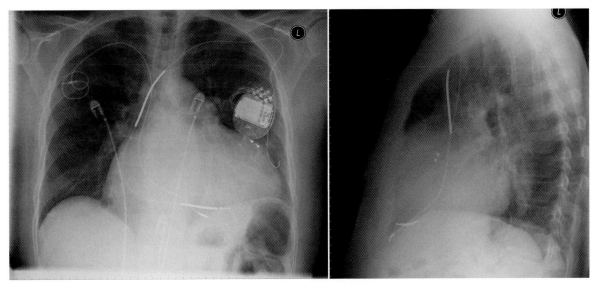

Figure 14-5. The cardiothoracic ratio is grossly increased, the heart shape is globular, and there are signs of multichamber enlargement. An implantable cardioverter defibrillator (ICD) and its lead, an old pacer wire, and a resynchronization wire are present. The difference between pacer leads and ICD leads is exemplified.

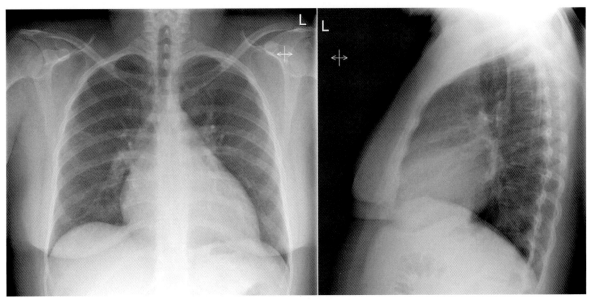

Figure 14-6. Posteroanterior and lateral radiographs demonstrating cardiomegaly with a flask/globular shape and prominence of all four cardiac chambers in nonischemic dilated cardiomyopathy with chronic heart failure, pretransplantation. The pulmonary veins are prominent.

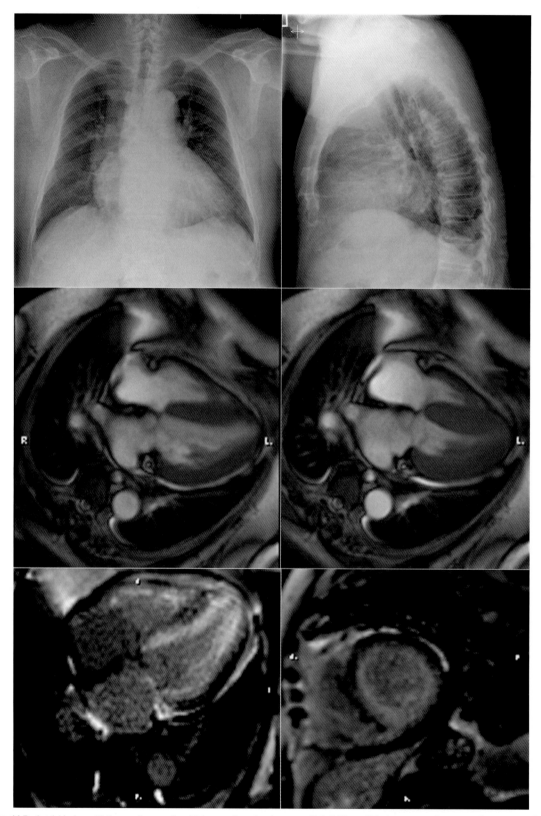

Figure 14-7. Amyloidosis restrictive cardiomyopathy. All four cardiac chambers are dilated. The middle images, cardiac magnetic resonance images (steady-state free precession), show mild-to-moderate right ventricular hypertrophy and right ventricular hypertrophy (*left image*: diastole) and normal systolic function (*right image*). In the inversion recovery (*lower images*), there is deep circumferential subendocardial late enhancement, consistent with amyloidosis.

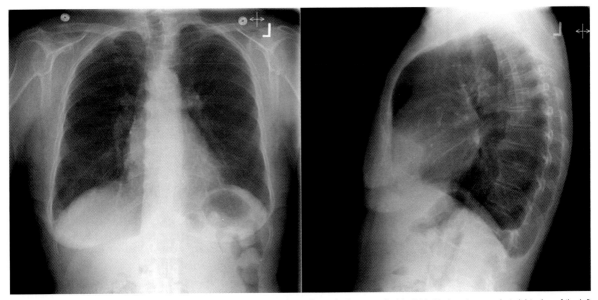

Figure 14-8. Amyloidosis restrictive cardiomyopathy. In the posteroanterior radiograph, there are double right-sided contours and straightening of the left upper heart border consistent with biatrial dilation. In the lateral radiograph, left atrial dilation is prominent. There are small pleural effusions but no overt signs of heart failure.

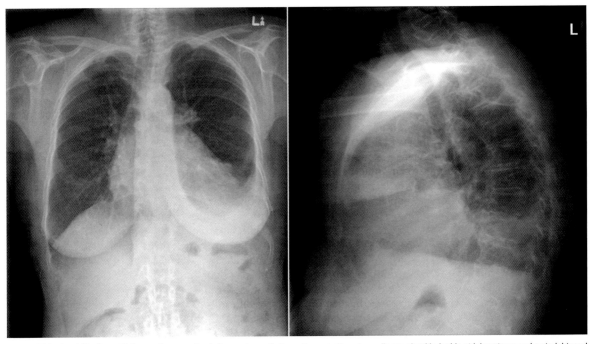

Figure 14-9. Amyloidosis restrictive cardiomyopathy. In the posteroanterior radiograph, there is cardiomegaly with double atrial contours and a straightened left upper heart border consistent with biatrial dilation. In the lateral radiograph, the moderate-sized left pleural effusion obscures much of the assessment of cardiac contours, but there clearly is cardiomegaly and interstitial pulmonary edema. The aortic arch is prominently calcified.

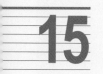

15 Radiographic Findings by Diagnosis: Valvular Heart Disease

ACQUIRED VALVULOPATHIES

Mitral Stenosis

The radiographic findings of mitral stenosis (Graphic 15-1; Figs. 15-1 to 15-16) reflect the pressure overload of the left atrium and pulmonary veins, and later of the right heart. As well, the commonly associated chronic atrial fibrillation contributes to (bi)atrial dilation. Associated rheumatic valvular lesions such as mitral regurgitation, tricuspid regurgitation, aortic insufficiency, and aortic stenosis/aortic insufficiency are common, and they alter the appearance of the heart.

Cardiac Findings of Mitral Stenosis on Chest Radiography

There is enlargement of the left atrium, disproportionate to other chamber enlargement, as the left atrium receives the principal hemodynamic burden of mitral stenosis. Left atrial appendage enlargement is usually the first sign. Later signs that develop when pulmonary hypertension ensues include enlargement of the right ventricle and atrium. One third of patients with severe mitral stenosis develop severe pulmonary hypertension.

A rheumatically distorted mitral valve may or may not be seen to be calcified on the plain chest radiograph but often is seen to be calcified on fluoroscopy. The likelihood of calcification depends more on the age of the patient than the degree of stenosis. Occasionally, calcification of the left atrial wall or of a left atrial thrombus may occur.

Vascular Findings of Mitral Stenosis on Chest Radiography

Findings include the following:
❐ Pulmonary venous hypertension (very common)
❐ Enlargement of the central pulmonary arteries. This is a later sign when pulmonary arteriolar hypertension ensues.
❐ Interstitial pulmonary edema and Kerley B lines (classic)
❐ Transient localized nodular shadows. These likely represent edema. Localized nodular shadows may also represent hemosiderosis (rare), and localized calcific nodules may be caused by pulmonary ossification (extremely rare).

The "mitralized heart" appearance is not specific for mitral valve disease. It may be seen with atrial septal defects and also with other forms of left atrial pressure overload such as a left atrial myxoma. The term is a classic and is used for the following features:
❐ Steep left heart border (indicating a normal-sized left ventricle)
❐ Straight mid-portion of the left heart border
❐ Mildly enlarged main pulmonary artery, consistent with pulmonary hypertension
❐ Slight convexity in the area of the pulmonary artery segment (left atrial appendage enlargement)
❐ Small aorta (no associated aortic valve disease)

Differentiating mitral stenosis from mitral insufficiency (see Graphic 15-1) on the basis of chest radiography is difficult unless it can be clearly determined that the left ventricle is normal-sized or enlarged. Left ventricular enlargement in the context of valvular heart disease suggests significant regurgitation and left ventricular volume overload. Left ventricular volume overload may also be secondary to aortic insufficiency, which is also commonly concurrent with mitral stenosis. Radiographic differentiation of left ventricular enlargement from right ventricular enlargement may be difficult.

Mitral Regurgitation

The radiographic findings of mitral regurgitation (Figs. 15-17 to 15-25; see also Figs. 15-12 to 15-14 and Graphic 15-1.) reflect the volume overload of the left

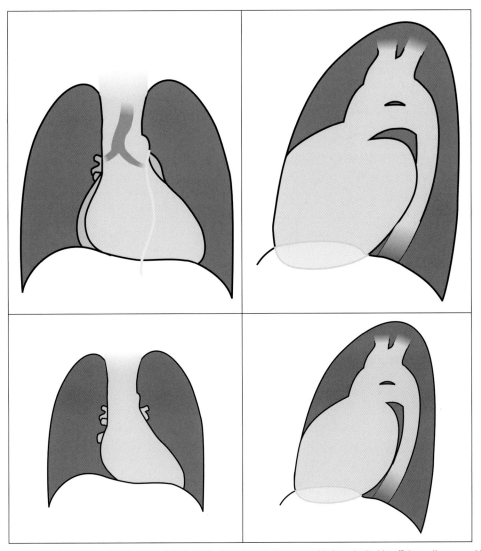

Graphic 15-1. Posteroanterior and lateral projections of findings of mitral stenosis (*upper graphics*), and mitral insufficiency (*lower graphics*). In mitral stenosis, the left atrium is dilated but the left ventricle is not. Often there is significant associated pulmonary hypertension. Associated right-sided heart enlargement is common, due to both pulmonary hypertension and associated tricuspid insufficiency. In mitral insufficiency, the volume overload dilates both the left atrium and the left ventricle.

ventricle and atrium and the secondary pressure over-load of the pulmonary vasculature and the right heart (see Graphic 15-1).

Cardiac Findings of Mitral Regurgitation on Chest Radiography
There is enlargement of the left ventricle and left atrium. Later signs that develop when pulmonary hypertension ensues include enlargement of the right ventricle and atrium.

A mitral valve that is insufficient because of rheumatic disease may or may not appear to be calcified on the plain chest radiograph but often is seen to be calcified on fluoroscopy. Myxomatous disease of the mitral valve is often associated with radiographically evident calcification of the annulus.

Vascular Findings of Mitral Regurgitation on Chest Radiography
Pulmonary venous hypertension is a late finding, and pulmonary arteriolar hypertension develops even later. Pulmonary edema may or may not be present.

Differentiating the chest radiographic findings of combined mitral stenosis and aortic insufficiency from those of mitral insufficiency may be impossible.

Aortic Valvular Stenosis
The radiographic findings of aortic stenosis (Graphic 15-2; Figs. 15-26 to 15-30; see also Graphic 15-1) primarily reflect the pressure overload of the left ventricle and secondarily the left atrium and pulmonary vasculature, as well as (often) poststenotic dilatation of the ascending aorta.

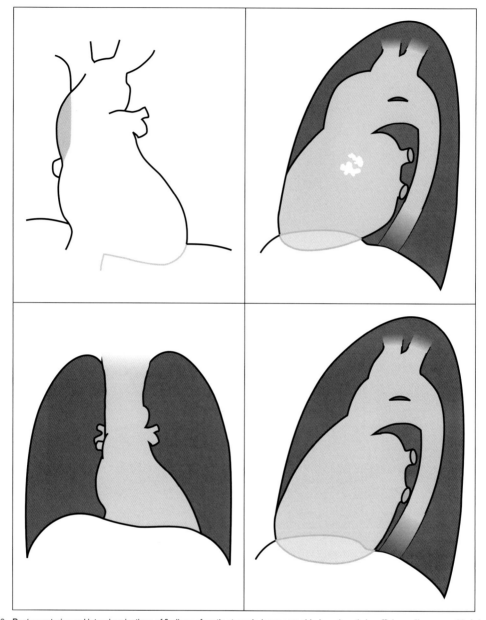

Graphic 15-2. Posteroanterior and lateral projections of findings of aortic stenosis (*upper graphics*), and aortic insufficiency (*lower graphics*). In aortic stenosis, there may be associated dilation of the ascending aorta apparent on the frontal radiograph. Calcification of the aortic valve, if heavy, is most apparent on the lateral radiograph. Typically, the effect of aortic stenosis on the left ventricle is concentric hypertrophy, which does not prominently enlarge the chamber. In aortic insufficiency, there may be generalized enlargement of the aorta secondary to the aortic insufficiency, or there may be underlying dilation of the aortic root causing the insufficiency. The volume load on the left ventricle results in dilation and lengthening.

Cardiac Findings of Aortic Stenosis on Chest Radiography

The aortic valve may or may not be calcified. Aortic stenosis in very young adults (e.g., 20 years of age) may occur without calcification. Aortic stenosis in middle-aged individuals often occurs with radiographically visible calcification. Aortic stenosis in older patients (e.g., 65+ years of age) is usually accompanied by radiographically evident calcification. Aortic stenosis in the elderly is almost invariably heavily calcific.

Age-related calcification of the aortic valve may occur without hemodynamically important stenosis, and therefore calcification in older individuals is not specific for stenosis. Calcification of the aortic valve or mitral valve or their annuli is far more easily appreciated on fluoroscopy than on plain chest radiographs.

Until late in the natural history of aortic stenosis, the cardiopericardial silhouette (CPS) is only mildly enlarged because concentric left ventricular hypertrophy results in a minimal or only a mild increase in the

CPS due to left ventricular hypertrophy and left atrial enlargement. Concentric left ventricular hypertrophy may round the left heart border, forming a "knuckle."

Late in the natural history of aortic stenosis, the left ventricle dilates as it decompensates from its "concentric hypertrophy." By this point, there are signs of pulmonary edema/congestive heart failure.

Vascular Findings of Aortic Stenosis on Chest Radiography

The ascending aorta is commonly but not invariably dilated in aortic stenosis ("poststenotic dilatation"). It is seen in both aortic stenosis due to congenitally bicuspid valves and also in aortic stenosis due to degenerative calcific disease.

In older patients with aortic stenosis, the aorta itself is often calcified. When the aortic wall calcification is confluent, it is referred to as a "porcelain aorta" and provides extreme technical difficulties at surgery. In addition, pulmonary edema is a common and important clinical occurrence in aortic stenosis.

Aortic Insufficiency

The radiographic findings of aortic insufficiency (Figs. 15-31 to 15-37) reflect the volume overload of the left ventricle and aorta. In addition, chest radiography indicates that the etiology of the valvular insufficiency is due to a root aneurysm.

Cardiac Findings of Aortic Insufficiency on Chest Radiography (see Graphic 15-2)

Enlargement of the left ventricle may occur posteriorly, laterally, or both posteriorly and laterally. In response to the volume overload of aortic insufficiency, the left ventricle elongates, and consequently the left ventricular border on the frontal chest radiograph is elongated. Of note, these findings are present only in chronic aortic insufficiency because remodeling of the heart to adapt to volume overload takes

months. Acute aortic insufficiency (e.g., from endocarditis) may occur with a normal or near-normal CPS. The aortic valve may or may not be calcified.

Vascular Findings of Aortic Insufficiency on Chest Radiography

Mild enlargement of the (entire) aorta takes place, and enlargement of the aortic root may occur as a result of the disease causing the aortic insufficiency (e.g., annuloaortic ectasia, syphilis, dissection, or aortitis). Aortic root calcification is unusual but may be seen after syphilis, aortitis, or Takayasu disease, as well as with atheromatous disease. There may or may not be pulmonary edema.

Tricuspid Valve Disease

The radiographic findings of tricuspid stenosis (Figs. 15-38 and 15-39) reflect pressure overload of the right atrium, and the radiographic findings of tricuspid insufficiency reflect the volume load on both right-sided cardiac chambers and often the pulmonary hypertension that causes most cases of tricuspid regurgitation.

Cardiac Findings of Tricuspid Valve Disease on Chest Radiography

In tricuspid stenosis, the right atrium is enlarged, often markedly, and the right ventricle and pulmonary arteries are normal-sized. In tricuspid insufficiency, the right atrium and ventricle are both dilated.

Vascular Findings of Tricuspid Valve Disease on Chest Radiography

The azygous vein is enlarged when the central venous pressure is increased by tricuspid valve disease. The pulmonary artery is normal-sized in tricuspid stenosis but may be increased in tricuspid insufficiency (when it is driven by pulmonary hypertension). Pulmonary edema is not encountered in the setting of primary tricuspid valve disease.

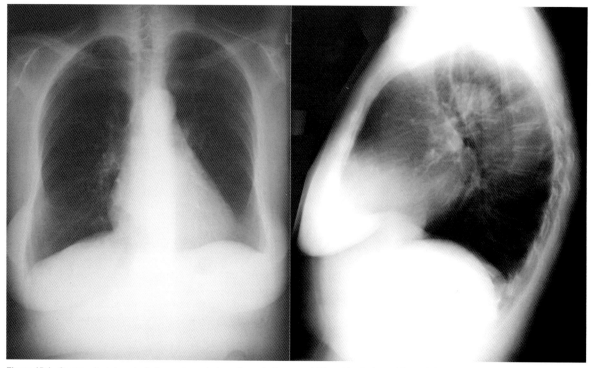

Figure 15-1. Severe mitral stenosis. In the posteroanterior radiograph, the upper left heart border is straightened due to left atrial appendage enlargement. In the lateral radiograph, prominent posterior left atrial dilation is apparent.

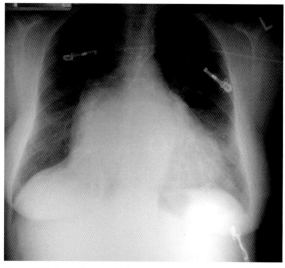

Figure 15-2. Several signs of left atrial enlargement persist in this case of post–mitral valve replacement for mitral stenosis: (1) the left upper heart border is full due to left atrial appendage enlargement; (2) the "carinal angle" is greater than 90°; and (3) the right (upper) heart border is displaced rightward, showing dilation of the left atrium.

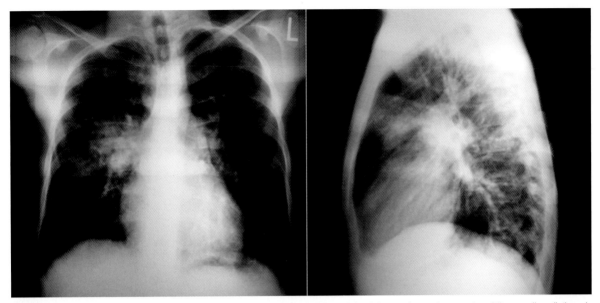

Figure 15-3. Severe mitral stenosis. The upper left heart border is straightened due to left atrial appendage enlargement, and the overall cardiothoracic ratio is normal. The left atrium is posteriorly enlarged on the lateral radiograph. The pulmonary arteries are enlarged. There is air-space infiltration within the mid-lung zones due to pulmonary (bronchial artery) hemorrhage.

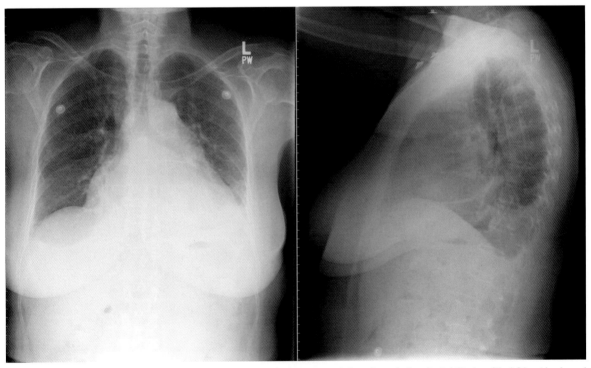

Figure 15-4. Severe mitral stenosis and severe tricuspid insufficiency. On the posteroanterior radiograph, there is straightening of the left heart border and fullness in the area of the left atrial appendage. As well, the lower left heart border is elongated, suggesting left ventricular enlargement, and there is right lower prominence consistent with right atrial enlargement.

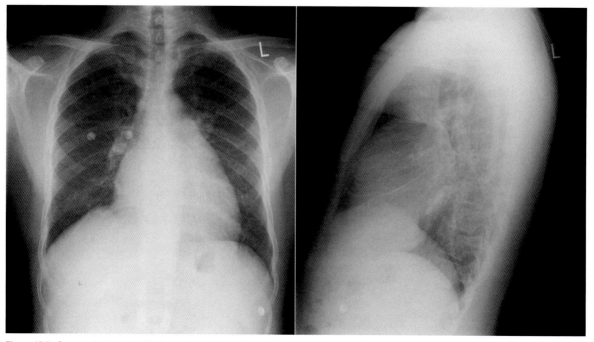

Figure 15-5. Severe mitral stenosis. On the posteroanterior radiograph, there is straightening of the upper left heart border and particular fullness in the area of the left atrial appendage. On the lateral radiograph, there is left atrial posterior displacement.

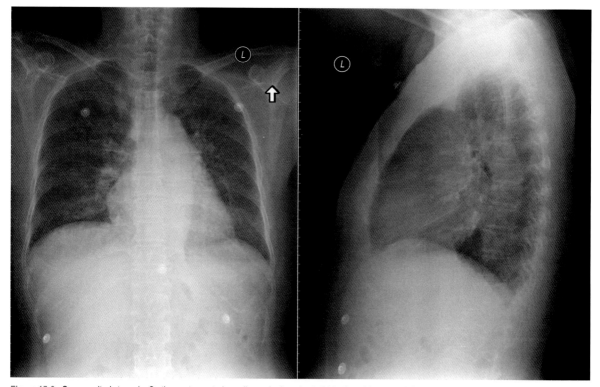

Figure 15-6. Severe mitral stenosis. On the posteroanterior radiograph, there is straightening of the upper left heart border and particular fullness in the area of the left atrial appendage. On the lateral radiograph, there is left atrial posterior displacement.

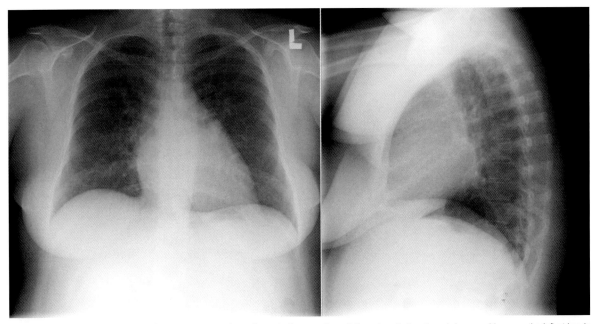

Figure 15-7. Severe mitral stenosis. On the posteroanterior radiograph, the overall cardiothoracic ratio is not much increased because the left atrium is not well represented on this projection. The left upper heart border is full/straightened due to left atrial appendage enlargement. There is pulmonary venous prominence. On the lateral radiograph, which depicts the left atrial size more directly, the heart size is obviously increased, mainly from posterior displacement of the left atrium.

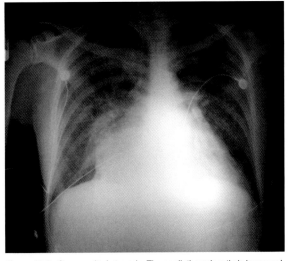

Figure 15-8. Severe mitral stenosis. The cardiothoracic ratio is increased, the left upper heart border is full/straightened, the carina is splayed, and there is a "double contour"/silhouette of the right heart border, all from left atrial enlargement. As well, there is enlargement of the pulmonary arteries and pulmonary edema.

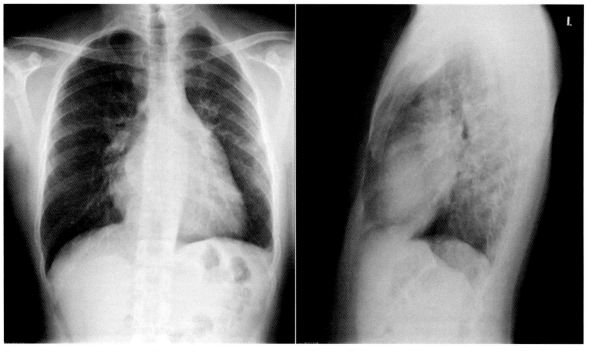

Figure 15-13. Severe mitral stenosis, with moderate pulmonary hypertension and 3+ tricuspid regurgitation (TR). The carina is splayed by left atrial dilation, the left upper heart border is moderately bulging due to left atrial appendage dilation, and there are definite double contours on the right side of the heart from left atrial dilation (upper bulge) and right atrial dilation (lower bulge). On the lateral radiograph, the left atrium is mildly enlarged and dilated posteriorly, and the heart is pressed against the sternum from both left atrial dilation and right ventricular dilation from TR and pulmonary hypertension.

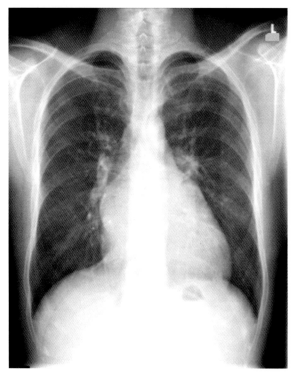

Figure 15-14. Severe mitral stenosis, with moderate pulmonary hypertension and 3+ tricuspid regurgitation. The carina is splayed by left atrial dilation, the left upper heart border is moderately bulging due to left atrial appendage dilation, and there are definite "double contours" on the right side of the heart from left atrial dilation (upper bulge) and right atrial dilation (lower bulge).

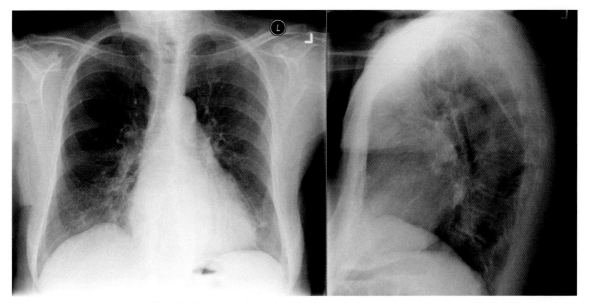

Figure 15-15. Severe mitral stenosis with moderately severe pulmonary hypertension. On the frontal radiograph, there is straightening of the left upper heart border due to dilation of the main pulmonary artery and of the left atrial appendage. The pulmonary veins are distended. On the lateral radiograph, the left atrium is dilated posteriorly, and the right ventricle is either enlarged or displaced anteriorly.

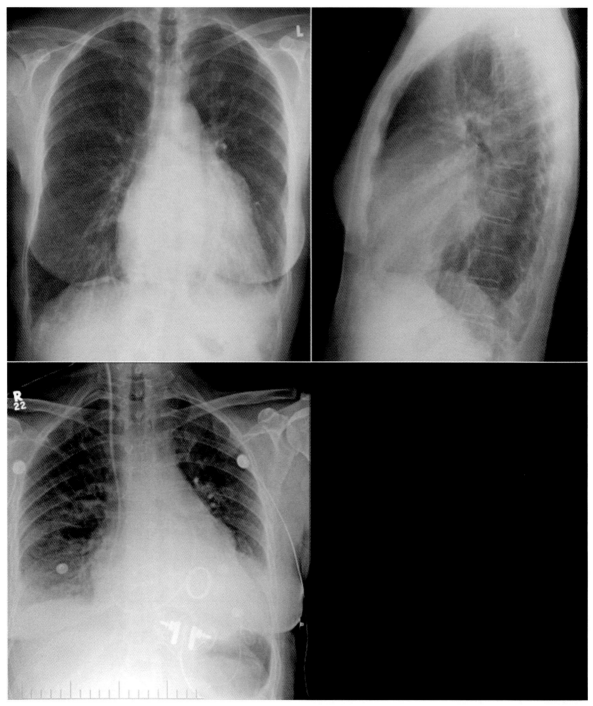

Figure 15-16. *Upper images:* Posteroanterior and lateral radiographs of severe mitral stenosis with pulmonary hypertension. Note the bulge of the left atrial appendage on the frontal radiograph. *Lower image:* Anteroposterior radiograph following mitral valve replacement with a bileaflet mechanical prosthesis.

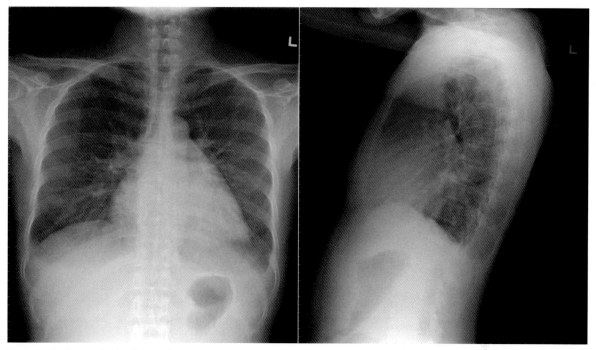

Figure 15-17. Severe mitral insufficiency. On the posteroanterior radiograph, the upper left heart border is straightened from left atrial appendage protrusion, the lower left heart border is lengthening due to lateral left ventricular enlargement. In addition, there is near carinal splaying. On the lateral radiograph, the left atrium and the left ventricle are both enlarged posteriorly. The pulmonary venous markings are increased. There are minor signs of right heart chamber dilation as well.

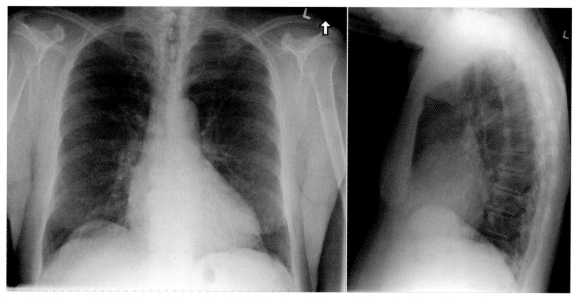

Figure 15-18. Severe mitral insufficiency. On the posteroanterior (PA) radiograph, the upper left heart border is straightened from left atrial appendage protrusion and the lower left heart border is lengthening due to lateral left ventricular enlargement. On the lateral radiograph, the left atrium and the left ventricle are both enlarged posteriorly (the left ventricle more so than what would be anticipated from the PA radiograph). The pulmonary venous markings are increased.

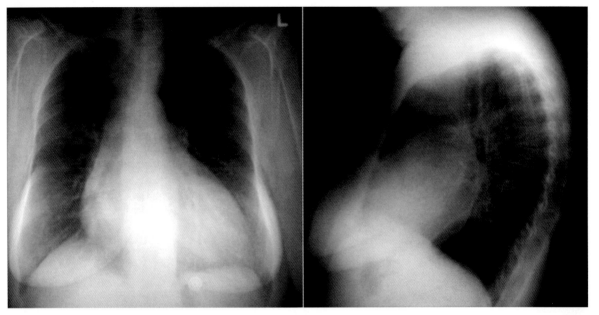

Figure 15-19. Severe mitral insufficiency. On the posteroanterior radiograph, the upper left heart border is straightened from left atrial appendage protrusion, and the lower left heart border is lengthening due to lateral left ventricular enlargement. On the lateral radiograph, the left atrium and the left ventricle are both enlarged posteriorly.

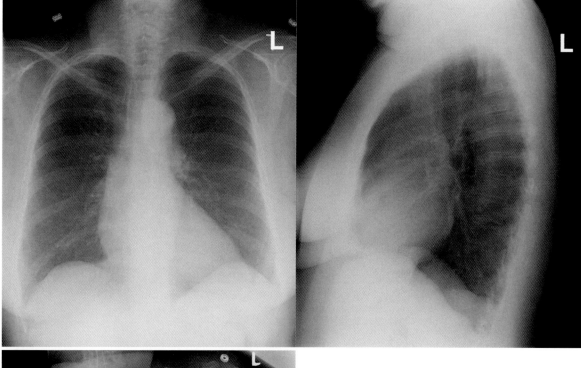

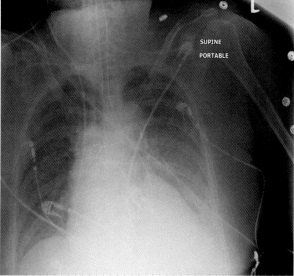

Figure 15-20. The upper films show severe chronic mitral regurgitation (MR) (and moderate left ventricular dysfunction due to coronary artery disease) pre–mitral valve repair. The left heart border is straightened and lengthened. The lateral radiograph reveals both left atrial and left ventricular enlargement. The lower film is following dehiscence of the mitral repair with acute massive MR and cardiogenic shock. Typical of acute valve insufficiency, the cardiothoracic ratio is not significantly increased (factoring in the anteroposterior versus posteroanterior projection and the lesser lung volumes). Intra-aortic balloon and pulmonary artery lines are in place.

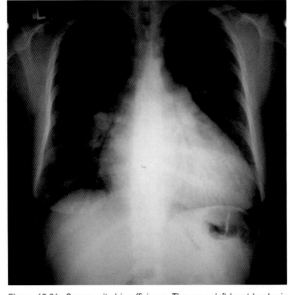

Figure 15-21. Severe mitral insufficiency. The upper left heart border is straightened from left atrial appendage protrusion, and the lower left heart border is lengthening due to lateral left ventricular enlargement. The main pulmonary artery is dilated, and there is a double (superior) right heart contour due to left atrial enlargement.

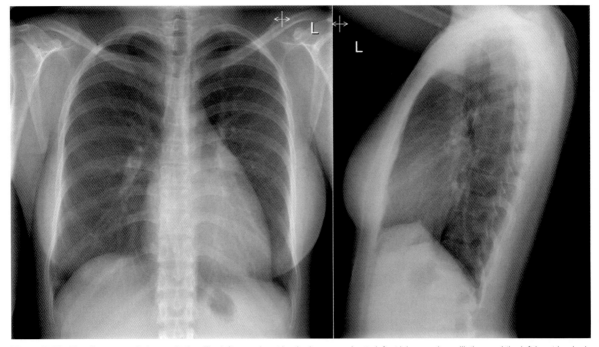

Figure 15-22. Chronic severe mitral regurgitation. The left upper heart border is convex due to left atrial appendage dilation, and the left heart border is elongated due to left ventricular elongation/dilation.

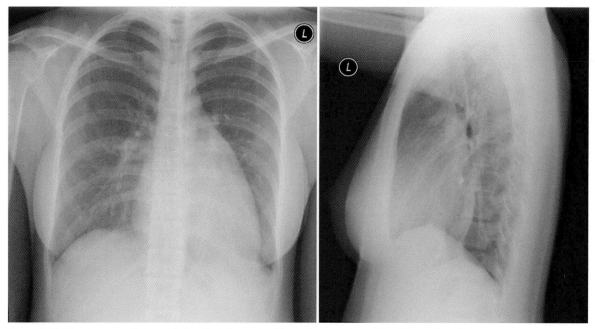

Figure 15-23. Chronic severe mitral regurgitation. The left upper heart border is convex due to left atrial appendage dilation, and the left heart border is elongated due to left ventricular dilation. It is dilated by the rule of Rigler as seen on the lateral radiograph.

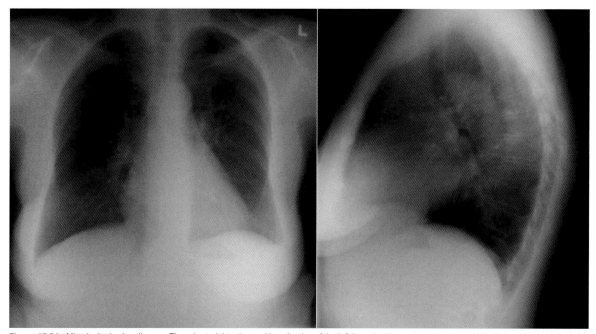

Figure 15-24. Mixed mitral valve disease. There is straightening and lengthening of the left heart border on the posteroanterior radiograph and enlargement of the left atrium and right ventricle on the lateral radiograph.

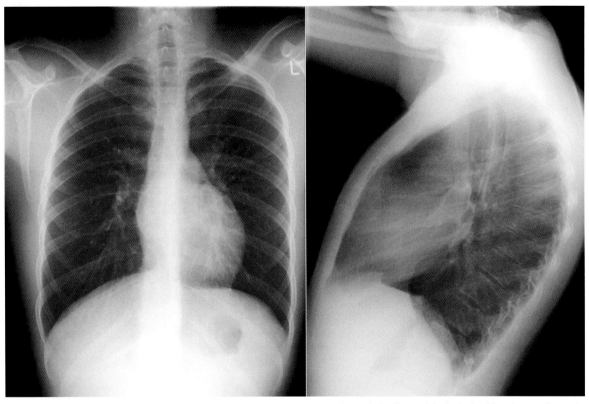

Figure 15-25. Posteroanterior and lateral radiographs showing moderate to severe mitral regurgitation from a cleft mitral valve. There is no cardiomegaly, but the heart contours are abnormal. The left upper heart border bulges due to enlargement of the left atrial appendage. On the lateral radiograph, there is increased right ventricular apposition to the sternum and posterior dilation of the left atrium. The left ventricle is not dilated, according to the rule of Rigler.

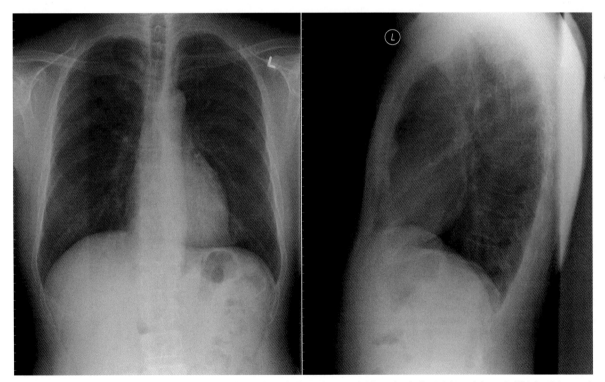

Figure 15-26. Severe aortic stenosis. The posteroanterior (PA) radiograph shows the upper left heart border is straightened due to (mild) left atrial appendage enlargement. The lower left heart border curvature is consistent with, but not specific for, left ventricular hypertrophy. The lateral radiograph reveals more posterior displacement (enlargement) than would be anticipated on basis of the PA radiograph.

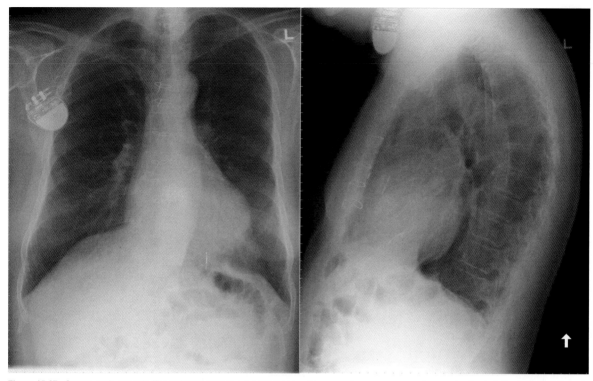

Figure 15-27. Severe aortic stenosis. The patient had previously undergone aortocoronary bypass surgery and pacemaker implantation. The cardiothoracic ratio is not increased, as it usually is not with concentric left ventricular hypertrophy. The lower left heart border is consistent with, but not specific for, LVH. The pulmonary venous vasculature is prominent. The lateral radiograph depicts borderline posterior dilation of the left ventricle, and frank dilation of the left atrium.

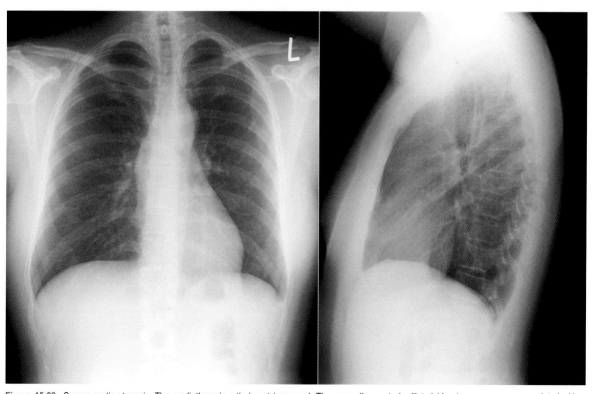

Figure 15-28. Severe aortic stenosis. The cardiothoracic ratio is not increased. The ascending aorta is dilated (due to an aneurysm associated with a bicuspid and stenotic aortic valve). The upper left heart border is borderline straightened due to (mild) left atrial appendage enlargement. The lower left heart border curvature is consistent with, but not specific for, left ventricular hypertrophy. The lateral radiograph reveals more posterior displacement (enlargement) than would be anticipated on basis of the posteroanterior radiograph.

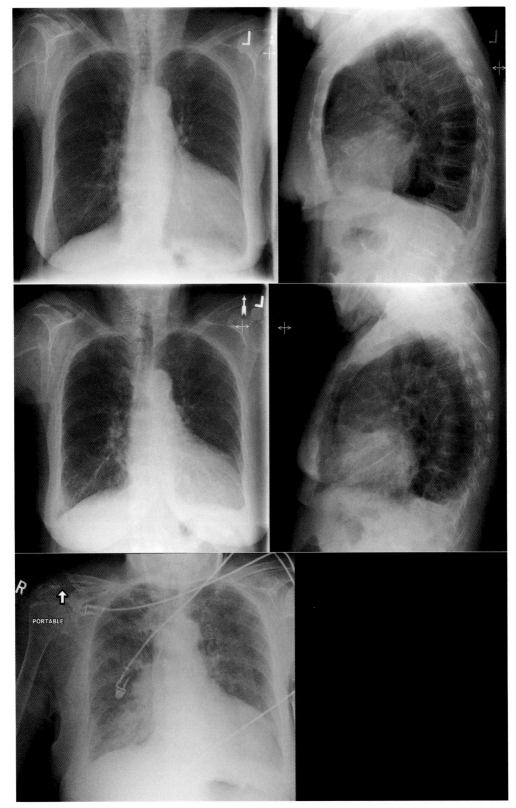

Figure 15-29. Aortic stenosis with worsening heart failure in a 90-year-old patient. On the upper images, there is cardiomegaly with prominence of the left ventricle and extensive calcification of both the aortic arch as seen on the posteroanterior radiograph and of the ascending aorta and arch, as seen on the lateral radiograph. The left atrium is also large. The pulmonary vasculature is prominent but there is no edema. On the middle images, there is mild pulmonary edema as seen by more prominent pulmonary vasculature and haziness of the hyla. On the lower image, there is frank interstitial and air space pulmonary edema.

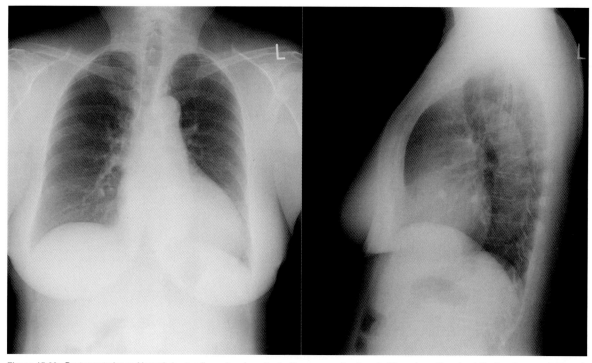

Figure 15-30. Posteroanterior and lateral chest radiographs of a patient with severe aortic stenosis. The valve, although calcific, is not apparent. There is cardiomegaly with enlargement to the left ventricle due principally to severe concentric left ventricular hypertrophy. There is also a mild heart failure. The S in the aorta is not prominently enlarged.

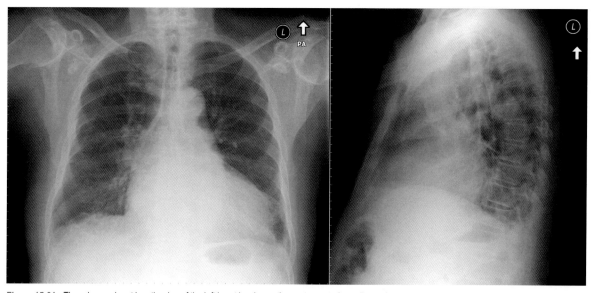

Figure 15-31. There is prominent lengthening of the left heart border on the posteroanterior radiograph and posterior displacement of the left ventricle on the lateral radiograph due to chronic severe aortic insufficiency. The ascending aorta is not convincingly enlarged. The descending aorta is tortuous.

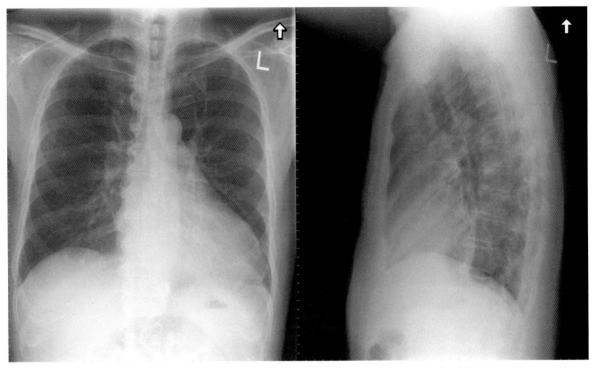

Figure 15-32. There is prominent lengthening of the left heart border on the posteroanterior radiograph and posterior displacement of the left ventricle on the lateral radiograph due to chronic aortic insufficiency. The ascending aorta is not convincingly enlarged.

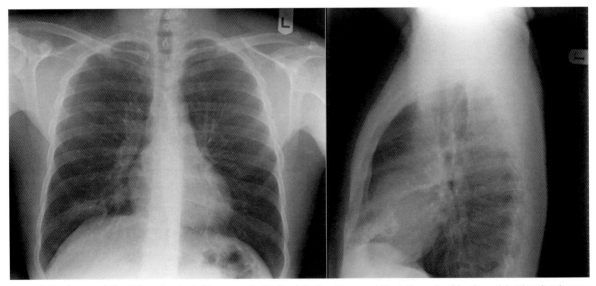

Figure 15-33. Acute aortic insufficiency from bacterial endocarditis. The heart size is not increased (due to the acuity of the disease), but there is pulmonary venous congestion consistent with mild heart failure.

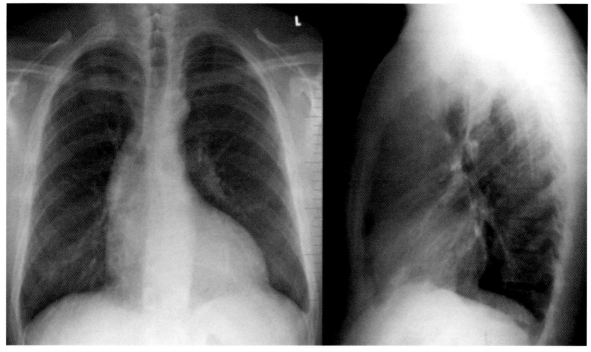

Figure 15-34. Chronic severe aortic insufficiency. Note the right hilar overlay sign of dilation of the ascending aorta and the cardiomegaly due mainly to left ventricular enlargement/elongation. The upper left heart border is slightly straightened from mild left atrial dilation.

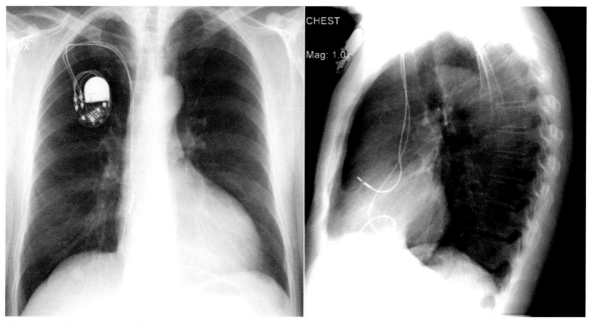

Figure 15-35. Chronic severe aortic insufficiency and dual chamber pacemaker leads. Note the cardiomegaly due mainly to left ventricular enlargement/elongation. The upper left heart border is slightly straightened from mild left atrial dilation. The aorta is mildly prominent.

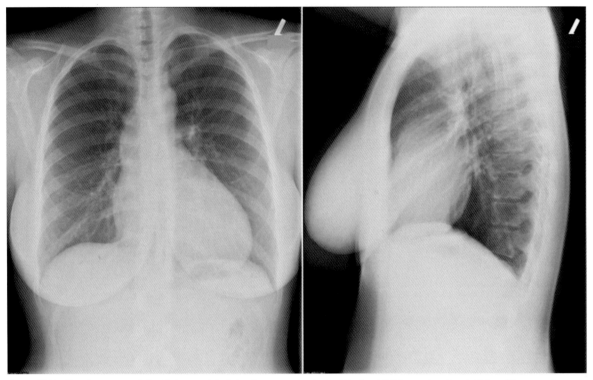

Figure 15-36. Chronic severe aortic insufficiency and dual chamber pacemaker leads. Note the right hilar overlay sign of dilation of the ascending aorta and the cardiomegaly due mainly to left ventricular enlargement/elongation. The upper left heart border is slightly straightened from mild left atrial dilation.

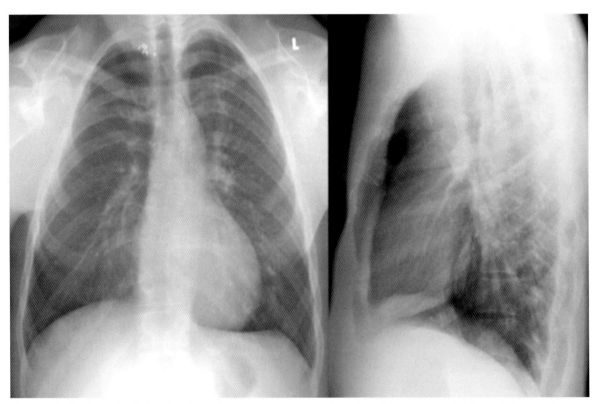

Figure 15-37. Chronic mixed aortic stenosis and insufficiency. The upper left heart border is slightly straightened from mild left atrial dilation. The left ventricle is more hypertrophied than dilated, resulting in a raised apex.

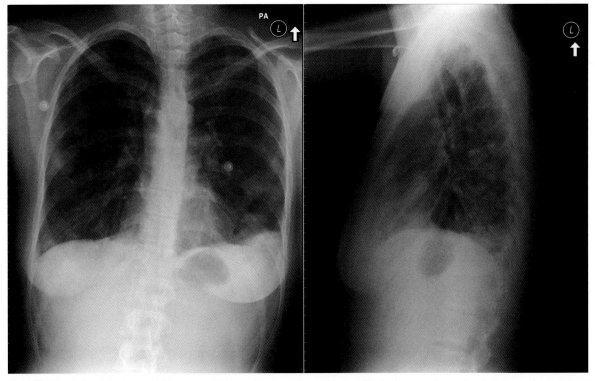

Figure 15-38. The heart size is normal. There are multiple rounded areas of consolidation within the lungs–septic emboli and abscesses due to rampant tricuspid endocarditis.

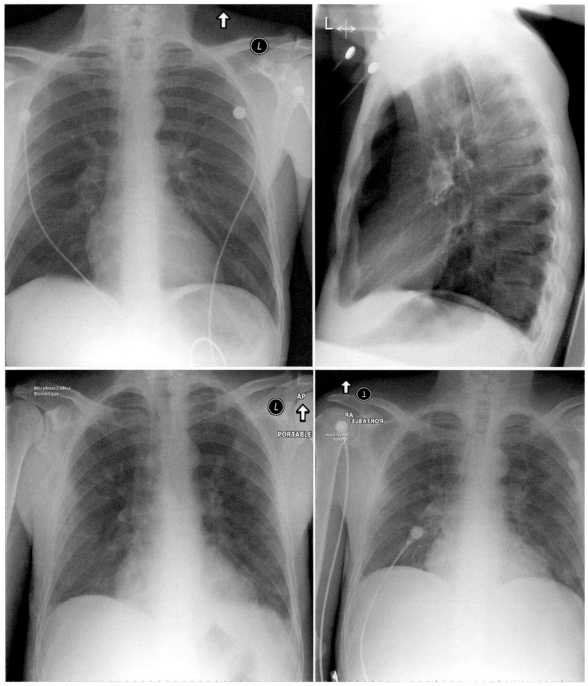

Figure 15-39. The upper chest radiographs were taken a year before the development of IV drug abuse–related tricuspid valve endocarditis. The lower chest radiographs depict the complications of this endocarditis. There has been enlargement of the cardiopericardial silhouette and a change in the right heart curvature with bulging of the right atrium due to complication of endocarditis by severe tricuspid insufficency. There are numerous areas of opacity within the lungs due to septic embolization to the lungs. The tricuspid valve was massively insufficient due to a multiple-centimeter tear resulting from the endocarditis.

ACQUIRED PERICARDIAL DISEASE

Pericardial Effusion

A pericardial effusion (Figs. 16-1 to 16-15) is often suggested on the frontal chest radiograph by a smoothly distended, "flasklike" CPS. More than 500 mL of fluid must be present before the change in the CPS is fairly obvious. A flasklike appearance may be caused by myocardial disease as well; scrutiny of the hilar vessels may distinguish the two. In the presence of pericardial effusion, the hilar vessels are covered (the pericardium runs up onto them and obscures them). In the presence of myocardial disease, the hilar vessels are unusually prominent as they are distended under higher than usual pressure.

In a minority of patients with pericardial effusion, on the lateral radiograph, a stripe of radiolucent epicardial fat, a "fat line," may be visible anteriorly, suggesting fluid in the pericardial space. A stripe greater than 2 mm is abnormal. This "pericardial stripe sign" is more easily seen in adults than children (more fat!).

A prominent azygous vein, superior vena cava, or inferior vena cava suggests cardiac tamponade.

Echocardiography is the diagnostic test of choice for the evaluation of pericardial effusions. Pericardial tamponade remains a clinical diagnosis, strengthened by supportive echocardiographic findings.

Constrictive Pericarditis

In constrictive pericarditis (Graphic 16-1; Figs. 16-16 to 16-23), the CPS is usually nonspecifically and mildly enlarged. Occasionally, the heart is normal or small in size. The left atrium is the most frequently enlarged chamber, because its enlargement is less restricted by pericardium. The right atrial contour on the frontal chest radiograph may be flattened. Calcification of the pericardium suggests past tuberculosis, but since tuberculosis has become uncommon at most centers, 90% of cases of constrictive pericarditis are currently noncalcified. Calcification, especially diaphragmatic, is not specific for constrictive physiology; it may be seen in the absence of cardiac compression. The apical surface is less frequently calcified than the interventricular and atrioventricular grooves. The apex seldom calcifies prominently in constrictive pericarditis; this finding suggests a calcified apical aneurysm rather that constrictive pericarditis.

Pericardial Cysts

Pericardial cysts may be congenital or acquired (Figs. 16-24 to 16-31). Most are located at the cardiodiaphragmatic angles (right-to-left: 3:1). A few are located more superiorly and lie against the upper heart or medial mediastinum. A wide range of sizes may occur. The celomic variety seldom calcifies. Calcification suggests a bronchogenic cyst, teratoma, or echinococcal cyst.

Pneumopericardium

Pneumopericardium (Figs. 16-32 to 16-42) may occur for several reasons, including the tracking of mediastinal air along pulmonary venous sheaths into the pericardial space, erosion of an esophageal or colonic carcinoma into the space, gas-forming or iatrogenic infection from barotrauma or pericardiocentesis/catheter/drainage misadventure. The parietal pericardium is projected away from the heart and appears as a 1- to 2-mm line—a thin stripe. Air and fluid may coexist in the pericardium; hence, an air-fluid level may occur.

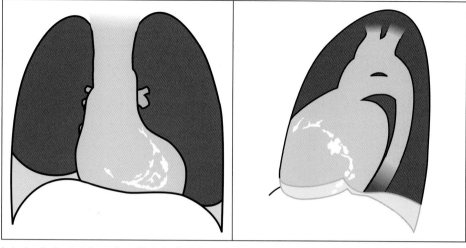

Graphic 16-1. Lateral projection depicting radiographic finds of calcific constrictive pericarditis. Note the mildly enlarged cardiac silhouette and the presence of plaquelike patches of pericardial calcification principally seen in the atrioventricular grooves. Pleural effusions are also depicted. Posteroanterior projection showing calcific constrictive pericarditis. Note the plaquelike pericardial calcification, which spares the left ventricular apex, mild cardiomegaly, and pleural effusion.

Congenital Absence of the Pericardium

Congenital absence of the pericardium is a rare condition that may involve partial or complete absence of the parietal pericardium (Figs. 16-43 to 16-46). Partial absence of the pericardium may involve smaller or large defects. Larger defects allow the heart to rotate or displace laterally into the (usually left) chest, with the trachea remaining midline. The main pulmonary artery is prominent. Very rarely, small defects may result in herniation of the left atrial appendage. The presence of aerated lung into recesses that it is normally excluded from by normally present parietal pericardium offers the diagnosis, which is more easily made by computed tomography scanning or cardiac magnetic resonance imaging. A "tongue" of aerated lung entering between the main pulmonary artery and the aorta or under the left ventricle may be seen, but generally, only the leftward displacement of the heart is apparent. The left heart border interface with the lung is often hazy and indistinct, probably due to excess motion enabled by the pericardial absence or the irregular heart surface blurring it.

Pleural Effusion

Pleural effusions (Figs. 16-47 to 16-52) are common among cardiac patients, especially those with predominantly right heart or pericardial disease burden. Pleural fluid generally descends uniformly to the costodiaphragmatic recesses, imparting a meniscus that is apparent on the frontal radiograph and obvious on the lateral radiograph. However, pleural fluid may localize (e.g., within a fissure), occasionally producing a "pseudotumor" lesion that resolves with correction of heart failure. The larger the pleural effusion, the more difficult it becomes to resolve the heart size due to silhouetting of the heart borders.

Pneumothorax

Pneumothoraces may occur for several reasons (Figs. 16-53 to 16-56). They are apparent as abnormal lucency without lung markings, with the lateral margin of the lung generally providing a brighter line. A false-positive diagnosis of pneumothorax may arise from a prominent posterior skin fold, which may superimpose a plausible line similar to that of a pneumothorax. However, the line is usually dark rather than bright, and lung markings are still present lateral to it. Pneumothoraces are larger during expiration than inspiration and are far more apparent on erect radiographs versus supine ones. A pneumothorax may be apparent on a supine film by the "deep sulcus sign," where the costodiaphragmatic recess/sulcus depresses abnormally.

Pleural Plaques/Fibrothorax

Pleural plaques (Figs. 16-57 and 16-58) may result from several disorders but are typical of prior asbestos exposure, especially when they calcify. When seen enface (head-on), they are less apparent, but when seen tangentially, they are obvious. Extensive calcification of the visceral and parietal pleura, especially when unilateral, is typical of a fibrothorax (Fig. 16-59). Causes include prior tuberculous disease, prior empyema, or hemothorax.

Other abnormal lucencies within the chest may occur for a number of reasons, and their anatomic location and shape usually suggests one the following causes:

❏ Epicardial fat adjacent to a pericardial effusion (Graphic 16-2)
❏ Pneumopericardium (Graphic 16-3)
❏ Pneumomediastinum (Fig. 16-60)
❏ Pneumothorax (Fig 16-61)
❏ Subcutaneous emphysema

❏ Hiatal hernia (see Figs. 16-39 to 16-42)
  • Localization of air by the lateral radiograph within the hiatus hernia to be posterior to the heart. This readily distinguishes a hiatal hernia from a pneumopericardium.
  • Hyperinflation of one lung

❏ A unilateral lucent lung (Fig. 16-62): bronchiolitis obliterans/Swyer-James syndrome of unilateral lucent lung, a smaller hemithorax, and air trapping on expiratory series
❏ Free air in the abdomen, which is apparent as well on the chest radiograph (Fig. 16-63)

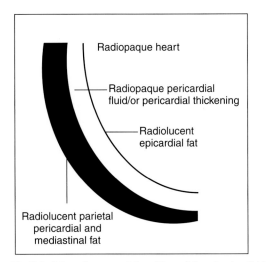

Graphic 16-2. Schematic representation of the radiolucent pericardial fat stripe seen best on a lateral radiograph.

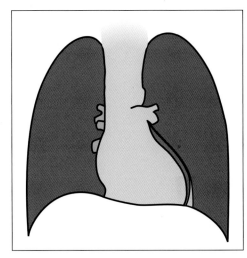

Graphic 16-3. Posteroanterior projection of a pneumopericardium. Note the lucency caused by air within the pericardium.

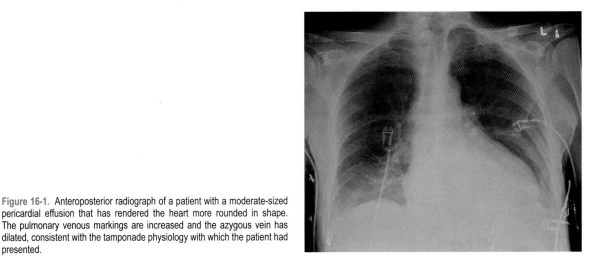

Figure 16-1. Anteroposterior radiograph of a patient with a moderate-sized pericardial effusion that has rendered the heart more rounded in shape. The pulmonary venous markings are increased and the azygous vein has dilated, consistent with the tamponade physiology with which the patient had presented.

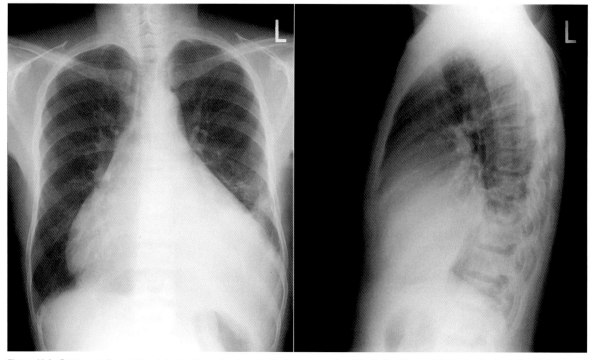

Figure 16-2. Posteroanterior and lateral chest radiographs of a patient with a large pericardial effusion. The cardiothoracic ratio is prominently increased, and the shape is globular, with flasklike tapering superiorly as the pericardial effusion has run up the pericardial sleeve over the aorta and pulmonary artery.

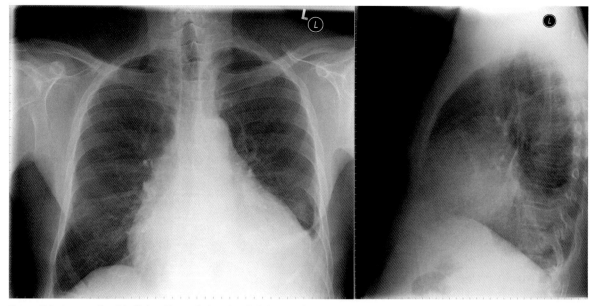

Figure 16-3. Large pericardial effusion. The cardiothoracic ratio is increased, and the shape, although partially obscured by a large left-sided pleural effusion, is globular.

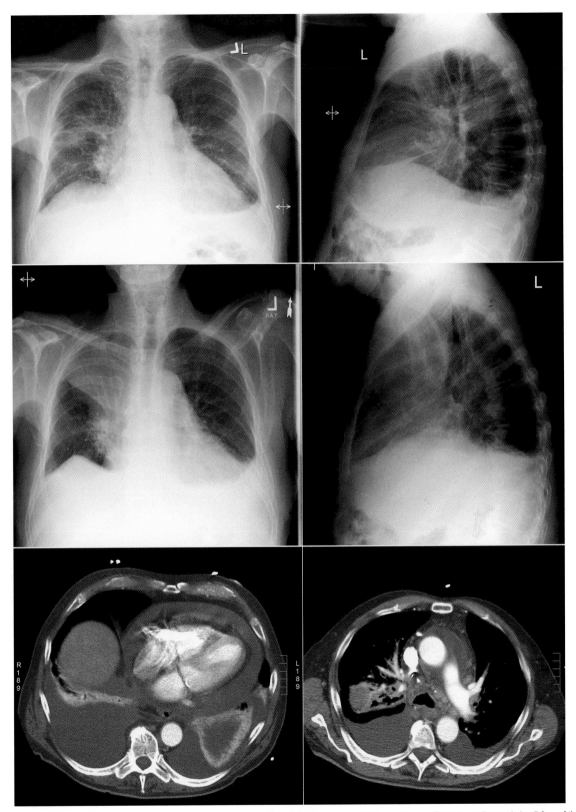

Figure 16-4. Chest radiographs and corresponding contrast-enhanced computed tomography (CT) axial images. There is cardiomegaly in all four of the chest radiographs. Between the upper and the lower chest radiographs, there has been collapse of the right upper lobe. The CT scans reveal that the cardiomegaly is due to a moderate-sized pericardial effusion that can be seen both around the heart on the left lower image and extending up the pericardial sleeve of the great vessels along the aorta and the pulmonary artery seen on the right lower image. Bronchogenic carcinoma with right upper lobe collapse and malignant pericardial and pleural effusions is seen.

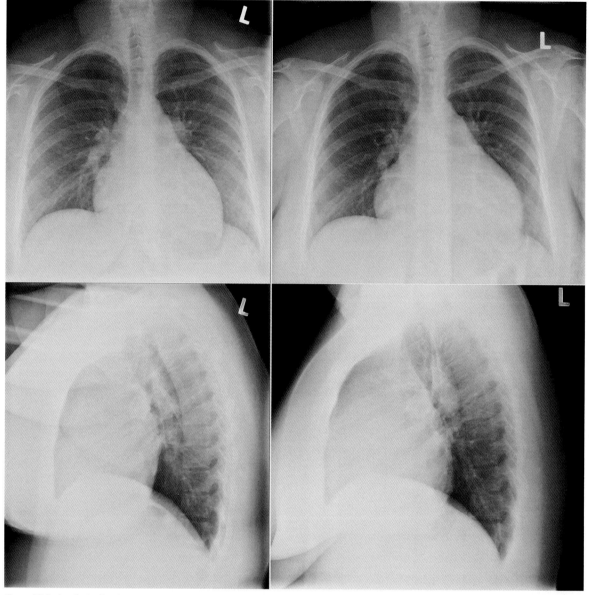

Figure 16-5. A patient with advanced pulmonary hypertension. The left images are prior to the development of a pericardial effusion. Note the prominent pulmonary arteries and large right atrium and ventricle. The right images reveal the development of a moderate-sized pericardial effusion; the cardiopericardial silhouette has increased in size.

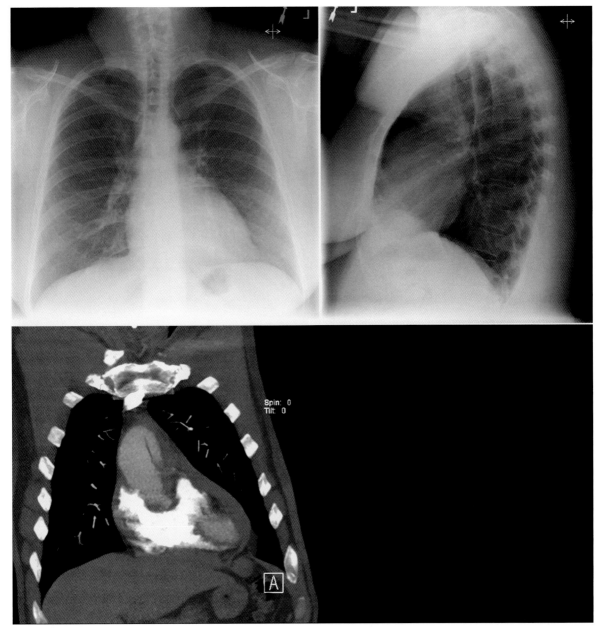

Figure 16-6. There is mild rounding of the heart silhouette on the chest radiographs. The flasklike shape of the heart due to the moderate-sized pericardial effusion extending up the vascular sleeves of the pericardial space is more apparent on the coronal computed tomography image.

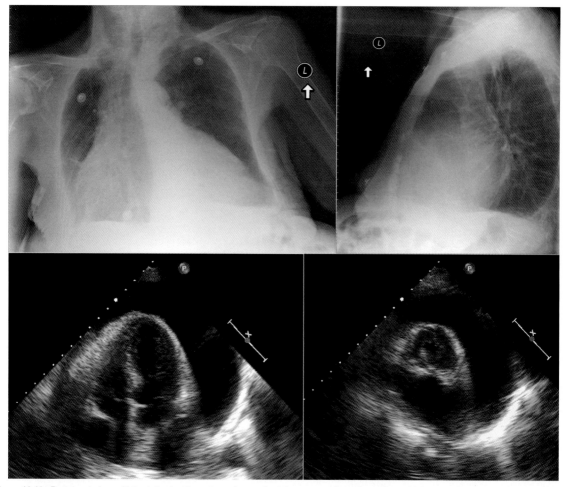

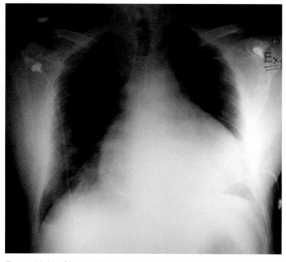

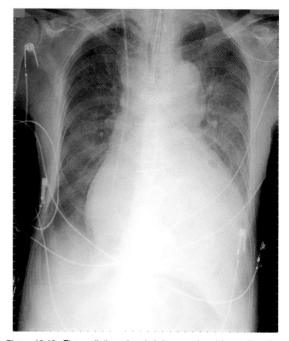

Figure 16-10. Posteroanterior and lateral chest radiographs and approximately corresponding echocardiographic images of a patient with pericardial tamponade. The cardiothoracic ratio is prominently increased, and the shape is globular. The echocardiographic images depict the proportion of the cardiomegaly that is due to fluid.

Figure 16-11. Chest radiograph of a patient with pericardial tamponade. The cardiothoracic ratio is prominently increased, and the shape is globular. There is a double shadow superiorly on the left due to fluid within the pericardial space at the arch level.

Figure 16-12. The cardiothoracic ratio is increased, and the cardiopericardial silhouette shape is globular due to hemopericardium. The pulmonary artery catheter is within the right heart.

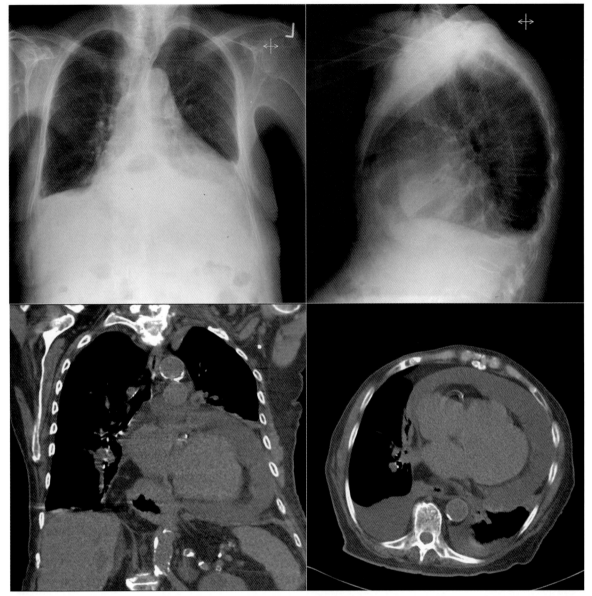

Figure 16-13. Posteroanterior and lateral chest radiographs and non–contrast-enhanced computed tomography coronal and axial views of a female patient with prior bilateral mastectomies (note axillary dissection clip) who presented with pleural effusions and pericardial tamponade due to metastatic bowel carcinoma. Note the rounded or flasklike shape of the cardiopericardial silhouette and the prominent azygous vein/superior vena cava, consistent with raised central venous pressure due to tamponade.

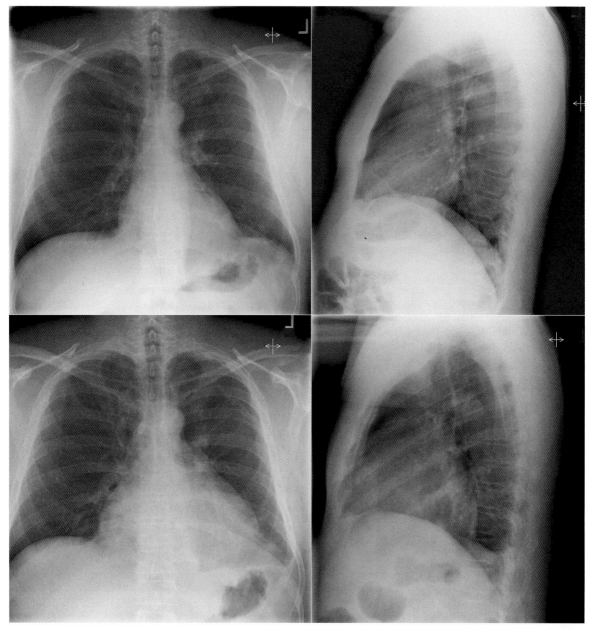

Figure 16-14. *Upper images:* Posteroanterior and lateral chest radiographs during a presentation with acute pericarditis. The lower images are at a later date during subsequent re-presentation to hospital with dyspnea and fatigue. The heart size has visibly increased within a 3-week period, with the shape becoming more globular on both the frontal and lateral radiographs. As well, the azygous vein is plethoric consistent with raised central venous pressure. The second presentation was associated with the hemodynamics of tamponade.

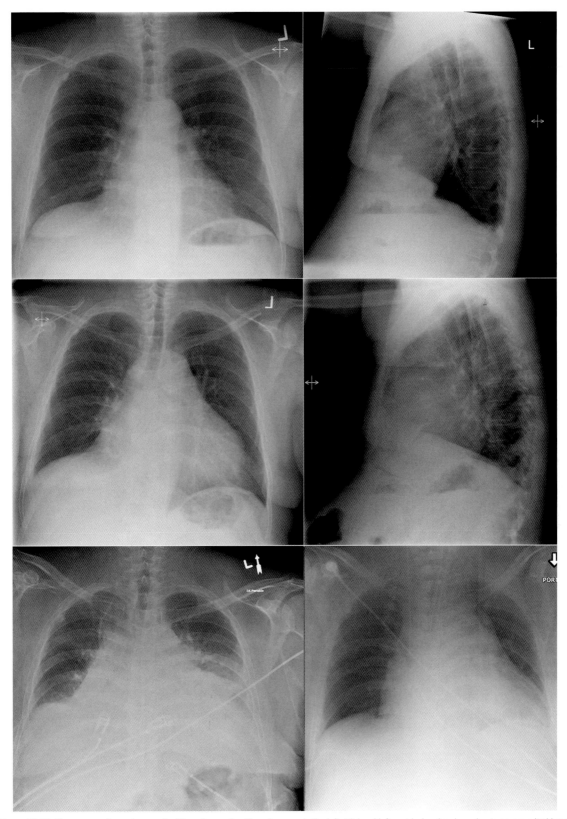

Figure 16-15. The upper radiographs reveal mild cardiomegaly with an increase in the left atrial and left ventricular chambers due to severe mitral insufficiency without heart failure. The middle radiographs, taken 3 months later while the patient was awaiting mitral valve surgery, reveal an increase in the size of the cardiopericardial silhouette. This was due to the development of malignant tamponade in the intervening period. The left lower radiograph is post–pigtail catheter insertion into the pericardial space. The right lower radiograph is post–pigtail catheter insertion into both pleural spaces to drain malignant pleural effusions.

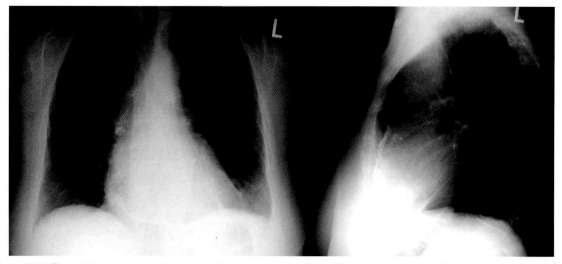

Figure 16-16. The cardiothoracic ratio is not increased, and there is no particular abnormality to the cardiopericardial silhouette. The lung fields are clear, although the film is overpenetrated. The left costophrenic angle is blunted. There is an extensive plate of pericardial calcification present under the heart on the posteroanterior (PA) film. The lateral radiograph reveals that the pericardial calcification is also anterior to the right ventricle and is not appreciable on the PA radiograph, where it is "en-face."

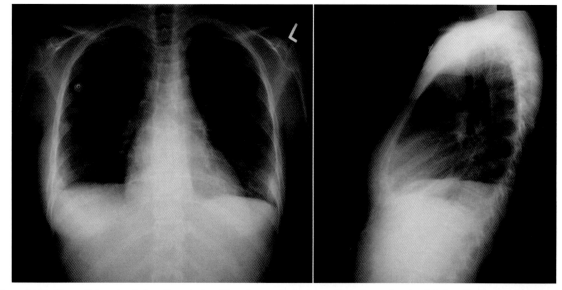

Figure 16-17. The cardiothoracic ratio is not increased, and there is no particular abnormality to the cardiopericardial silhouette. The lung fields are clear, although the film is overpenetrated. The azygous vein is bulging over the right mainstem bronchus due to the elevation of central venous pressure from acute tamponade.

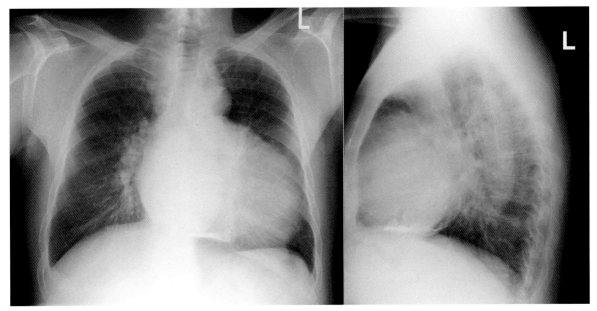

Figure 16-18. Calcified chronic organized intrapericardial hematoma. The cardiothoracic ratio is increased. There is an extensive plate of pericardial calcification present under the heart, seen on both the posteroanterior and lateral radiographs.

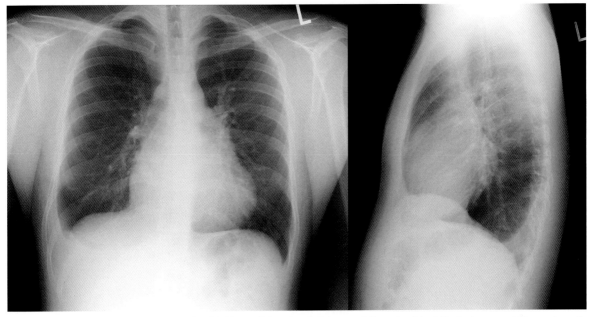

Figure 16-19. Surgically proven constrictive pericarditis. The cardiothoracic ratio is increased. No pericardial calcification is apparent. The most specific abnormality of the cardiopericardial silhouette is that of left atrial (and appendage) enlargement.

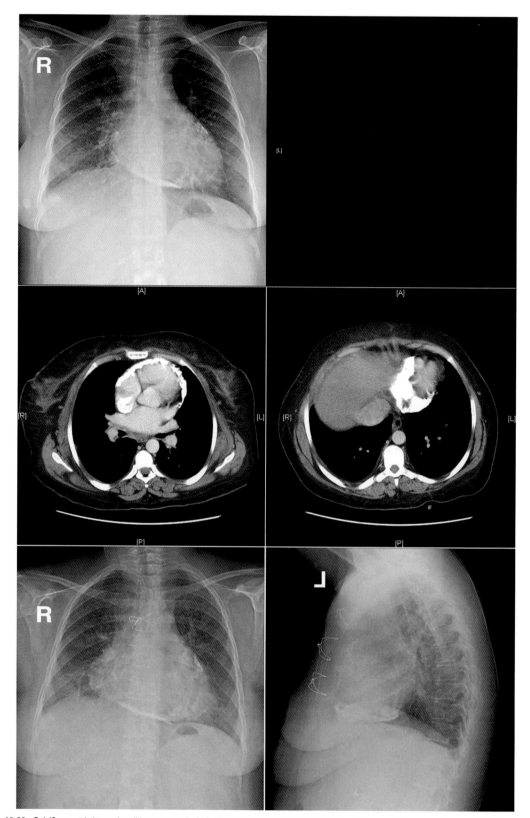

Figure 16-20. Calcific constrictive pericarditis, preoperatively, is shown in the upper radiograph and axial computed tomography scans. Note the dense thick plates of calcium over the right heart free wall and along the diaphragmatic surface, as well as the diaphragmatic plates of calcification seen well on the frontal radiograph. The plates over the right heart free wall, which are projected "en-face", are not well depicted. Conversely, both are seen tangentially and well on the lateral radiograph. The lower radiographs were taken years later, revealing the incompleteness of the pericardial resection.

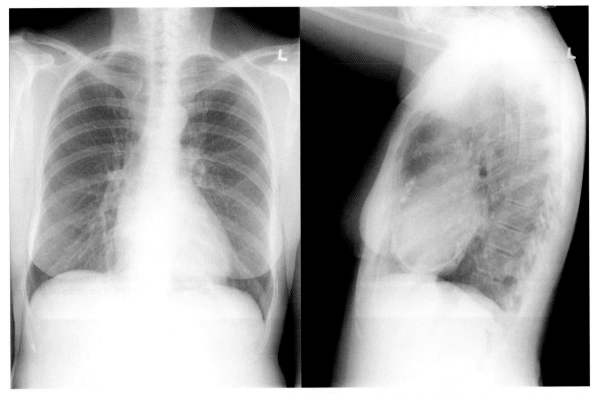

Figure 16-21. Posteroanterior and lateral chest radiographs of a patient with extensive pericardial calcification that is far better seen on the lateral radiograph. Despite the calcification, there was no evidence of contrictive physiology.

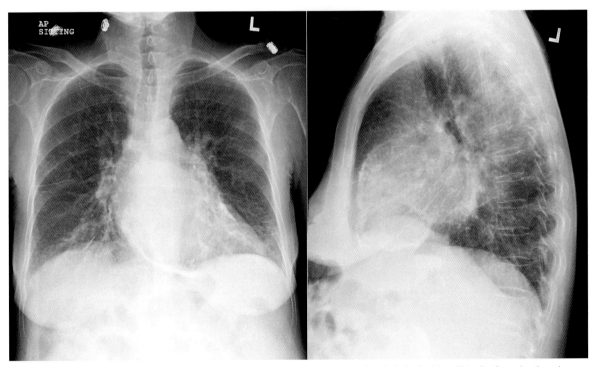

Figure 16-22. Note the cardiomegaly, increased left atrial size, platelike calcification seen well on both the frontal and lateral radiographs, the pulmonary venous congestion, and prominent azygous vein in this patient with calcific constrictive pericarditis.

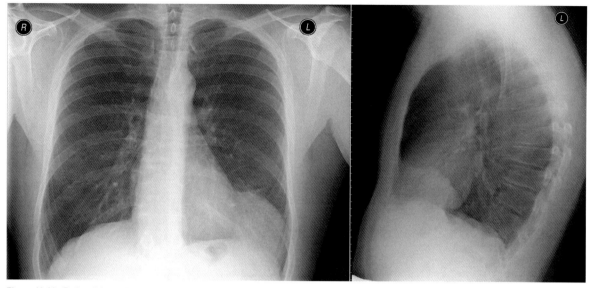

Figure 16-28. Pericardial cyst. There is a rounded mass at the left cardiophrenic angle, a less common site of pericardial cysts. The fluid-filled nature of the mass is not apparent on plain film radiography.

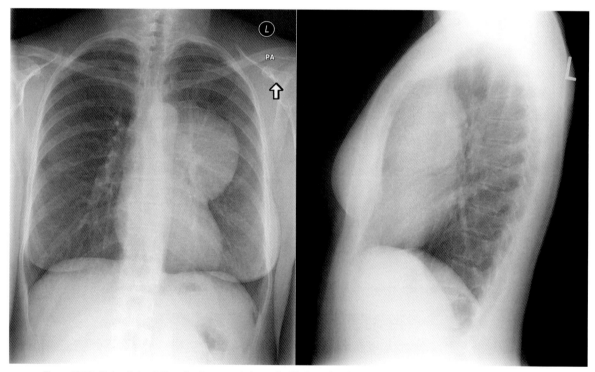

Figure 16-29. Pericardial cyst. There is a large rounded mass beside the main pulmonary artery, a less frequent site of pericardial cysts.

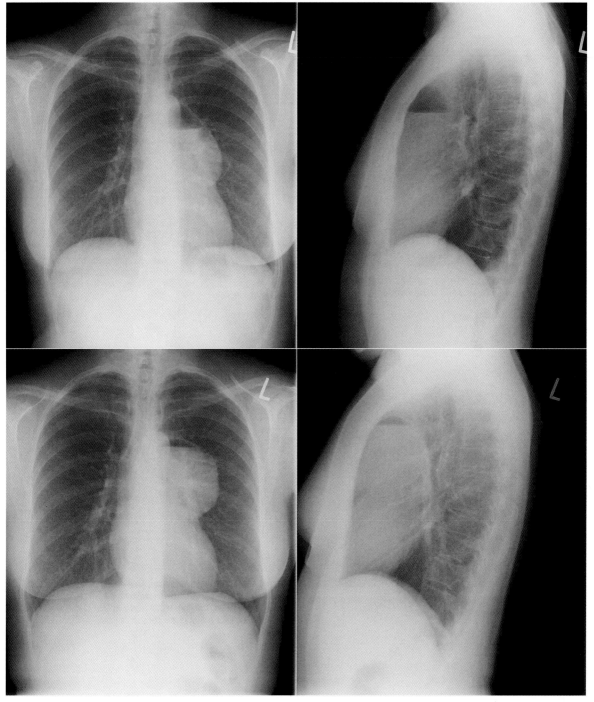

Figure 16-30. Posteroanterior and lateral radiographs following pericardial cyst drainage. There is an air-fluid level within the cyst. With time (*lower images*), the volume of fluid increases and the air-fluid level rises. Eventually, the cyst completely refills with fluid.

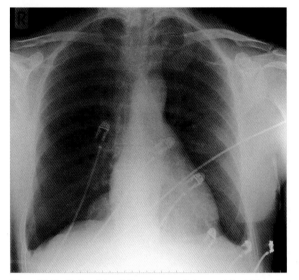

Figure 16-31. Pericardial cyst. There is a rounded mass at the right cardiophrenic angle, the most common site of pericardial cysts.

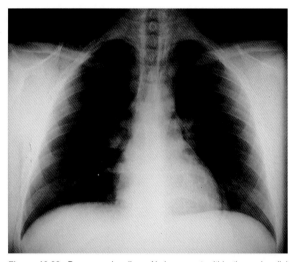

Figure 16-32. Pneumopericardium. Air is present within the pericardial space, and the parietal pericardium is apparent as a thin stripe. The parietal pericardial fat pad, near the diaphragm, renders the pericardial stripe thicker in that area.

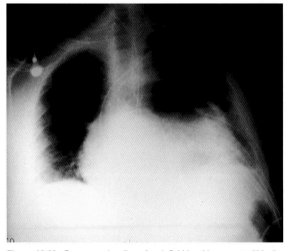

Figure 16-33. Pneumopericardium. An air-fluid level is present within the pericardial space (purulent pericarditis/fistula).

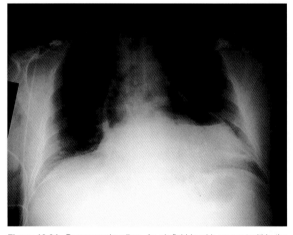

Figure 16-34. Pneumopericardium. An air-fluid level is present within the pericardial space. The parietal pericardium, when seen edge-on, is apparent as a thin stripe. The right lateral aspect of the ascending aorta is obvious. The superior extent of the parietal pericardium to the aortic arch is apparent.

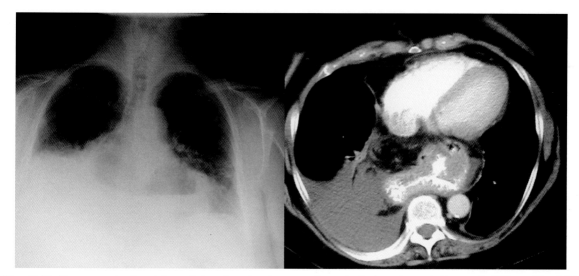

Figure 16-35. No pneumopericardium. Anteroposterior radiograph and corresponding contrast-enhanced computed tomography (CT) scan. The air-fluid level is located within a hiatal hernia posterior to the heart, as confirmed by the CT scan.

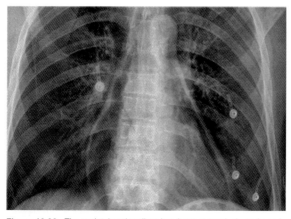

Figure 16-36. The parietal pericardium has been extensively and nearly symmetrically lifted off the heart by pneumopericardium. The full anatomic extent of the pericardium superiorly is revealed in this case. (From Karoui M, Bucur PO: Pneumopericardium. *N Engl J Med* 359[14]:e16, 2008. Used with permission.)

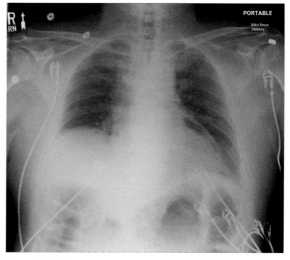

Figure 16-37. Pneumopericardium. Note the air stripe as seen on this anteroposterior chest radiograph over the left heart border demarcating the parietal pericardium over the left heart, which when seen tangentially (edge-on) appears as a thin stripe. Note as well the sternal wires and small lung volumes. This patient, recently post–aortic coronary bypass grafting, had re-presented with tamponade, which had been drained percutaneously. Air had entered the pericardial space through the percutaneous drain, which had a poor air seal.

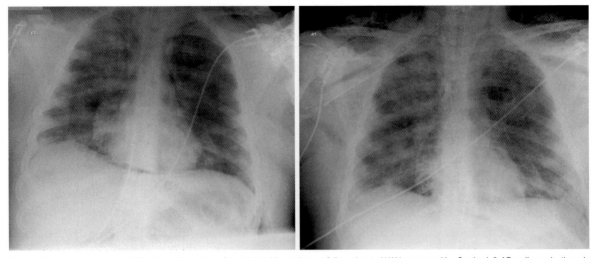

Figure 16-38. Anteroposterior (AP) chest radiographs of a patient with respiratory failure due to H1N1 pneumonitis. On the left AP radiograph, there is clearly pneumopericardium with air underneath the heart and between the heart and the diaphragm. On the right AP radiograph, the thin stripe of the parietal pericardium is more evident. As well, there is evolved extensive subcutaneous emphysema.

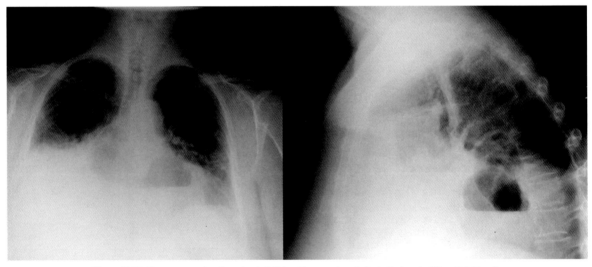

Figure 16-39. No pneumopericardium. An air-fluid level is present posterior to the heart within a hiatal hernia.

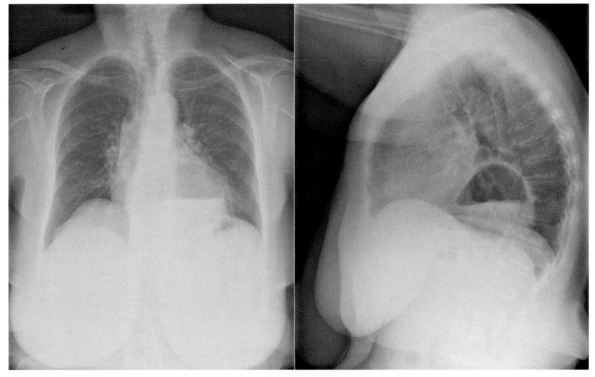

Figure 16-40. An air-fluid level is present posterior to the heart in a hiatal hernia, whose margins are particularly well seen on both the posteroanterior and lateral radiographs.

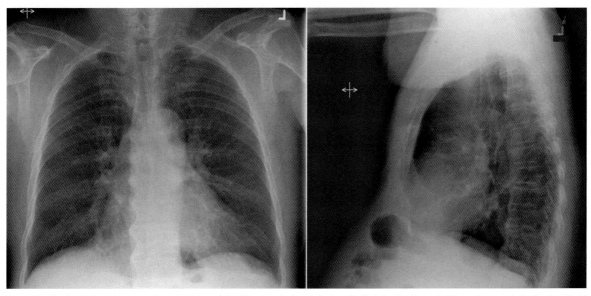

Figure 16-41. On the frontal radiograph, note the two air bubbles over the heart shadow. On the lateral radiograph, this can be seen to be due to a hiatal hernia posteriorly and a loop of bowel anteriorly.

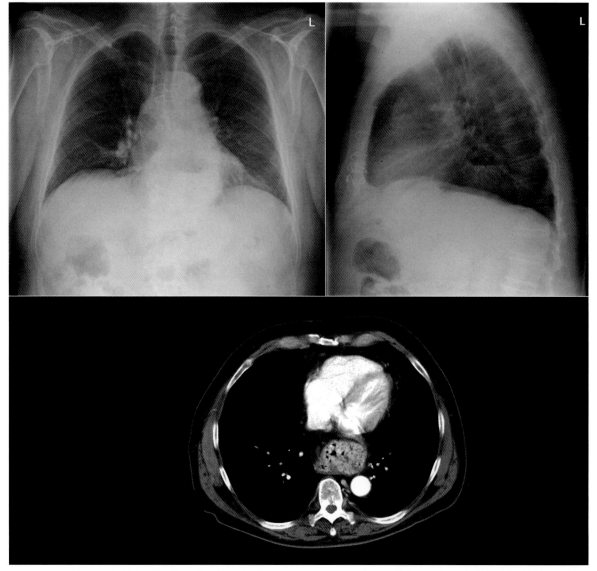

Figure 16-42. The posteroanterior chest radiograph shows an air-fluid level in line with the heart shadow. The lateral chest radiograph clearly establishes that this is retrocardiac and consistent with a hiatal hernia. The contrast-enhanced computed tomography scan reveals a periesophageal hernia in this case.

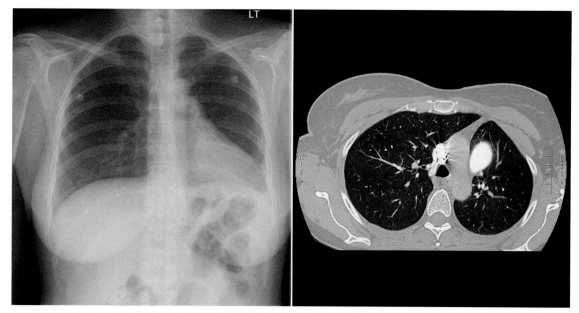

Figure 16-43. Posteroanterior radiograph and corresponding contrast-enhanced computed tomography scan showing absence of the left pericardium. The heart is displaced into the left chest; the right border of the heart shadow is projected over that of the spine. There is a "tongue" of aerated lung tissue interposed between the aortic arch and the main pulmonary artery.

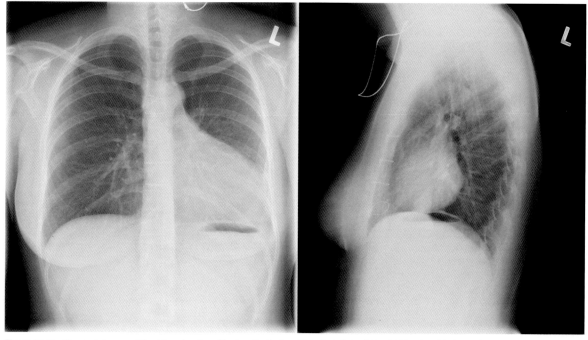

Figure 16-44. Repaired absence of the left pericardium. The heart is displaced into the left chest; the right border of the heart shadow is projected over that of the spine. There is a "tongue" of aerated lung tissue interposed between the aortic arch and the main pulmonary artery.

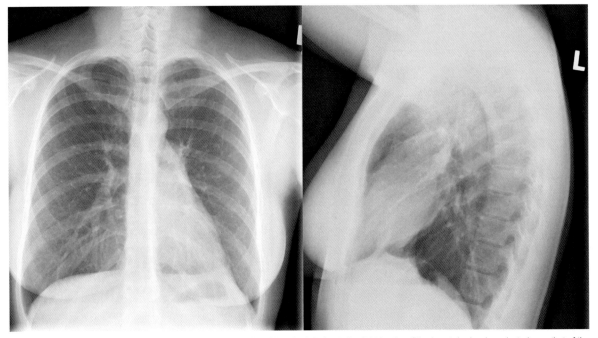

Figure 16-45. Absence of the left pericardium. The heart is displaced into the left chest; the right border of the heart shadow is projected over that of the spine. There is a "tongue" of aerated lung tissue interposed between the aortic arch and the main pulmonary artery and also under heart between the left ventricle and diaphragm.

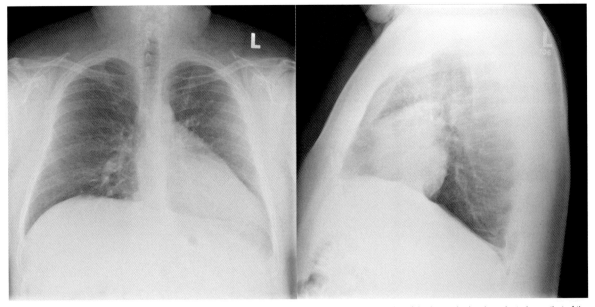

Figure 16-46. Absence of the left pericardium. The heart is displaced into the left chest; the right border of the heart shadow is projected over that of the spine.

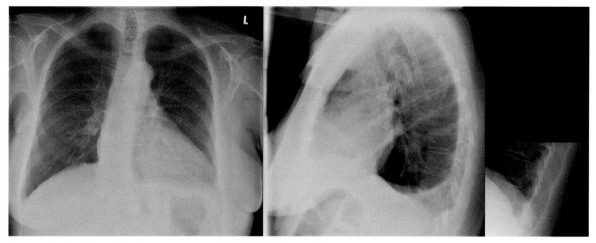

Figure 16-47. Small pleural effusions apparent as a meniscal blunting of the costodiaphragmatic recesses. They are best seen on the lateral radiograph. By way of contrast, on the far right a normal set of posterior costodiaphragmatic recesses is depicted.

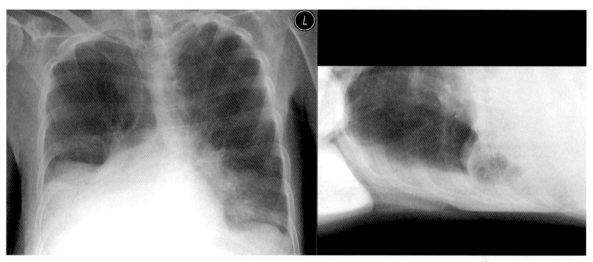

Figure 16-48. The amount of pleural fluid may be more evident on a lateral decubitus radiograph than on a posteroanterior radiograph.

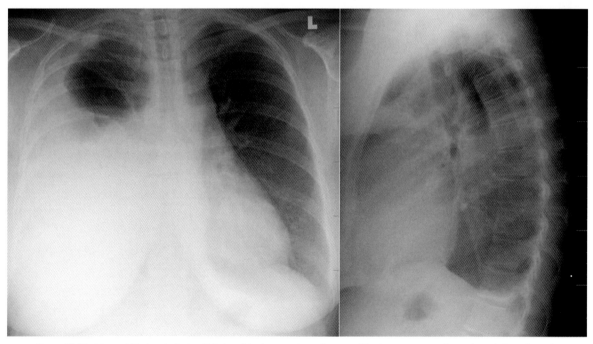

Figure 16-49. A large right pleural effusion. Note how it tracks up and over the apex of the lung, as seen on the posteroanterior radiograph.

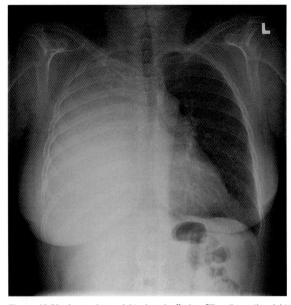

Figure 16-50. A very large right pleural effusion filling the entire right hemithorax.

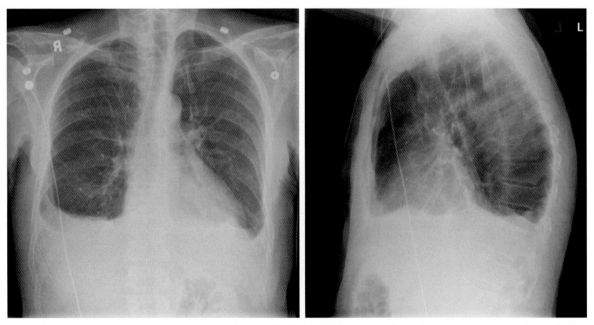

Figure 16-51. Prominent pulmonary venous vasculature, peribronchial "cuffing," and bilateral pleural effusions (right greater than left) consistent with heart failure.

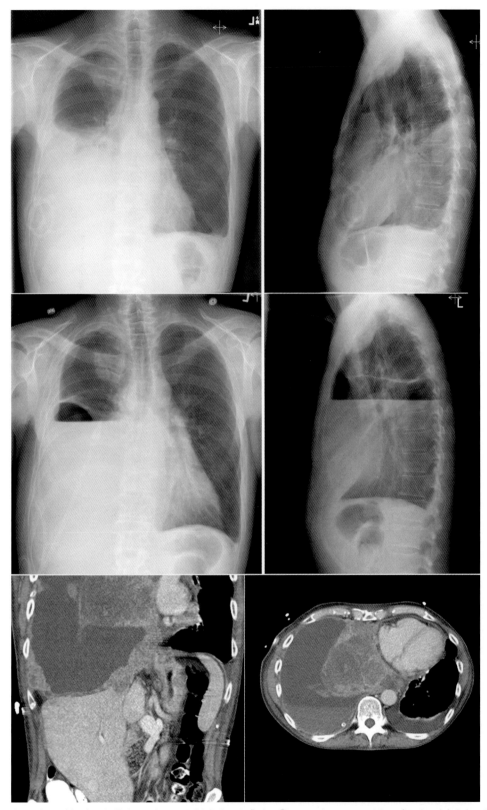

Figure 16-52. A very large right pleural effusion and very small left pleural effusion. The upper images were taken after pleural drain insertion. Note the meniscus. The middle images were taken after air was inadvertently admitted through the pleural drain. Note the air-fluid level. The lower images are contrast-enhanced computed tomography images. In the left lower image, note the depression of the right hemidiaphragm and liver by the weight of the pleural fluid. Note as well the large pleural metastases (non–small cell lung cancer). In the right lower image, note the hematocrit level due to the blood content settling by gravitation.

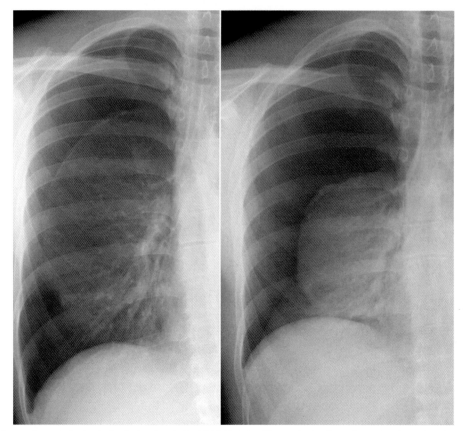

Figure 16-53. Pneumothorax during inspiration *(left)* and expiration *(right)*. Note the difference in size depending on the phase of respiration. Positive pressure ventilation would simulate expiration.

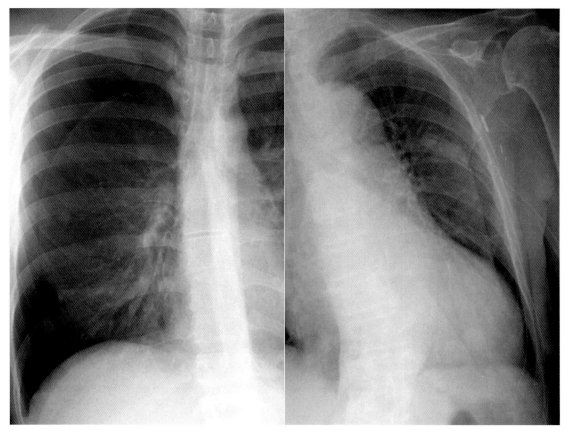

Figure 16-54. Pneumothorax *(left)*. Note the bright line of the visceral pleura and the absence of lung markings lateral to it. Posterior skin fold *(right)*. Note the darkness of the line and the presence of lung markings lateral to it.

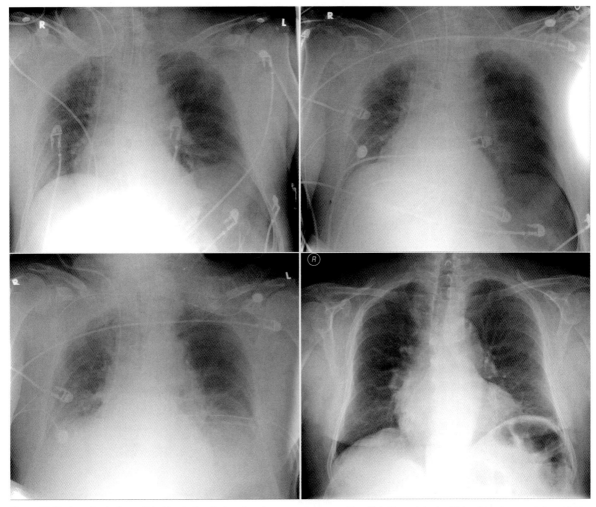

Figure 16-55. A mechanically ventilated (supine) patient post–aortocoronary bypass grafting. Note the endotracheal tube, the pulmonary artery catheter, and epicardial pacing leads. In the left upper image, there is a "deep sulcus sign" of a depressed left hemidiaphragm. Note the absence of lung markings. In the right upper image, there has been progression of the left-sided pneumothorax, which is apparent by the "deep sulcus sign" and also now by the line of the visceral pleura. Note the absence of lung markings lateral to it. In the left lower image, note the chest tube. In the right lower image (postextubation and follow-up), note by way of contrast, the level of the left hemidiaphragm and the lung markings now present in all lung fields.

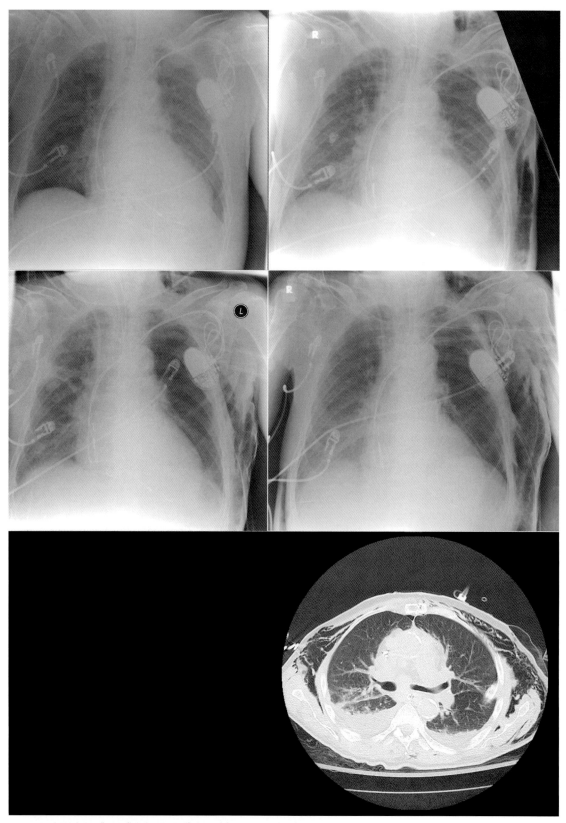

Figure 16-56. A mechanically ventilated patient with heart failure, a dual-chamber pacemaker, a central venous line, and a nasogastric tube. In the left upper image, note the questionable reduction of lung markings at the left lung base and the deeper sulcus. In the right upper image, note the deep sulcus sign and the subcutaneous emphysema. In the middle images (post–chest tube insertion), note the higher diaphragm and normalization of the sulcus. In the lower image (computed tomography scan, also post–chest tube insertion) there is elimination of the pneumothorax but considerable residual subcutaneous emphysema.

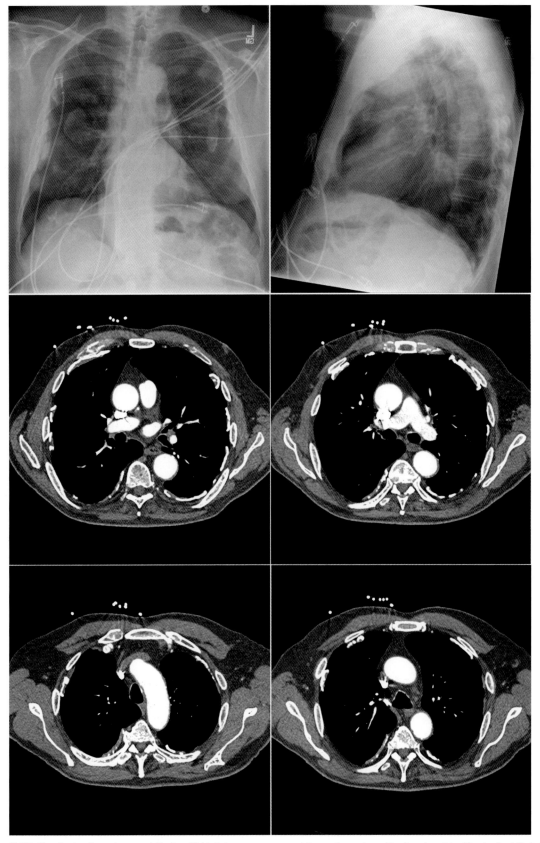

Figure 16-57. The chest radiographs are notable for a highly tortuous or aneurysmal descending aorta and for discrete potato chip–sized calcified pleural plaques that are seen both en-face and tangentially. The contrast-enhanced computed tomography scans reveal the numerous calcified pleural plaques from previous asbestos exposure.

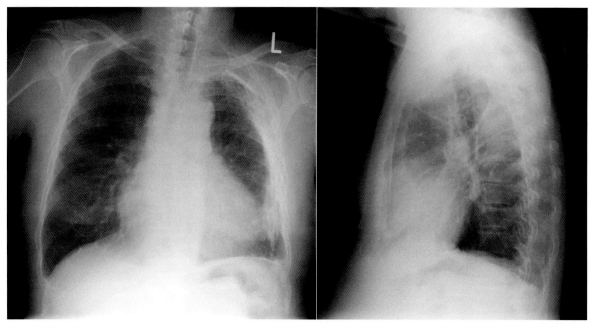

Figure 16-58. Left pleural disease from prior tuberculosis. There are thick pleural plaques in the left chest cavity, with calcification. The effect is to reduce left lung volume.

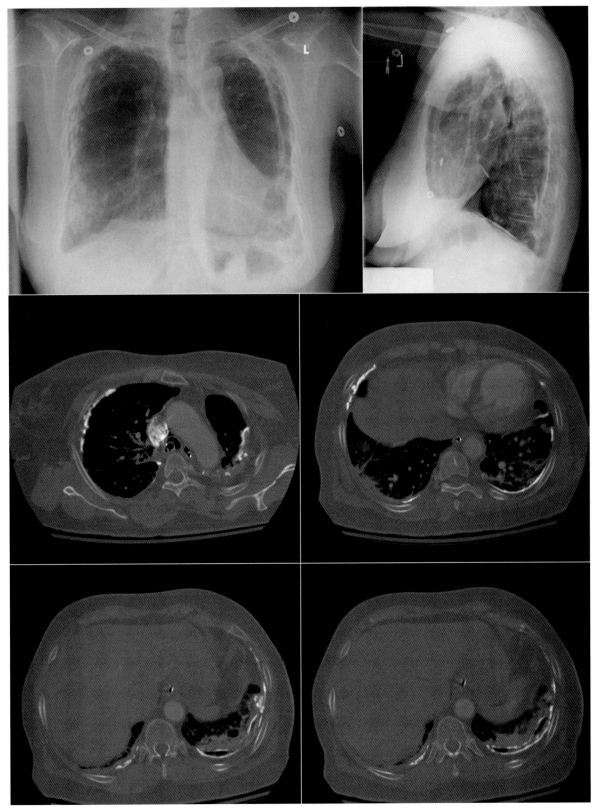

Figure 16-59. Bilateral fibrothorases. Note the thickened pleural plaques, with calcification is seen both on the posteroanterior and lateral chest radiographs and also on the computed tomography images. The left fibrothorax, with its thicker peel, is associated with lesser lung volume.

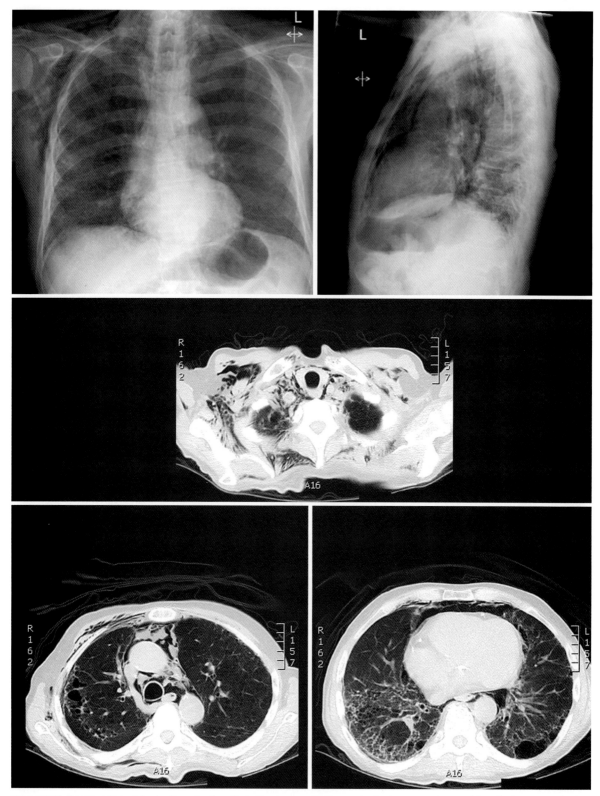

Figure 16-60. Frontal and lateral chest radiographs of a patient with pneumomediastinum and subcutaneous emphysema. The subcutaneous emphysema is predominantly right-sided. The pneumomediastinum on the lateral radiograph beautifully outlines the heart and aorta. Axial computed tomography images confirm the right-sided subcutaneous emphysema and the pneumomediastinum around and thereby outlining the aorta and the heart itself.

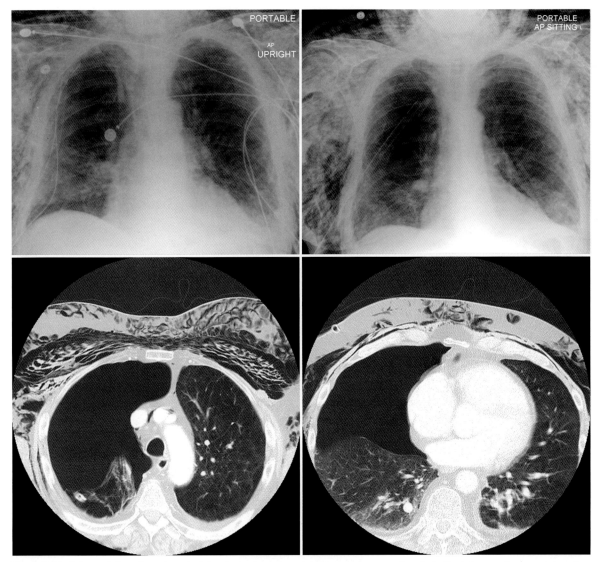

Figure 16-61. Anteroposterior radiographs and axial contrast-enhanced computed tomography scans of a patient with a left pneumothorax, massive subcutaneous emphysema, and pneumomediastinum, despite multiple left chest tubes.

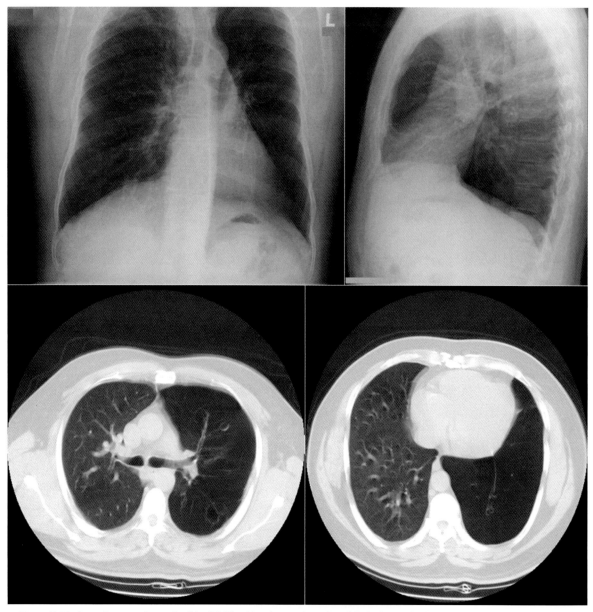

Figure 16-62. Swyer-James syndrome of unilateral (left lung) lung lucency due to hyperinflation imparted by bronchiolitis obliterans. Note the bullae.

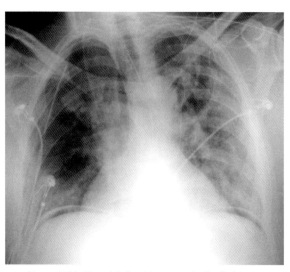

Figure 16-63. Free air in the abdomen, under the diaphragm.

17 Radiographic Findings by Diagnosis: Coronary Artery Disease—Complications of Infarction

Key Points

- Chest radiography in all subsets of patients with myocardial infarction increases the sensitivity and specificity of determination of left-sided heart failure.
- A false aneurysm of the anterior, apical, or lateral wall may be apparent by a bulging contour of the left ventricular silhouette.
- Postinfarction ruptures of papillary muscle result in severe left-sided heart failure.
- Ventricular septal ruptures result in pulmonary vascular plethora.

LEFT VENTRICULAR ANEURYSM

Signs include the following:
- Bulge of the left ventricular contour
- Calcification of the aneurysm (Graphic 17-1; Figs. 17-1 and 17-2)

An aneurysm of the left ventricle may occur on any wall that has experienced a transmural infarction, but radiographically, the ones most commonly seen are on the anterolateral wall; they appear as a "bump" on the left heart border, usually well below the left atrial appendage area. The left ventricle is enlarged; the left atrium commonly is as well, and overall cardiomegaly is also common. Signs of associated left heart failure may be present. Calcification is often, but not always, seen in the area of the aneurysm and may represent either calcification of the aneurysm itself or of an organized thrombus within it. Overpenetration of the chest radiograph may make the calcification more apparent. A calcified aneurysm of the anteroseptum may rarely be seen on an overexposed posteroanterior view. The paradoxical nature of the motion of the aneurysm is best appreciated on fluoroscopy.

PAPILLARY MUSCLE RUPTURE

Papillary muscle rupture (Figs. 17-3 and 17-4) is invariably associated with severe mitral insufficiency and much greater left-sided heart failure than is seen with ventricular septal rupture.

VENTRICULAR SEPTAL RUPTURE

Ventricular septal rupture (Figs. 17-5 to 17-8) typically results in a greater than or equal to doubling of pulmonary blood flow versus systemic blood flow. There is a generalized increase of the pulmonary vascularity.

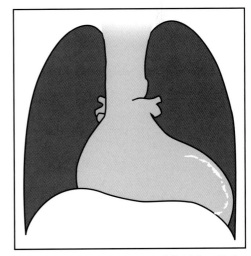

Graphic 17-1. Posteroanterior projection: calcified left ventricular aneurysm. Note a thin and well-defined line of calcification toward the left ventricular apex/free wall, as well as cardiomegaly.

257

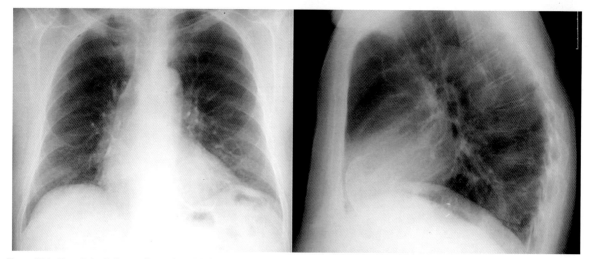

Figure 17-1. There is borderline cardiomegaly and definite calcification of a left ventricular aneurysm. There is increased pulmonary venous vascular prominence due to heart failure associated with the left ventricular aneurysm and systolic dysfunction.

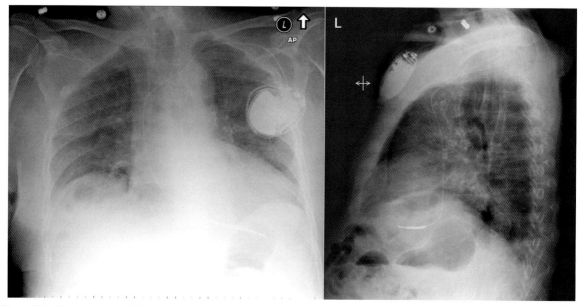

Figure 17-2. Cardiomegaly, heart failure, and an implantable cardioverter defibrillator lead. The left heart border is elongated and elevated in this patient with an anteroapical aneurysm.

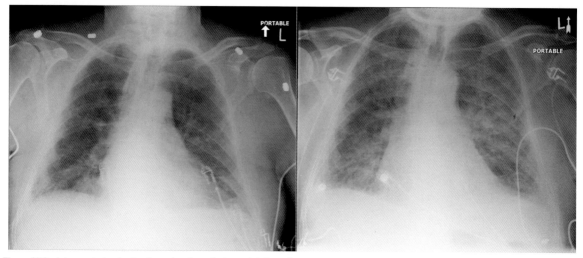

Figure 17-3. Anteroposterior chest radiographs of a patient post–inferior wall myocardial infarction. Initially, the patient was in right-sided heart failure due to an associated right ventricular infarct (admission chest radiograph on the left). Two days later, the patient went into abrupt and overwhelming pulmonary edema due to a confirmed postremedial papillary muscle rupture (radiograph on the right).

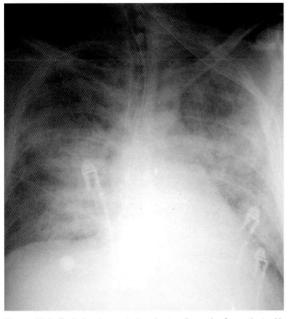

Figure 17-4. Typical anteroposterior chest radiograph of a patient with papillary muscle rupture, fulminant mitral regurgitation, and left-sided heart failure.

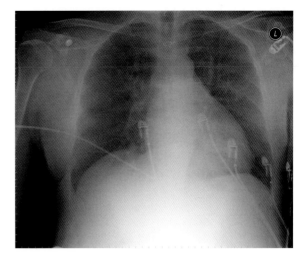

Figure 17-5. Post-infarction septal rupture. Mild cardiomegaly and generalized increase in pulmonary vasculature.

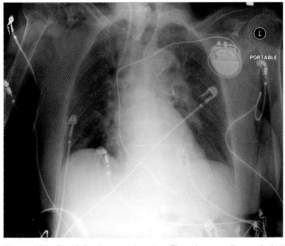

Figure 17-6. Post-infarction septal rupture. There is no cardiomegaly, but there is left-sided heart failure and a generalized increase in pulmonary vascularity. An intra-aortic balloon tip in the descending aorta is denoted by the radiopaque marker tip.

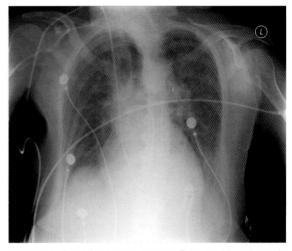

Figure 17-7. Post-infarction septal rupture. There is mild cardiomegaly, left-sided heart failure, and a generalized increase in pulmonary vascularity. An intra-aortic balloon tip in the descending aorta is denoted by the radiopaque marker tip.

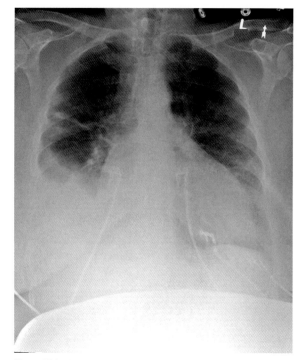

Figure 17-8. Cardiomegaly with lengthening and straightening of the left heart border due to left-sided chamber enlargement, post–late presentation anterior infarction, and ventricular septal rupture. The hilar borders are indistinct consistent with interstitial pulmonary edema, and the lung vessels are prominent. There is a moderate-sized right pleural effusion.

Radiographic Findings by Diagnosis: Congenital Heart Disease—Shunts and Closure Devices

Key Points

■ The chest radiograph is predominantly useful to detect/characterize the pulmonary vascularity as influenced by congenital shunt lesions, such as pulmonary vascular shunt plethora of larger shunts and signs of pulmonary hypertension complicating large shunts.

■ Small shunt lesions are not evident on chest radiography, other than pulmonary arteriovenous malformations.

■ A minority of shunt lesions are directly suggested by chest radiography, such as the vertical vein of left-sided anomalous pulmonary venous return, the "scimitar sign" of the scimitar variant of right-sided anomalous pulmonary venous return, and ductal calcification.

Left-to-right shunts initially result in volume overload of the chambers carrying the shunt volume, causing enlargement of the volume-overloaded chambers and an increase in pulmonary blood flow. If the amount of pulmonary blood flow is sufficiently high, obliterative disease of the pulmonary arterioles develops ("pulmonary vascular disease"), resulting in pulmonary hypertension. The chest radiographic appearance of pulmonary hypertension is one of centralization of pulmonary flow and accelerating enlargement of the right-sided chambers.

The size of a shunt is represented best by the shunt ratio (volume of blood through the pulmonary circuit vs. the systemic circuit, such as 2:1, 3:1, 4:1) and by the degree of elevation of the pulmonary pressures.

PATENT FORAMEN OVALE

A patent foramen ovale is present in 25% to 30% of the adult population (Figs. 18-1 to 18-4). Any magnitude of shunting across it in normal circumstances is undetectable radiographically. Percutaneous patent foramen ovale closure devices are fairly commonly inserted and are radiographically evident.

ATRIAL SEPTAL DEFECT

See Figures 18-5 to 18-31. Possible findings are discussed in the following sections.

Cardiac Findings on Chest Radiography
(Graphic 18-1)
❑ An enlarged right atrium, right ventricle, and left atrium
❑ Enlargement of the left atrium, which is seen with primum atrial septal defects that have significant mitral insufficiency from an associated cleft mitral valve
❑ Enlarged cardiopericardial silhouette (CPS) in 80% of secundum atrial septal defects

Vascular Findings on Chest Radiography
❑ Enlarged pulmonary arteries and engorgement of vasculature (enlarged veins)
❑ Centralization of flow and peripheral pruning (late findings)
❑ Tendency for primum atrial septal defect hearts to be larger than secundum atrial septal defect hearts (with primum atrial septal defects, there is a higher incidence of significant mitral and tricuspid insufficiency)
❑ Atrial versus ventricular septal defects: by adulthood, the peripheral vascular pattern is almost always pruned somewhat in patients with ventricular septal defects, but it may not be in patients with atrial septal defects.
❑ Chest radiographs of atrial septal defects may look very similar to those of mitral stenosis, except the lung vasculature is more engorged in the case of the atrial septal defect. However, with the development of pulmonary hypertension, the two conditions look very similar radiographically.

VENTRICULAR SEPTAL DEFECT

See Figures 18-32 to 18-37. Possible findings are discussed in the following sections.

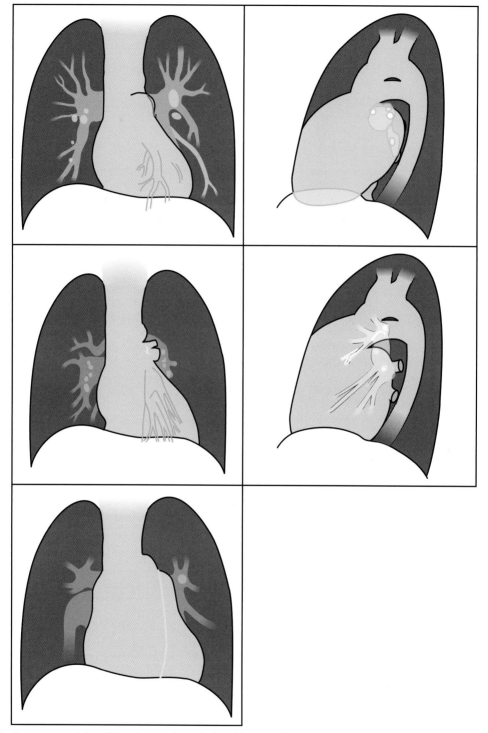

Graphic 18-1. Graphic representations of shunt lesions and complications. *Upper graphics:* Posteroanterior and lateral projections of an atrial septal defect. On the posteroanterior projection, note the prominence of the right atrial contour of the left atrial appendage and of the central peripheral pulmonary arteries. On the lateral projection, note the enlargement of the left atrium and right ventricle, as well as the pulmonary arteries. The left ventricle and aorta are normal size. *Middle graphics:* Posteroanterior and lateral projections of patent ductus arteriosus. On the frontal projection, note the enlargement of the pulmonary arteries, the calcified ductus, and cardiomegaly. On the lateral projection, note the enlargement of the right heart and left ventricle, as well as of the pulmonary vasculature. *Lower graphic:* Posteroanterior chest radiograph of Eisenmenger syndrome. Note the marked dilation of the central pulmonary arteries with distal pruning. Note also cardiomegaly due to predominantly right heart enlargement.

Cardiac Findings on Chest Radiography
❑ No cardiomegaly with small ventricular septal defects
❑ Left atrial, left ventricular, and right ventricular enlargement with larger defects and shunts

Vascular Findings on Chest Radiography
❑ Pulmonary artery enlargement
❑ Centralization and peripheral pruning (see Graphic 18-1) (late findings)
❑ Right-sided chamber enlargement
❑ Pulmonary artery calcification (very late)

PATENT DUCTUS ARTERIOSUS

See Figures 18-38 to 18-43. Possible findings are discussed in the following sections.

Cardiac Findings on Chest Radiography
(see Graphic 18-1)
There is left atrial and ventricular enlargement with or without right ventricular enlargement if there is pulmonary hypertension.

Vascular Findings on Chest Radiography
❑ Large pulmonary artery
❑ Large ascending aorta and aortic arch
❑ Pulmonary vascular engorgement until there is pulmonary hypertension
❑ Centralization of pulmonary blood flow (later sign)
❑ Overt calcification of a patent ductus arteriosus is uncommon, but the distinct pattern and location of a calcified patent ductus arteriosus is pathognomonic for its presence. Calcification of ductus

arteriosus usually means patency of the structure (aortopulmonary communication).
❑ Possibly evident ductal diverticulum that fills in the aorticopulmonary window or causes an abnormal bulging outward of the window

PARTIAL ANOMALOUS PULMONARY VENOUS RETURN (Figs. 18-44 and 18-45)

Anomalous return of pulmonary veins may involve the right lung, the left lung, or both. Partial anomalous return of the right-sided pulmonary veins usually returns to the superior vena cava or right atrium, and partial anomalous return of the left pulmonary veins usually enters the innominate vein by a "vertical" vein.
Chest radiographic findings are as follows:
❑ Partial anomalous return of the right lung: an absence of the shadow of the right upper lobe pulmonary vein, with medial displacement of the superior vena cava and prominent confluence of veins at the drainage site (superior vena cava and right atrium)
❑ Partial anomalous venous return of the left lung: an oblique linear shadow rising to the innominate vein

SCIMITAR SYNDROME

Scimitar syndrome (pulmonary venolobar syndrome) is a congenital disorder of partial or total anomalous venous return from the right lung (Figs. 18-46 to 18-54). The radiographic appearance of the anomalous return to the inferior vena cava or other infradiaphragmatic vein receiving pulmonary venous discharge from the right lung generates the analogy of the broad and curved scimitar sword.

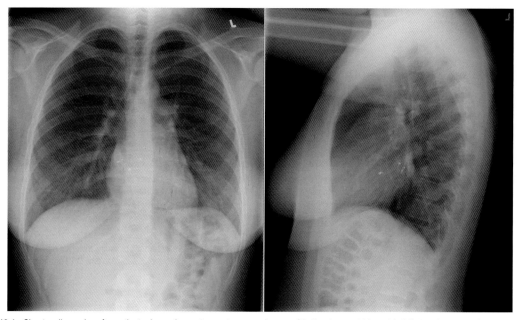

Figure 18-1. Chest radiographs of a patient who underwent percutaneous closure of both a large atrial septal defect and a patent foramen ovale with Amplatzer devices.

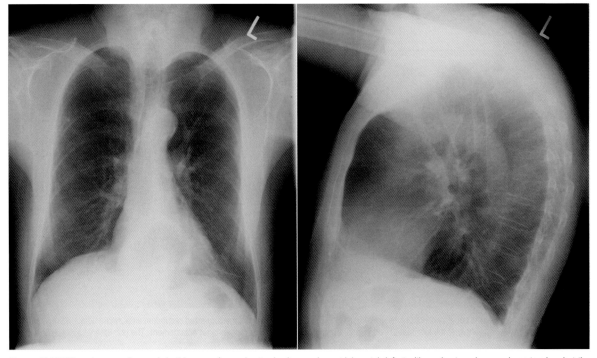

Figure 18-13. There is no cardiomegaly in this case of a moderate-sized secundum atrial septal defect with moderate pulmonary hypertension, but the lungs appear enlarged, and there has been obstructive lung disease to render plausible lung hyperinflation. The left upper heart border is straightened from left atrial (appendage) enlargement, and there is increased apposition of the right ventricle to the sternum. The central pulmonary arteries are enlarged and the peripheral vasculature is accentuated.

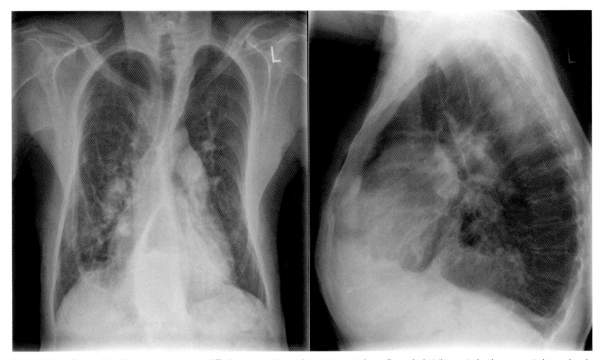

Figure 18-14. The cardiac silhouette contours are difficult to recognize on the posteroanterior radiograph, but the central pulmonary arteries and main pulmonary arteries are considerably dilated. The lateral chest radiograph is suggestive of right ventricular dilation. There is a large atrial septal defect in this patient, with extensive thoracic skeletal deformities and pulmonary disease associated with Marfan syndrome.

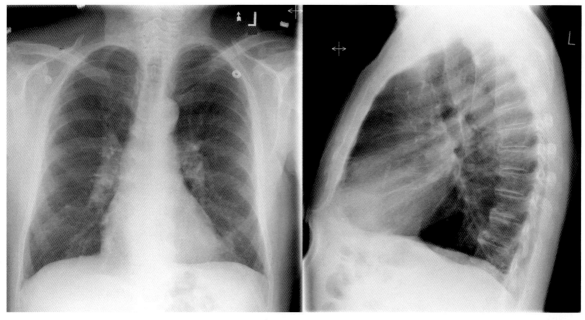

Figure 18-15. The frontal radiograph does not give the impression of cardiomegaly, but the lateral radiograph does in this patient with an atrial septal defect with moderate pulmonary hypertension. The left atrium in particular is dilated. The main and central pulmonary arteries are dilated, but there is only mild extenuation of the pulmonary vasculature.

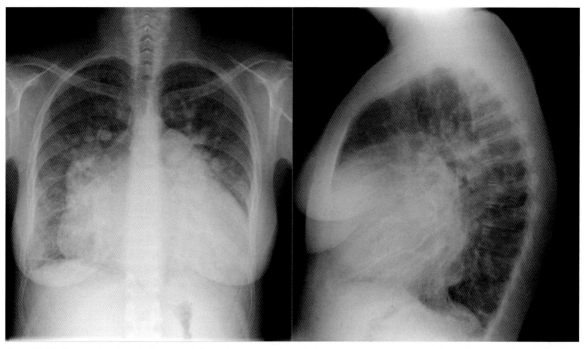

Figure 18-16. Prominently enlarged pulmonary arteries and veins, as well as a dilated main pulmonary artery from advanced pulmonary hypertension from a large secundum atrial septal defect. In addition, there is severe cardiomegaly, mainly from right and left atrial and right ventricular chamber enlargement.

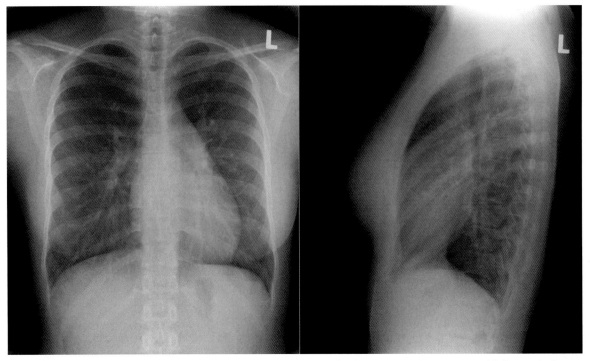

Figure 18-17. Mild cardiomegaly, straightening of the left upper heart border due to left atrial appendage enlargement, and mildly increased pulmonary vascularity due to a medium-sized secundum atrial septal defect.

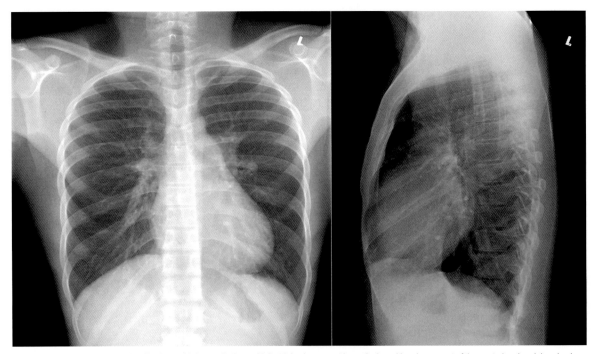

Figure 18-18. Mild cardiomegaly with signs of right ventricular and left atrial enlargement in particular, with enlargement of the central and peripheral pulmonary arteries, as well as veins, due to a sinus venosus atrial septal defect and right-sided anomalous pulmonary venous return.

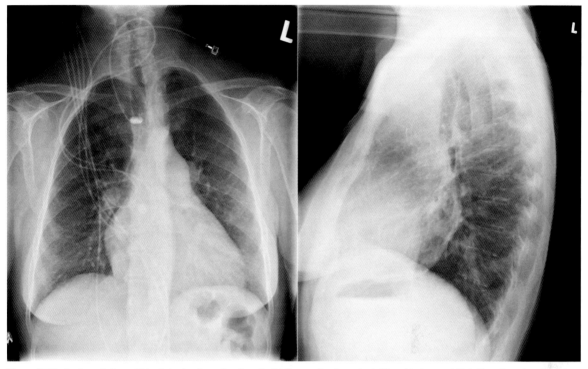

Figure 18-19. Posteroanterior and lateral chest radiographs of a patient with a previously repaired atrioventricular canal. Note the enlarged central pulmonary arteries, the right ventricular and right atrial prominence, and the left atrial and left ventricular enlargement.

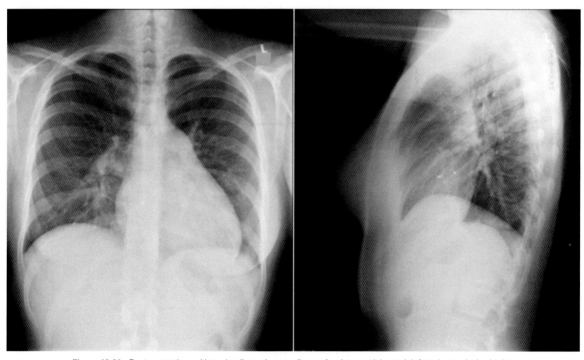

Figure 18-20. Posteroanterior and lateral radiographs revealing an Amplatzer atrial septal defect closure device in situ.

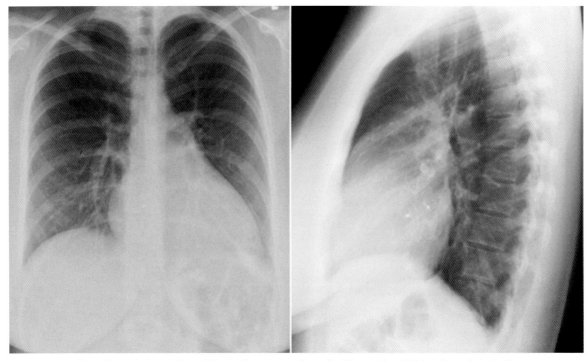

Figure 18-21. Posteroanterior and lateral radiographs revealing an Amplatzer atrial septal defect closure device in situ.

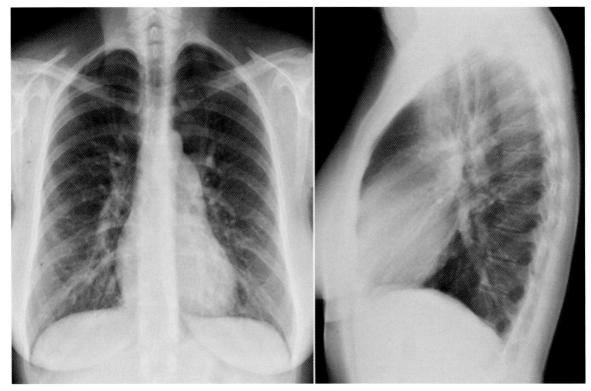

Figure 18-22. Posteroanterior and lateral chest radiographs in a patient with a large secundum atrial septal defect.

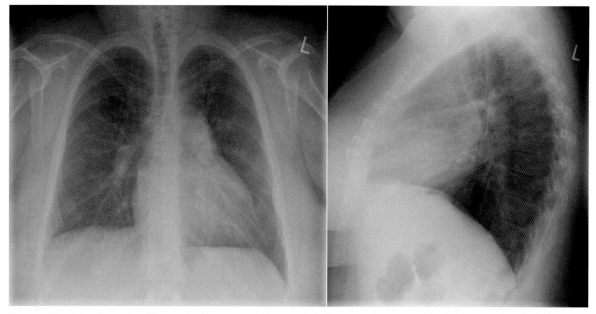

Figure 18-23. Mild cardiomegaly and increased pulmonary vascularity in a patient with an Amplatzer atrial septal defect closure device. The device is more readily seen on the lateral radiograph, particularly in this case; it is lost among the sternal wires on the frontal radiograph.

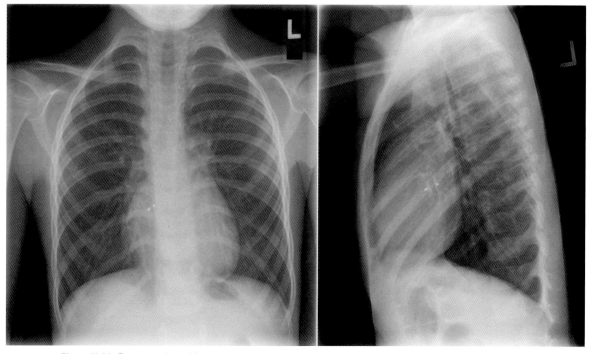

Figure 18-24. Posteroanterior and lateral chest radiographs of a patient with an Amplatzer atrial septal defect closure device.

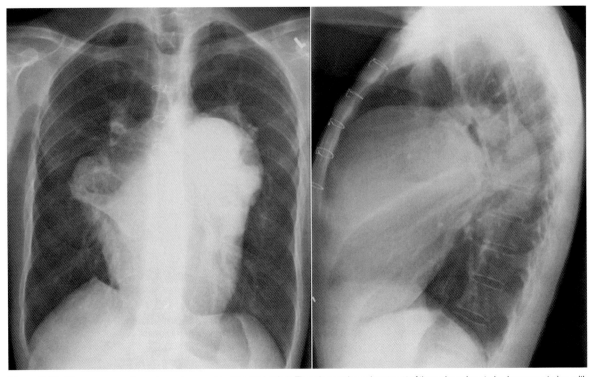

Figure 18-25. Eisenmenger syndrome from a large ventricular septal defect. There is massive enlargement of the main and central pulmonary arteries, with severe pruning. The right ventricle is enlarged as well.

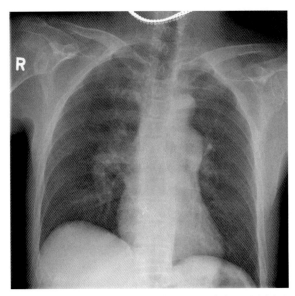

Figure 18-26. Eisenmenger syndrome due to a ventricular septal defect. Note the severely enlarged main and central pulmonary arteries, with peripheral vascular pruning–centralization of flow.

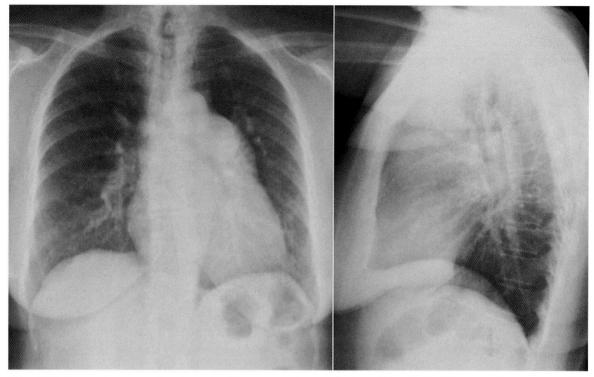

Figure 18-27. Severe pulmonary artery hypertension/pre–Eisenmenger syndrome due to a large atrial septal defect. There is prominent enlargement of the main and central pulmonary arteries. The pulmonary vascularity is still increased.

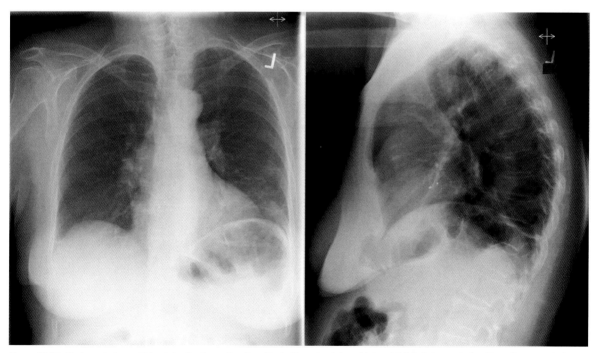

Figure 18-28. Posteroanterior and lateral chest radiographs of a patient with an Amplatzer atrial septal defect closure device. The pulmonary arteries are prominently enlarged due to moderately severe pulmonary hypertension from pulmonary vascular disease.

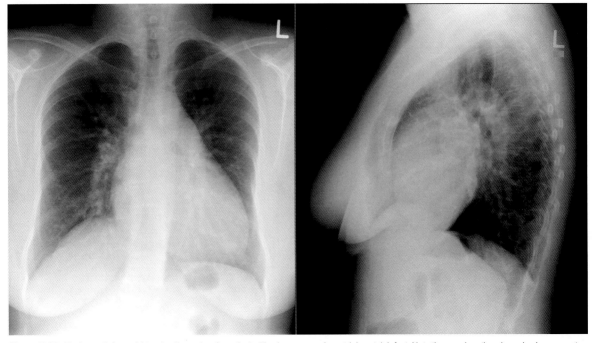

Figure 18-29. Posteroanterior and lateral radiographs of a patient with a large secundum atrial septal defect. Note the prominently enlarged pulmonary arteries and generalized (pulmonary arterial and venous) prominence. Note the right atrial border prominence on the frontal radiograph, as well as the upper left heart border straightening due to left atrial appendage enlargement. On the lateral radiograph, note the right ventricular, left atrial enlargement, and central pulmonary artery enlargement.

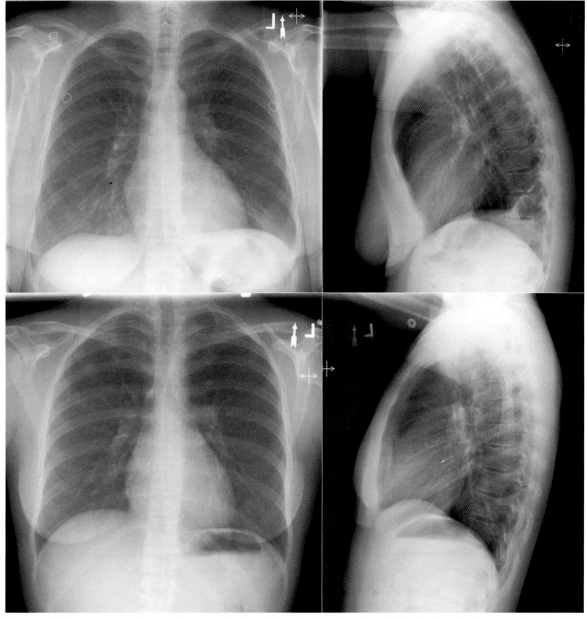

Figure 18-30. Posteroanterior and lateral radiographs, before (*upper images*) and after (*lower images*), of an Amplatzer device closure of a medium-sized secundum atrial septal defect.

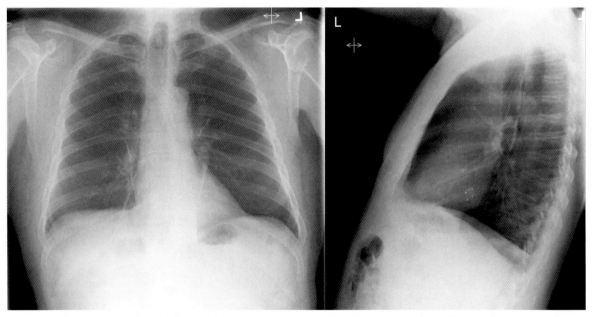

Figure 18-31. Posteroanterior and lateral radiographs after Amplatzer device closure of a medium-sized secundum atrial septal defect and a patent foramen ovale.

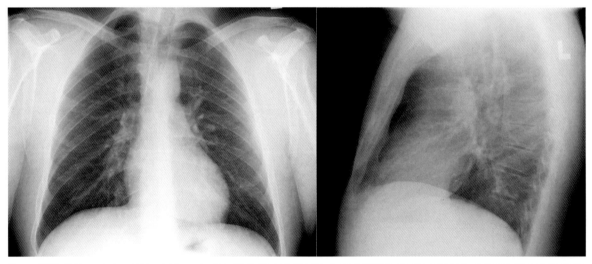

Figure 18-32. Posteroanterior and lateral radiographs of a patient with a small ventricular septal defect without pulmonary hypertension. There is no cardiomegaly, but the cardiac contours are abnormal. There is straightening of the left heart border and increased right ventricular apposition to the sternum. There is a generalized increase in the pulmonary vasculature.

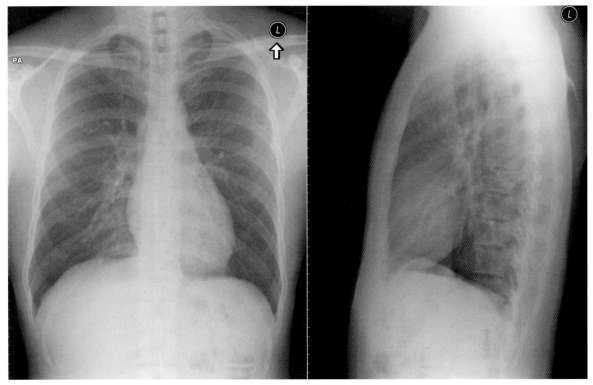

Figure 18-33. Posteroanterior and lateral radiographs of a patient with a small ventricular septal defect without pulmonary hypertension. There is no cardiomegaly. The only signs of specific chamber enlargement are the straightening of the left heart border and questionable increased right ventricular apposition to the sternum. There is a generalized increase in the pulmonary vasculature and enlargement of the central pulmonary artery.

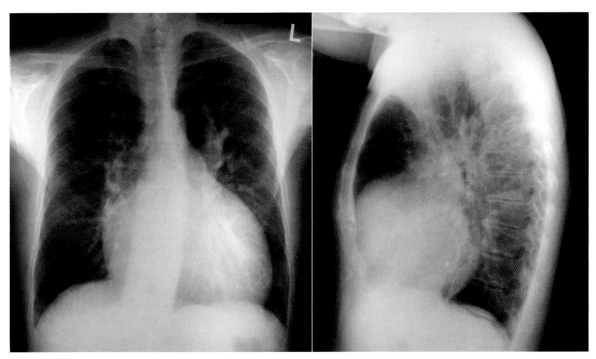

Figure 18-34. Posteroanterior and lateral radiographs of a patient with a large ventricular septal defect with pulmonary hypertension. There is cardiomegaly with signs of multichamber enlargement. The main pulmonary artery and central pulmonary arteries are enlarged. The peripheral pulmonary vessels are markedly diminished, consistent with advancing pulmonary vascular disease.

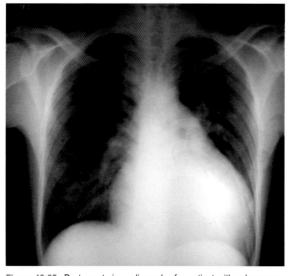

Figure 18-35. Posteroanterior radiograph of a patient with a large ventricular septal defect with pulmonary hypertension. There is cardiomegaly with signs of multichamber enlargement. The main pulmonary artery and central pulmonary arteries are enlarged. The peripheral pulmonary vessels are markedly diminished.

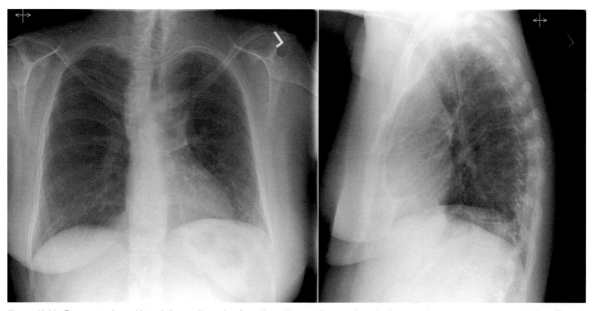

Figure 18-36. Posteroanterior and lateral chest radiographs of a patient with a small- to medium-sized perimembranous ventricular septal defect. There is no cardiomegaly, but there is generalized prominence of the pulmonary vasculature. The aortic arch is right-sided. Notice the "vertical vein" draining into the innominate vein.

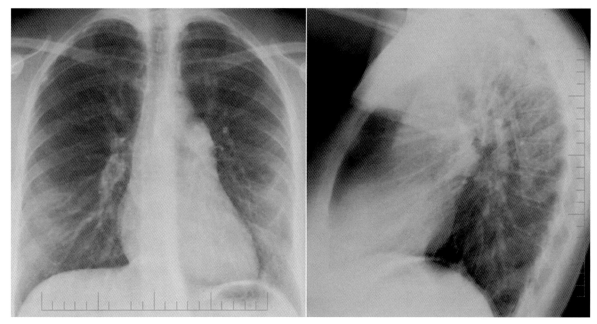

Figure 18-37. Eisenmenger syndrome due to a large ventricular septal defect. There is prominent enlargement of the main and central pulmonary arteries. The pulmonary vascularity is still increased.

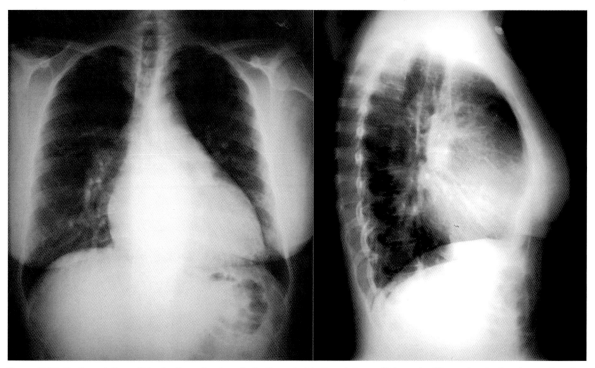

Figure 18-38. Posteroanterior and lateral radiographs of a patient with a patent ductus arteriosus with large shunt flow and moderate pulmonary hypertension. There is gross cardiomegaly, with straightening of the left heart border consistent with left atrial (appendage) enlargement, elongation of the left heart border, posterior displacement of the left ventricular (LV) silhouette consistent with LV enlargement, and enlargement of the central pulmonary arteries. The pulmonary vasculature is prominent. No calcification of the ductus is apparent.

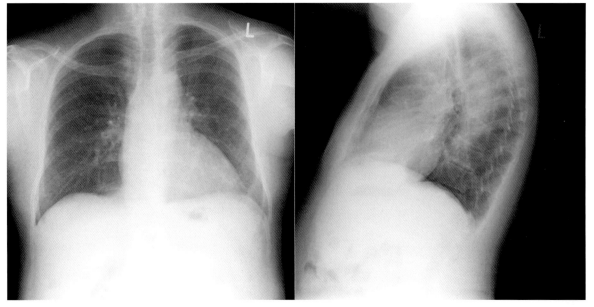

Figure 18-39. Posteroanterior and lateral radiographs of a patient with a patent ductus arteriosus with moderate shunt flow. There is no definite cardiomegaly, but the cardiac silhouettes are abnormal. The posterior border of the left ventricle is posteriorly displaced, and there is increased apposition to the sternum. The pulmonary vascularity is accentuated. No calcification of the ductus is apparent.

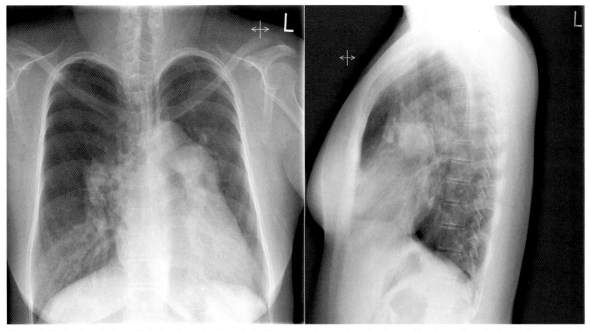

Figure 18-40. Posteroanterior and lateral radiographs of a patient with severe pulmonary hypertension resulting from a large ductus arteriosus. There is cardiomegaly with striking dilation of the main and central pulmonary arteries. The peripheral pulmonary vessels are diminished.

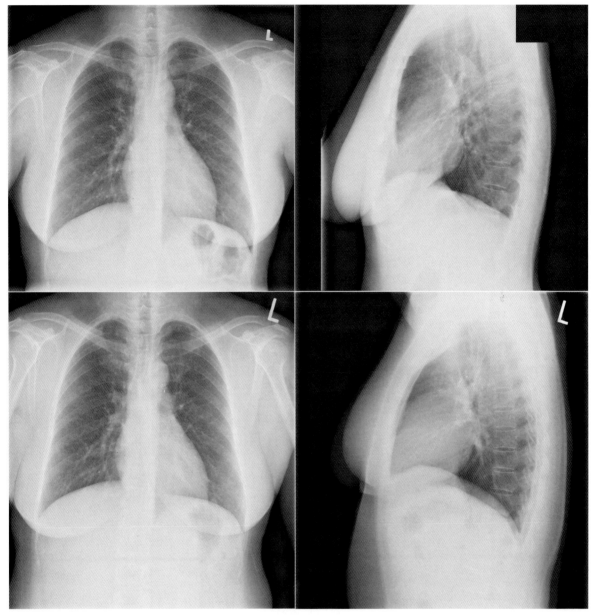

Figure 18-41. The upper images are chest radiographs before Amplatzer device closure of a patent ductus arteriosus, and the lower images are chest radiographs immediately after closure. Note the signs of enlargement of the left atrium and left ventricle. The change of the radiographic appearance of the pulmonary vasculature following device closure is underwhelming.

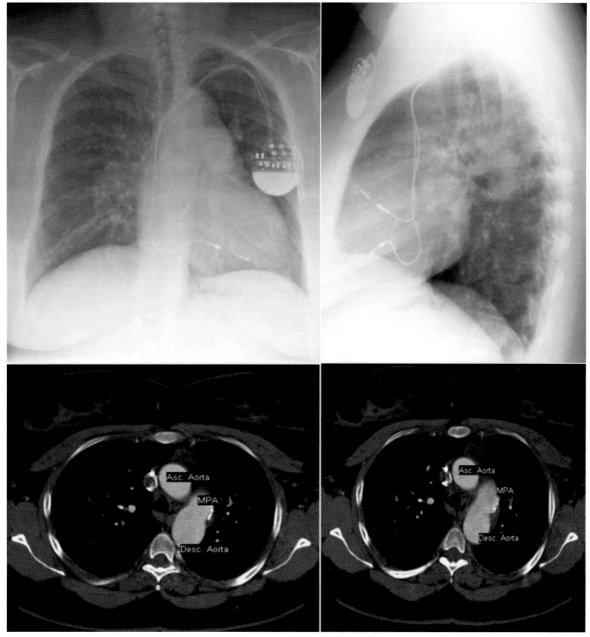

Figure 18-42. Eisenmenger syndrome due to a large patent ductus arteriosus (PDA). The calcification of the PDA is far more apparent on computed tomography scans than it is on radiographic plain films.

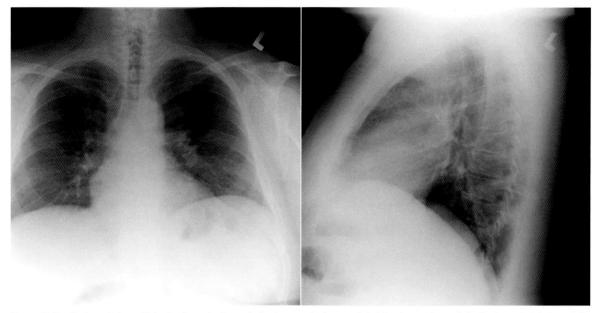

Figure 18-43. Posteroanterior and lateral radiographs demonstrating increased pulmonary (arterial and venous) vascularity due to a patent ductus arteriosus (PDA). The PDA is not overtly calcified and is not apparent radiographically.

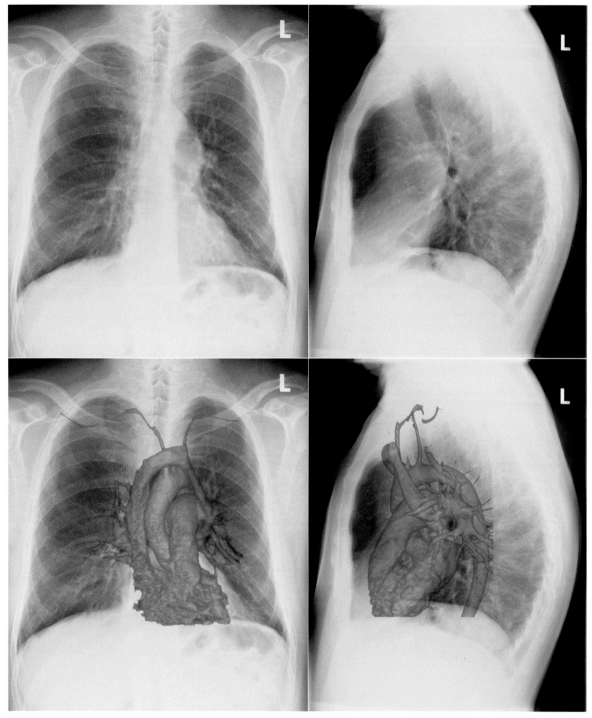

Figure 18-44. Chest radiographs (*upper images*) of a patient with partial left anomalous venous return (left vertical vein) with superimposed three-dimensional volume-rendered contrast-enhanced computed tomography images (*lower images*).

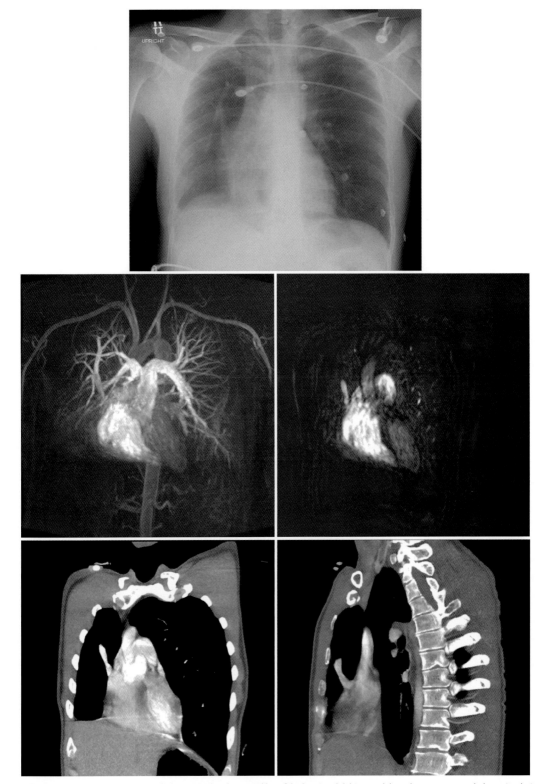

Figure 18-45. Posteroanterior chest radiograph demonstrating dextroposition of the heart and right upper lobe pulmonary venous drainage to what appears to be the right atrium (*upper image*); magnetic resonance angiography revealing the anomalous right upper lobe pulmonary vein draining toward the right atrium (*left middle image*); magnetic resonance angiography with a slice at a different level showing/confirming the entry of the anomalous right upper lobe pulmonary vein to the right atrium (*right middle image*); and frontal and sagittal projections of a contrast-enhanced computed tomography scan showing the entry of the anomalous right upper lobe pulmonary vein to right atrium (*lower images*).

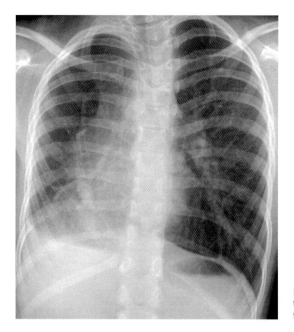

Figure 18-46. There is rotation of the radiograph. On the right side of the heart, there is the "scimitar" appearance of anomalous right pulmonary venous return to the inferior vena cava.

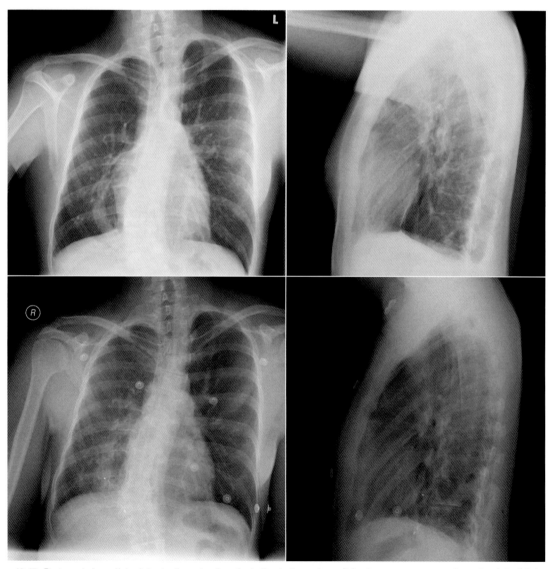

Figure 18-47. Posteroanterior and lateral chest radiographs of a patient with scimitar syndrome (left pulmonary venous anomalous return to the inferior vena cava), with before (upper images) and after (lower images) of Amplatzer device closure(s) of the anomalous pulmonary vein.

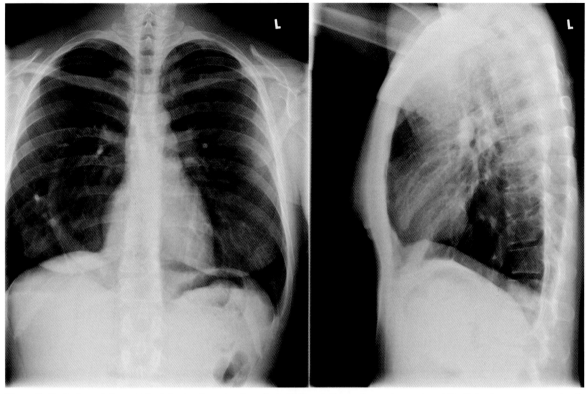

Figure 18-48. Posteroanterior and lateral chest radiographs of a patient with the scimitar syndrome of anomalous right-sided pulmonary venous return to the inferior vena cava.

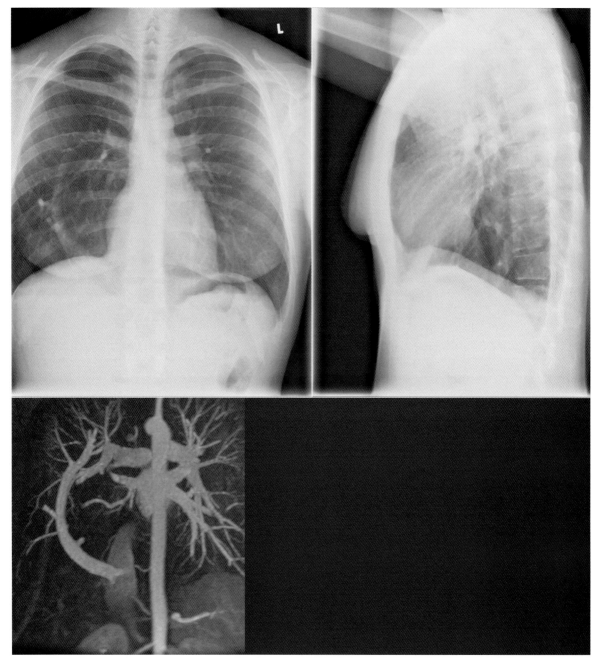

Figure 18-49. Posteroanterior and lateral chest radiographs and magnetic resonance angiogram demonstrating anomalous venous return of the right lung to the inferior vena cava, the scimitar syndrome. Note the off-take of the bridging veins seen on the magnetic resonance angiogram.

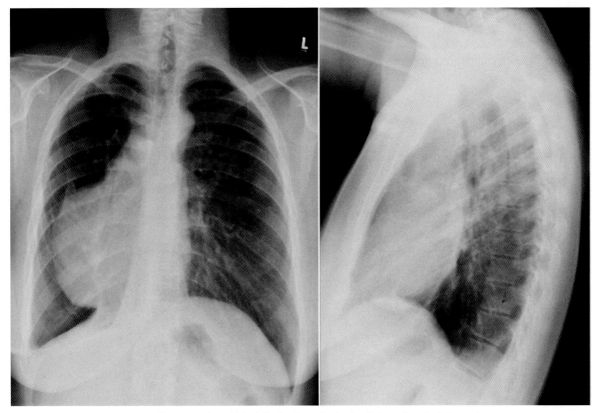

Figure 18-50. Posteroanterior and lateral chest radiographs showing dextrocardia and scimitar syndrome.

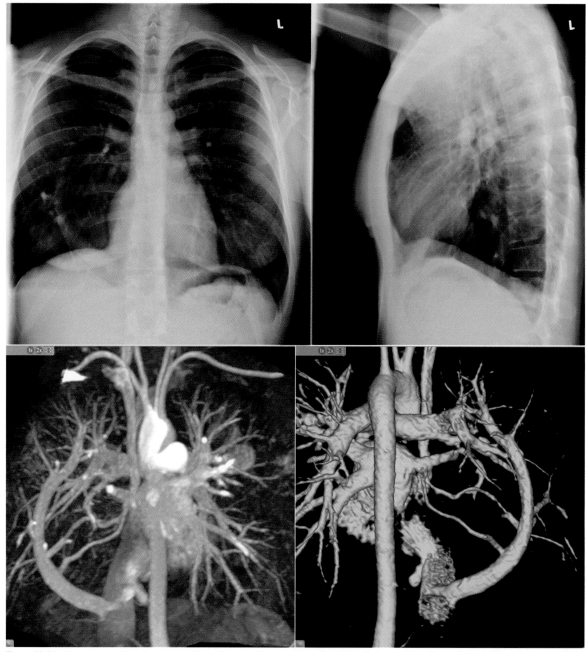

Figure 18-51. *Upper images:* Posterioanterior and lateral chest radiographs of a patient with scimitar syndrome. *Lower images:* MR contrast angiography demonstration of the anomalous pulmonary venous return to the inferior vena cava and the bridging veins to the left atrium.

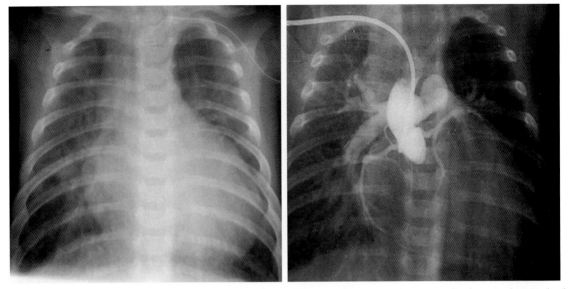

Figure 18-52. Chest radiograph of an infant with an aortopulmonary window (*left*) and contrast aortography demonstrating the aortopulmonary shunting (*right*).

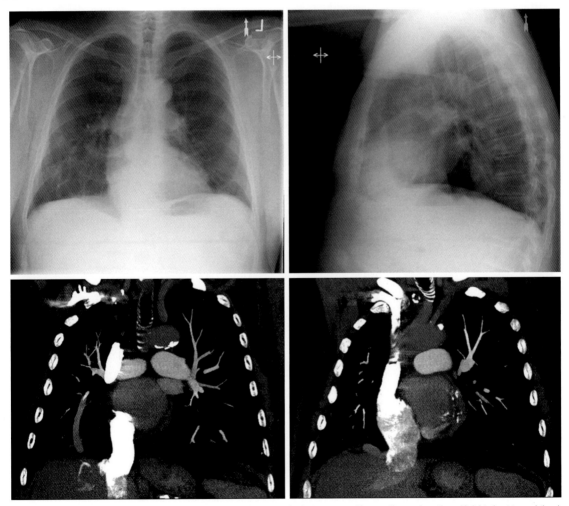

Figure 18-53. Scimitar syndrome of an anomalous right-sided pulmonary vein that courses with a gentle arc, from the mid-right chest toward the dome of the right diaphragm. The path of the anomalous vein is more obvious on the frontal radiograph than on the lateral one. The contrast-enhanced coronal computed tomography scans reveal the course of the anomalous pulmonary vein (*left lower image*) and the insertion of the anomalous vein (drainage) into the infradiaphragmatic inferior vena cava (*right lower image*). The central pulmonary arteries are dilated.

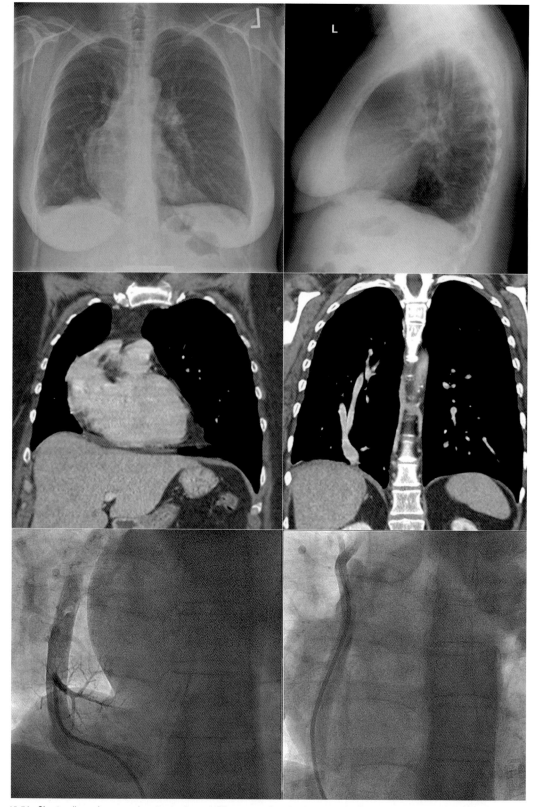

Figure 18-54. Chest radiographs, coronal contrast-enhanced CT scans, and contrast venography fluoroscopic images of a patient with partial anomalous venous return. The left hemithorax is notably smaller than the right one, consistent with one of the other names for this disorder—"hypogenetic lung syndrome." There is cardiomegaly, prominence of the central pulmonary arteries, and enlargement/displacement of the right atrial and right ventricular silhouettes. Posterior to the lateral aspect of the right atrium on the frontal radiograph, there is an arcing structure with nearly the same curvature as that of the right atrial freewall—the scimitar shape of anomalous pulmonary venous return, seen also in the posterior chest on the lateral radiograph. The CT scan images depict confluence of anomalous veins, and their crossing of the diaphragm. The venography images show the elegant tributaries of the anomalous drainage in finer detail.

19 Radiographic Findings by Diagnosis: Congenital Abnormalities and Obstructions—Pulmonary Stenosis and Coarctation of the Aorta

CONGENITAL HEART DISEASE: OBSTRUCTIONS

Pulmonary Valvular Stenosis
See Graphic 19-1 and Figures 19-1 to 19-13. Possible findings are discussed in the following sections.

Cardiac Findings on Chest Radiography
❐ Right ventricular enlargement
❐ Possible right atrial enlargement

Vascular Findings on Chest Radiography
(see Graphic 19-1)
Poststenotic dilation of the main and left pulmonary artery is seen with valvular pulmonary stenosis but seldom with subvalvular pulmonary stenosis. Because the jet is usually directed into the left pulmonary artery, the left pulmonary artery is usually larger than the right pulmonary artery. A prominent left pulmonary artery alone (without prominence of the main pulmonary artery) is usually spurious and results from elevation of the left hilum by a shrunken left upper lobe. The peripheral vasculature is usually normal.

Coarctation of the Aorta
See Graphic 19-2 and Figures 19-14 to 19-17. See also Graphic 19-1 and Figures 19-6 to 19-13. There is further text discussion of coarctation of the aorta in Chapter 7 (pp. 85–86).

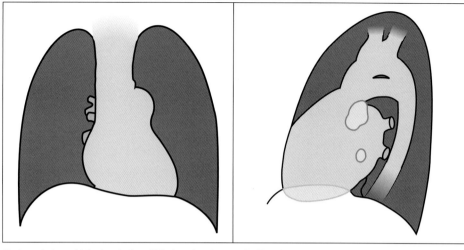

Graphic 19-1. Posteroanterior and lateral projections: Valvular pulmonic stenosis. Note dilated main pulmonary artery seen on the frontal projection, and slight accentuation of the right atrial curvature. On the lateral projection, note the indirect sign of right ventricular dilation—increased apposition of the heart to the sternum, and dilation of the right main pulmonary artery, seen end-on.

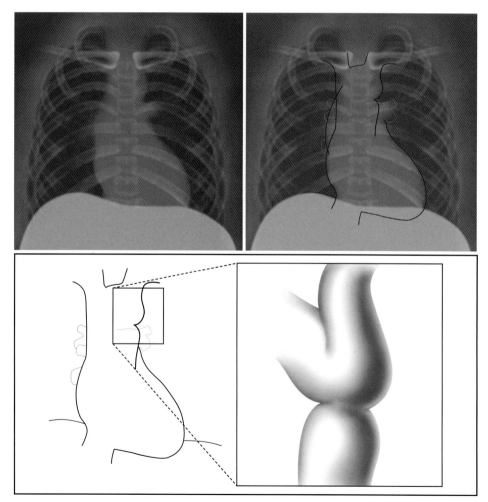

Graphic 19-2. Radiographic appearance of coarctation of the aorta. Note the "figure of 3" sign (the coarctation itself causes the indentation of the aorta; the proximal aorta/left subclavian artery provides the upper half of the "3," and the poststenotic dilation of the aorta provides the lower half), rib notching, and associated dilation of the ascending aorta, which may be caused by an associated bicuspid aortic valve.

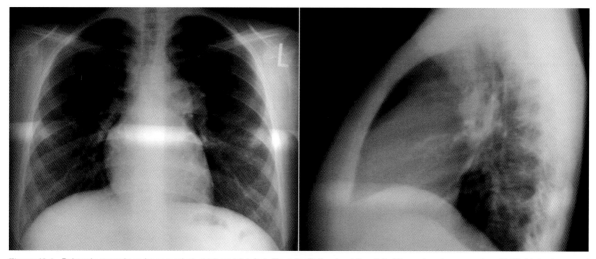

Figure 19-1. Pulmonic stenosis and a secundum atrial septal defect. There is dilation (poststenotic) of the main pulmonary artery. Right atrial enlargement is suggested by the right heart contour on the posteroanterior radiograph, and right ventricular enlargement is suggested by the sternal apposition on the lateral radiograph.

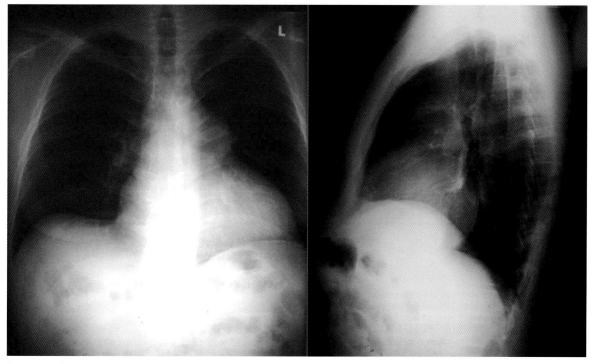

Figure 19-2. Pulmonic stenosis and dilated cardiomyopathy. The cardiothoracic ratio is increased, and the cardiac contour is globular with multichamber enlargement. There is dilation (poststenotic) of the main pulmonary artery.

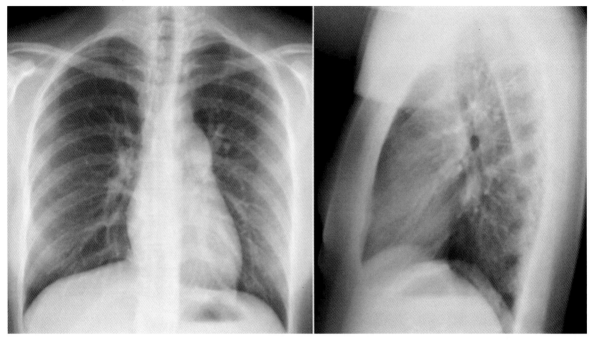

Figure 19-5. Valvular pulmonary stenosis with poststenotic dilation of the main pulmonary artery and with right ventricular enlargement.

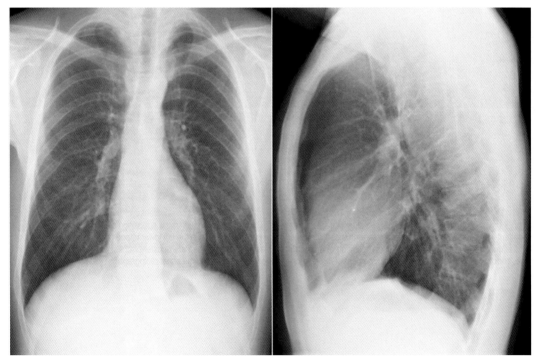

Figure 19-6. Coarctation of the aorta. There is rib notching and prominence of the left subclavian artery.

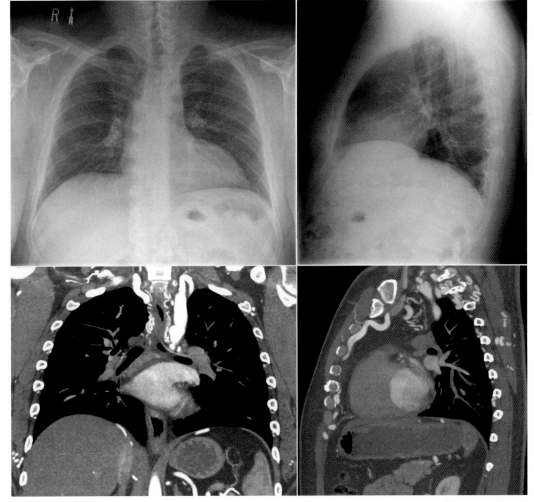

Figure 19-7. Coarctation of the aorta. There is slight cardiomegaly and prominence of the ascending aorta. Rib notching is present, and the left subclavian artery is dilated. A "figure of 3" contour of the descending aorta/left subclavian artery is debatably present. The lower coronal and sagittal computed tomography images demonstrate the waist of the coarctation of the aorta, the dilated left subclavian artery, prominent collaterals within the mediastinum throughout the scapular area, prominent subcostal arteries and chest wall collaterals, and an enormous left internal thoracic artery.

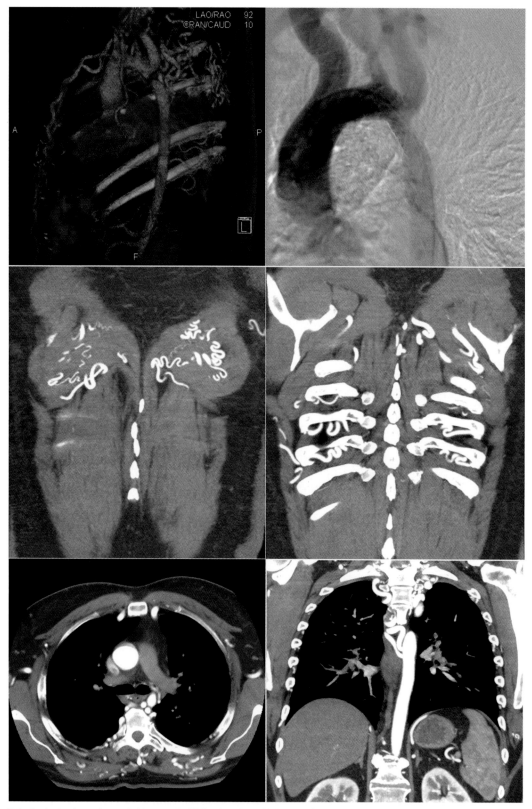

Figure 19-8. Contrast-enhanced computed tomography (CT) and angiographic images of a patient with recurrent coarctation of the aorta. The CT images reveal the abundant collaterals through several pathways, including the intercostal arteries, whose dilation results in rib notching.

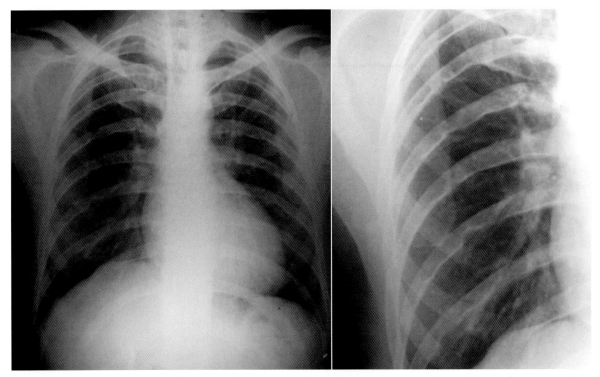

Figure 19-9. The cardiothoracic ratio is mildly increased. There is prominent rib notching due to intercostal collaterals. Otherwise, there are no particular features of coarctation in this proven case of coarctation.

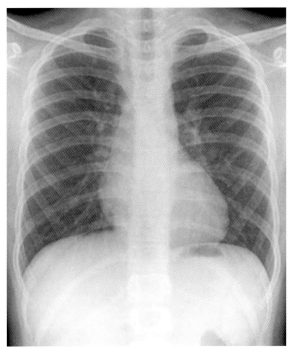

Figure 19-10. There is no frank cardiomegaly or abnormal contour to the descending aorta. There is bilateral rib notching present in this case of coarctation.

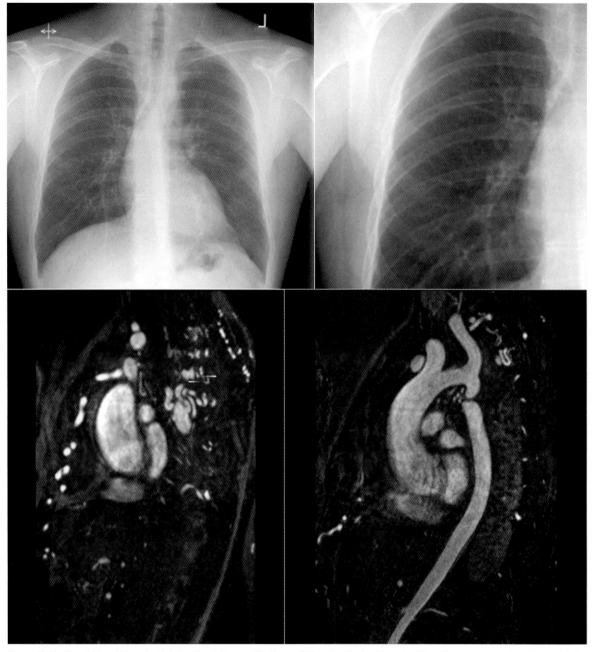

Figure 19-11. Coarctation of the aorta. Note the rib notching and the "figure of 3" on the chest radiographs. Magnetic resonance angiography reveals the abundant associated collaterals and the coarctation itself.

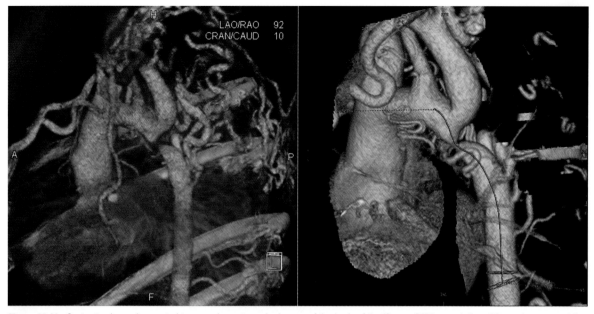

Figure 19-12. Contrast-enhanced computed tomography aortography images of the basis of the "figure of 3" in coarctation of the aorta: precoarctation dilation of the left subclavian artery, the waist of the coarctation, and resumption of the aorta. Note as well the strikingly dilated collateral vessels, including subscapular plexus and internal mammary/thoracic arteries.

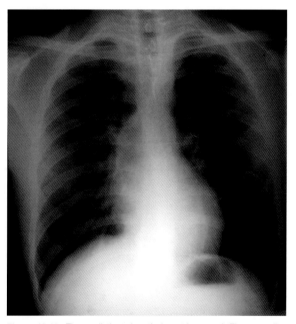

Figure 19-13. The cardiothoracic ratio is not increased. The ascending aorta is dilated due to an aneurysm of the ascending aorta associated with a bicuspid aortic valve. There is rib notching with the typical appearance of erosions and sclerosis.

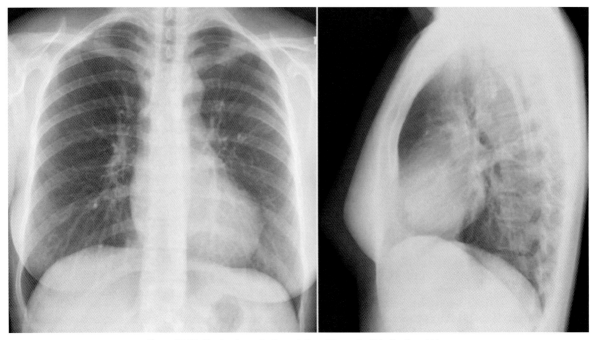

Figure 19-14. Previously repaired coarctation of the aorta. Note the rib notching.

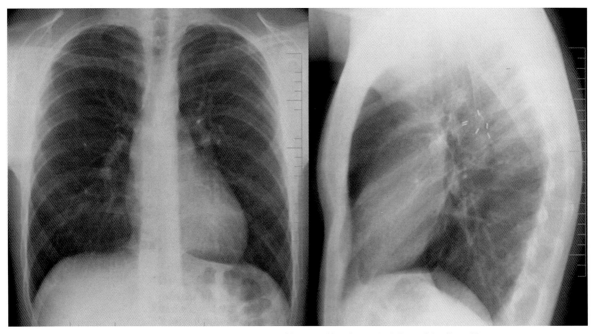

Figure 19-15. Previously repaired coarctation of the aorta. Note the surgical clips and the rib notching.

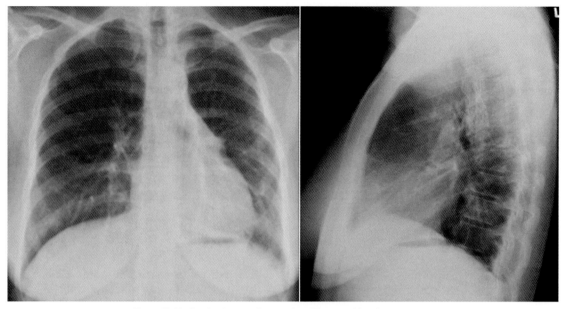

Figure 19-16. Previously stented coarctation of the aorta. Note the rib notching.

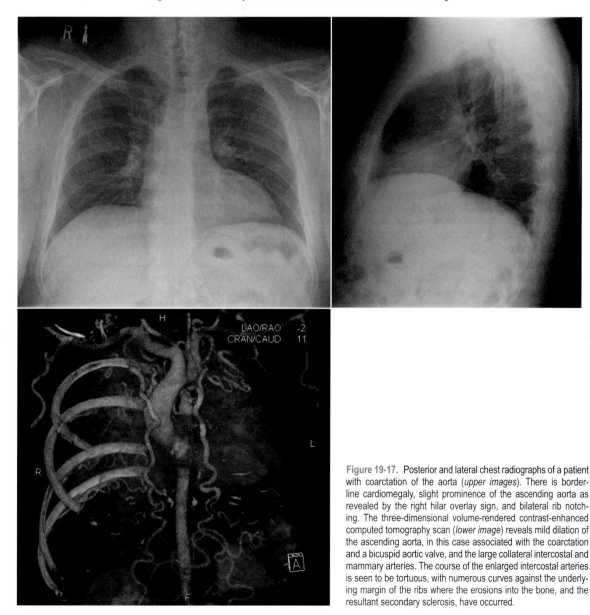

Figure 19-17. Posterior and lateral chest radiographs of a patient with coarctation of the aorta (*upper images*). There is borderline cardiomegaly, slight prominence of the ascending aorta as revealed by the right hilar overlay sign, and bilateral rib notching. The three-dimensional volume-rendered contrast-enhanced computed tomography scan (*lower image*) reveals mild dilation of the ascending aorta, in this case associated with the coarctation and a bicuspid aortic valve, and the large collateral intercostal and mammary arteries. The course of the enlarged intercostal arteries is seen to be tortuous, with numerous curves against the underlying margin of the ribs where the erosions into the bone, and the resultant secondary sclerosis, have occurred.

20 Radiographic Findings by Diagnosis: Situs and Complex Congenital Abnormalities

---

Key Points

- The chest radiograph can assist with establishing "situs" by identifying the orientation of the apex, the side of the aortic arch, and the stomach (gastric air bubble).
- The chest radiographic findings of complex disorders reflect not only the underlying abnormality but also often the interventions and their successes and complications.
- The classic physiology of Eisenmenger syndrome is represented on the chest radiograph by enlargement and centralization ("pruning") of the pulmonary arterial vasculature, diminished pulmonary venous vasculature, and right heart enlargement.

SITUS

Situs refers to the position/arrangement of the thoracic and abdominal organs (Figs 20-1 to 20-5). The posteroanterior/frontal chest radiograph is able to depict the location of the heart, the left ventricular apex, the aorta, and the gastric air bubble, and it may thereby determine situs.

There are three patterns of situs and one variable pattern:
1. Situs solitus
2. Dextrocardia
3. Situs inversus
4. Situs ambiguous/indeterminate situs/heterotaxy

Situs Solitus

Situs solitus is the term for the normal arrangement of thoracic and abdominal organs (Table 20-1).
- **Dextrocardia:** (where the apex is) heart in the right side of the chest; refers to "reversal of the heart" position in the chest or of its structures. The incidence is less than 1:10,000
- **DextroVERSION:** ventricular loop
- **Dextrocardia of embryonic arrest (situs solitus and a right-sided heart):** heart located rightward in the chest, with the other organs in

their normal positions (left gastric air bubble, left aortic arch). With dextrocardia of embryonic arrest/situs solitus with a right-sided heart, there is a 98% incidence of associated congenital heart disease, and 80% of affected individuals have anatomically corrected transposition of the great arteries. The next most frequent association of situs solitus and a right-sided heart is with a ventricular septal defect and pulmonary stenosis.
- **Dextrocardia situs inversus:** reversal/mirroring of the orientation of the heart chambers. The incidence is less than 1:30,000 (3.3% of cases of dextrocardia).
- **Dextrocardia situs inversus totalis:** reversal/mirroring of all visceral organs as well as the heart. Ninety to 95% of patients with situs inversus totalis do not have associated congenital heart disease, and they lead normal lives. Five to 10% of patients with situs inversus totalis have associated congenital heart disease, most commonly transposition of the great arteries. Primary ciliary dyskinesia/Kartagener syndrome is present in 25% cases of situs inversus totalis. The incidence is less than 1:15,000,000 (0.02% of cases of dextrocardia situs inversus).
- **Situs inversus:** left-right inversion/reversal of organ position
- **Situs inversus with levocardia:** 95% associated with congenital heart disease

Situs Ambiguous/Heterotaxy/Indeterminate Situs

The gastric air bubble and the aortic "knob" are on different sides; therefore, the situs is not predictable ("ambiguous"). Manifestations of ambiguous situs include the following:
- Errors of cardiac looping
  - Tetralogy of Fallot
  - Transposition of the great arteries
  - Pulmonic stenosis
  - Atrial septal defects and ventricular septal defects
- "Derangement" of abdominal organ symmetry
  - Isolated stomach or splenic reversal
  - Midline organs: stomach, liver, adrenal gland

❏ Organ malformation
- Asplenia/polysplenia
- Horseshoe kidney or adrenal gland

❏ Caval abnormalities
- Inferior vena caval interruption with azygous continuation (nearly always)
- Bilateral superior vena cava or inferior vena cava

Situs Determination by Chest Radiography

Appearance on chest radiography gives clues to the type of situs.

❏ Situs solitus (normal): left apex and left-sided stomach (Fig. 20-6)

❏ Situs inversus: right apex and right-sided stomach (Fig. 20-7)

❏ Levoversion: left apex and right-sided stomach

❏ Dextroversion: right apex and left-sided stomach (Fig. 20-8)

Tetralogy of Fallot

See Figures 20-9 to 20-22. Possible findings are discussed in the following sections.

Cardiac Findings on Chest Radiography

❏ Normal sized to mildly enlarged heart

❏ Boot-shaped heart ("coeur-en-sabot"); lifted apex (most common in childhood)

❏ Enlargement of the right ventricle

❏ Usually normal cardiac situs, but there may be associated dextrocardia

Vascular Findings on Chest Radiography

(Graphic 20-1)

❏ Normal or decreased pulmonary vasculature prominence (reduced pulmonary blood flow)

❏ Unrepaired tetralogy: usually underfilled main pulmonary artery/anteroposterior window region because the main pulmonary artery receives decreased blood flow due to the right ventricular outflow tract obstruction

❏ Repaired tetralogy, especially with transannular repair: commonly enlarged/dilated main pulmonary artery segment

❏ Small pulmonary arteries

❏ Possibly bronchial collaterals, which are equivalent to systemic to pulmonary artery collaterals

❏ Increased ("preferential") flow to the right side (10% of cases)

❏ With or without a diminutive hila

❏ With or without an absent pulmonary trunk

❏ Right-sided aortic arch in 20% to 30% of cases

❏ Prominent ascending aorta and arch, large superior vena cava

Note that there may be other associated abnormalities such as patent ductus arteriosus, atrial septal defect, congenitally corrected transposition of the great arteries, and left pulmonary artery stenosis.

Eisenmenger Syndrome (Figs. 20-23 to 20-27)

With large shunts, especially ventricular septal defect and patent ductus arteriosus, pulmonary vascular disease (obliteration) develops, resulting in pulmonary hypertension. The elevation of the pulmonary artery pressure reduces the shunting into the right heart or pulmonary artery. As a result of the pulmonary hypertension, right-sided chambers hypertrophy and enlarge. The pulmonary vascular findings are central artery dilation and peripheral artery pruning.

Complex Congenital Heart Disease

(Figs. 20-28 to 20-36)

With multiple lesions, congenital heart disease rapidly becomes complex conceptually and radiographically. The radiographic appearances vary according to the collection of lesions, stage of the natural history, development of complications, and interventions.

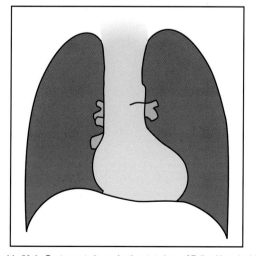

Graphic 20-1. Posteroanterior projection: tetralogy of Fallot. Note the high right ventricular apex, prominence of the right atrial contour, small aorta, and small pulmonary arteries.

TABLE 20-1 Situs Solitus	
RIGHT-SIDED	**LEFT-SIDED**
Thoracic Organ	
Right atrium	Left atrium
Trilobed lung	Bilobed lung
	Aorta
Abdominal Organ	
Liver	Stomach
Gallbladder	Spleen
Inferior vena cava	

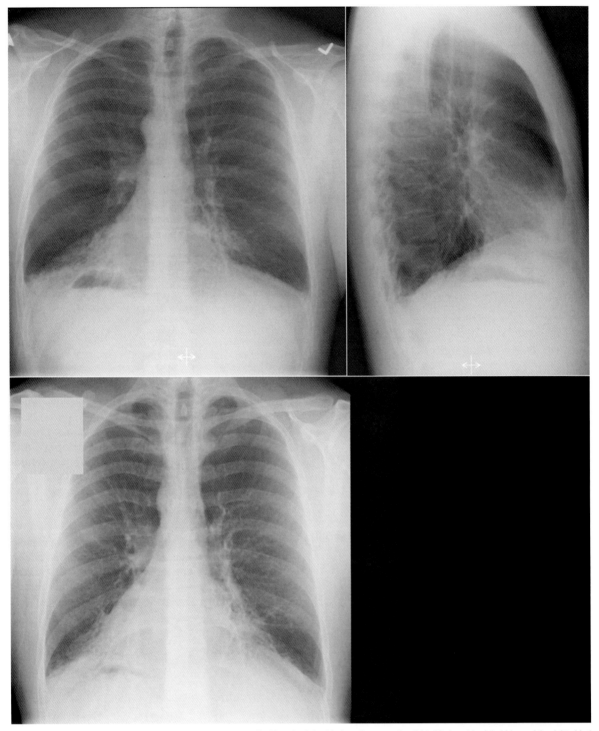

Figure 20-1. Kartagener syndrome: a subset of situs inversus totalis. Note the right-sided cardiac apex, the right-sided gastric air bubble, and the right-sided aortic arch.

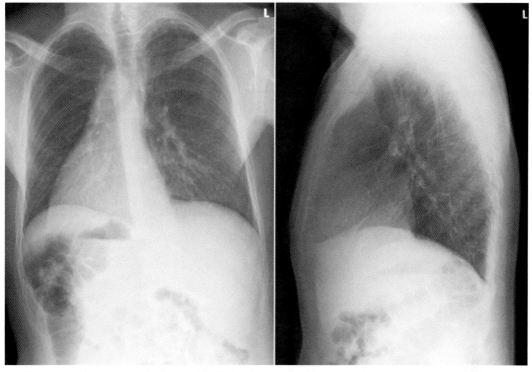

Figure 20-2. Situs inversus totalis. Note the right-sided cardiac apex, the right-sided gastric air bubble, and the right-sided aorta.

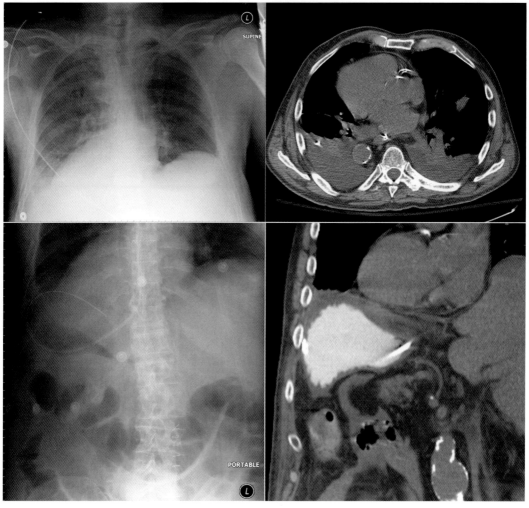

Figure 20-3. Situs inversus and L-transposition of the great arteries. Note the right-sided cardiac apex, the right-sided stomach, and the right-sided aortic arch. Although there is no gastric air bubble, the nasogastric tube and the computed tomography scans do localize the stomach to the right side.

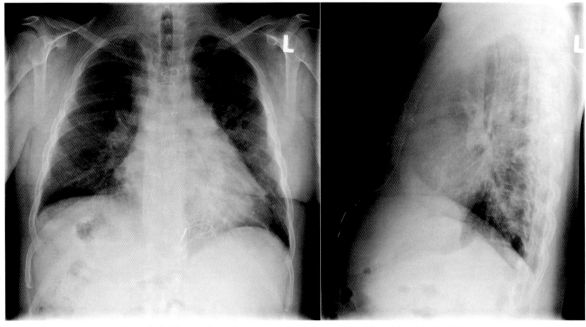

Figure 20-4. Situs ambiguous/heterotaxy: left-sided apex and a right-sided gastric air bubble.

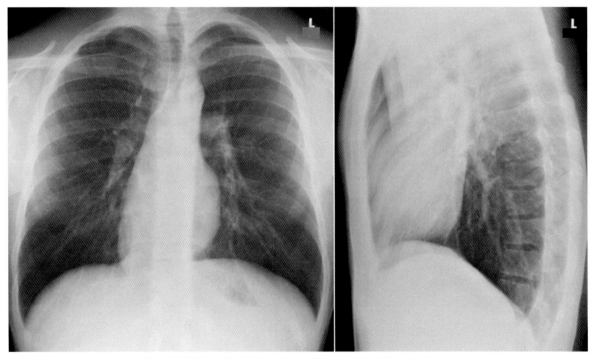

Figure 20-5. Situs solitus, dextroversion, and L-transposition of the great arteries.

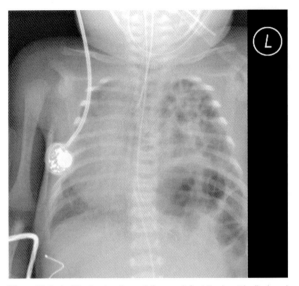

Figure 20-6. In this chest radiograph from an infant, the heart is displaced to the right side, not the apex. The position of the gastric air bubble is ambiguous. The responsible lesion is a large left-sided diaphragmatic hernia, with the stomach and bowel moved into the left chest, displacing the otherwise normal heart and rendering the gastric air bubble obscure.

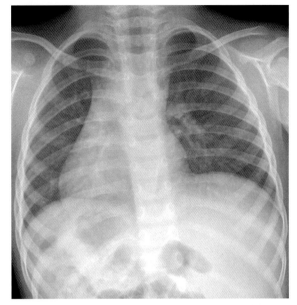

Figure 20-7. A right-sided apex and right-sided gastric air bubble attest to situs inversus.

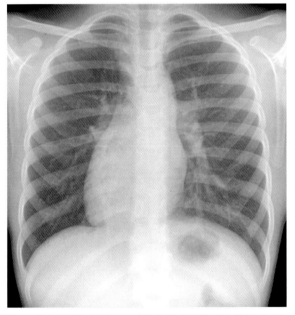

Figure 20-8. A right-sided apex and left-sided gastric air bubble attest to dextrocardia.

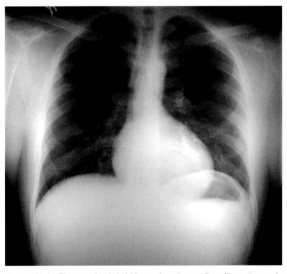

Figure 20-9. The gastric air bubble renders the cardiac silhouette nearly perfect for tetralogy of Fallot. The apex is elevated and the pulmonary arteries are small, consistent with obstruction of outflow to the lungs. The aortic arch is left-sided.

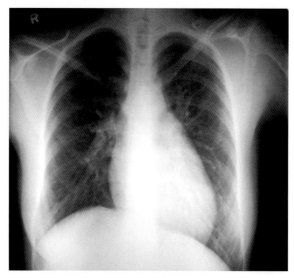

Figure 20-10. Tetralogy of Fallot. There is cardiomegaly, and the apex is elevated.

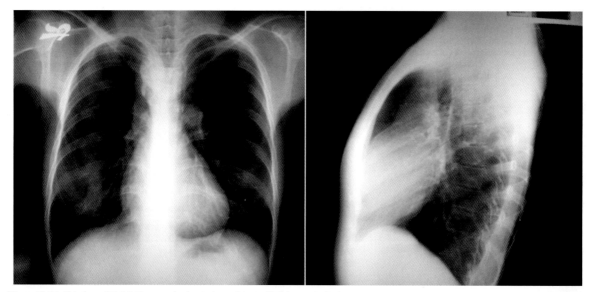

Figure 20-11. Tetralogy of Fallot. The apex is elevated, consistent with right ventricular hypertrophy, and the pulmonary arteries are small, consistent with obstruction of outflow to the lungs.

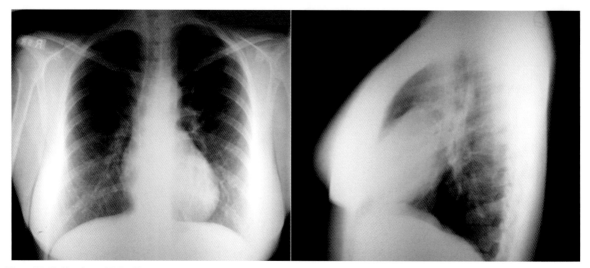

Figure 20-12. Tetralogy of Fallot. The apex is elevated, consistent with right ventricular hypertrophy, and the pulmonary arteries are small, consistent with obstruction of outflow to the lungs.

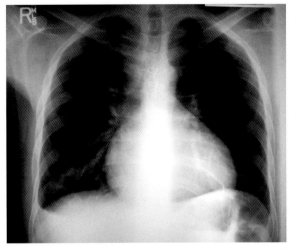

Figure 20-13. Tetralogy of Fallot. There is cardiomegaly with an elevated apex. The pulmonary arteries are small, consistent with obstruction of outflow to the lungs.

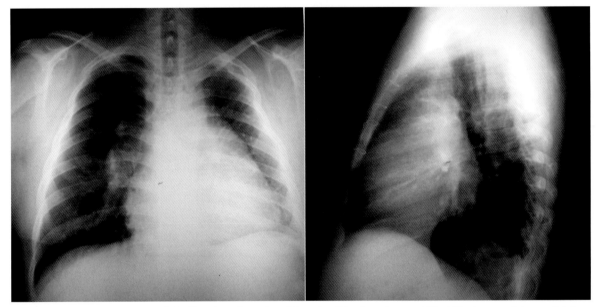

Figure 20-14. Repaired tetralogy of Fallot. There is cardiomegaly and signs of multichamber enlargement. The right pulmonary arteries are dilated.

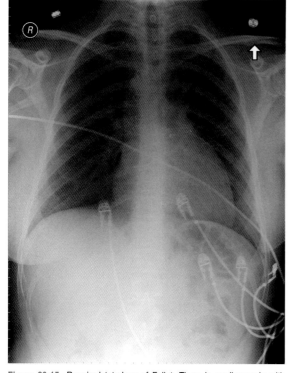

Figure 20-15. Repaired tetralogy of Fallot. There is cardiomegaly with signs of right atrial enlargement. A bioprosthesis is present in the pulmonic position.

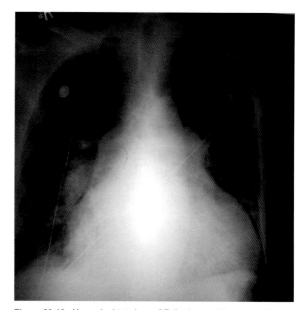

Figure 20-16. Unrepaired tetralogy of Fallot in an adult patient. There is gross cardiomegaly due to marked right heart chamber enlargement. The main pulmonary artery is dilated. The aortic arch is left-sided, and there is atheromatous calcification. There is azygous vein dilation due to the right heart failure.

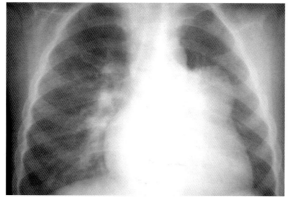

Figure 20-17. Tetralogy of Fallot in a young child with a right ventricular outflow tract aneurysm. In this anteroposterior film, there is cardiomegaly and an extensive bulging contour on the left superior aspect of the cardiac silhouette due to the outflow tract aneurysm.

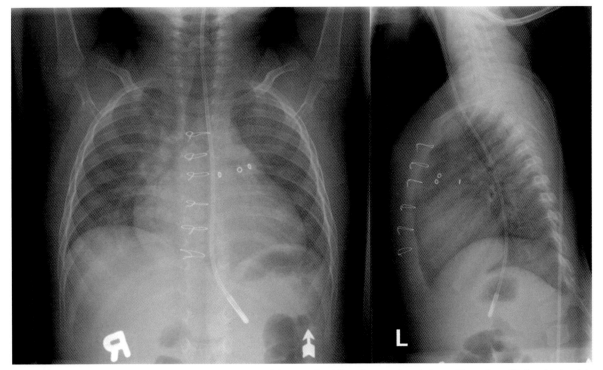

Figure 20-18. There is cardiomegaly with prominence of the right atrial contour. In addition, there are sternal wires and the radiographically evident eyelets of a bioprosthetic Hancock II conduit from the right ventricle to the pulmonary artery.

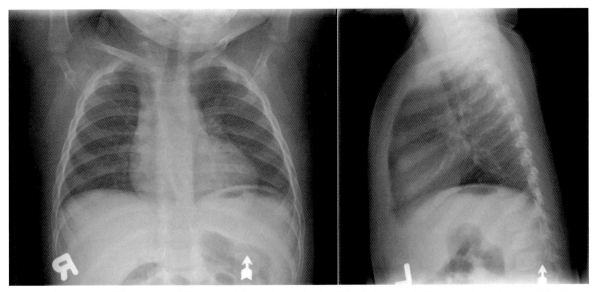

Figure 20-19. Tetralogy of Fallot, unoperated. There is borderline cardiomegaly with a high left-sided apex (which is more obvious because of visualization afforded through the gastric air bubble). The main pulmonary artery contours are diminished.

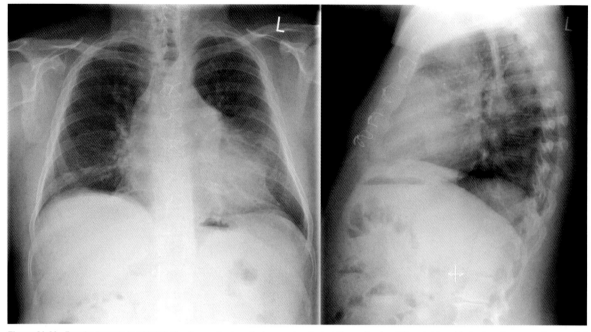

Figure 20-20. Repaired tetralogy of Fallot. Cardiomegaly, sternal wires, and a stented bioprosthesis within a right ventricular to pulmonary artery conduit are apparent.

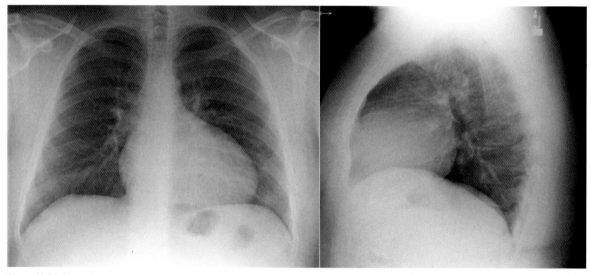

Figure 20-21. Unrepaired tetralogy of Fallot. There is prominence of the right atrial contour and an elevated apex to the heart seen on the posteroanterior radiograph and enlargement of the right ventricle as seen on the lateral radiograph.

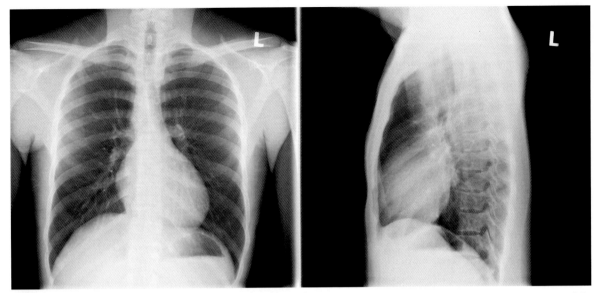

Figure 20-22. Unrepaired tetralogy of Fallot. Note the raised apex, the right atrial and right ventricular prominence, the small pulmonary artery, and the right-sided aortic arch.

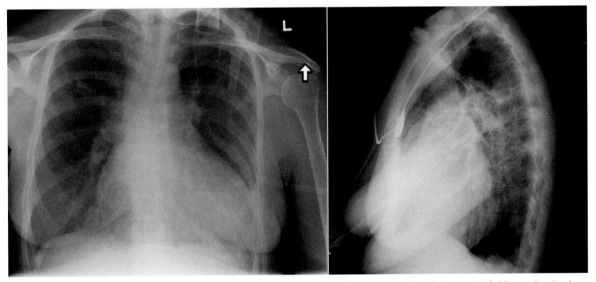

Figure 20-23. Eisenmenger syndrome due to a large ventricular septal defect. There is cardiomegaly, with signs of enlargement of all four cardiac chambers. The central pulmonary arteries are enlarged, but there is paucity of peripheral vessels—"pruning."

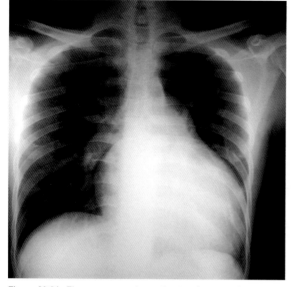

Figure 20-24. Eisenmenger syndrome due to a large ventricular septal defect. There is cardiomegaly, with signs of multichamber enlargement. The central pulmonary arteries are enlarged, but there is marked paucity of peripheral vessels—"pruning."

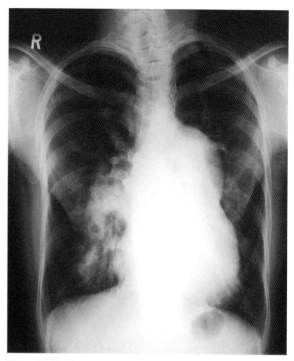

Figure 20-25. Eisenmenger syndrome due to a large ventricular septal defect: terminal. There is borderline cardiomegaly, with signs of multichamber enlargement. The central pulmonary arteries are markedly enlarged, and there is severe paucity of peripheral vessels—"pruning."

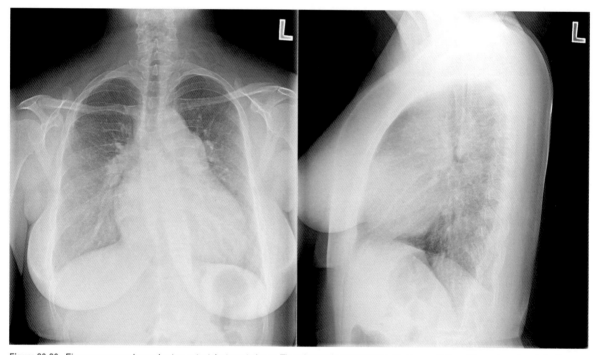

Figure 20-26. Eisenmenger syndrome due to a patent ductus arteriosus. There is prominent cardiomegaly, severe dilation of the main and central pulmonary arteries, and peripheral pulmonary arterial pruning ("centralization"). There is ductal or ductus-related calcification.

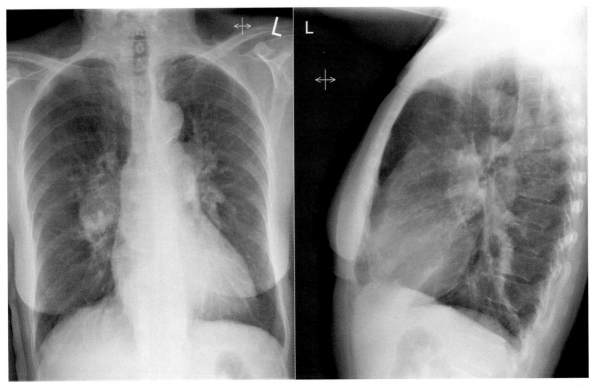

Figure 20-27. Posteroanterior and lateral chest radiographs of a patient with a large secundum atrial septal defect and severe pulmonary hypertension. Note the markedly enlarged central pulmonary arteries and their rapid peripheral "pruning," consistent with severe pulmonary vascular disease.

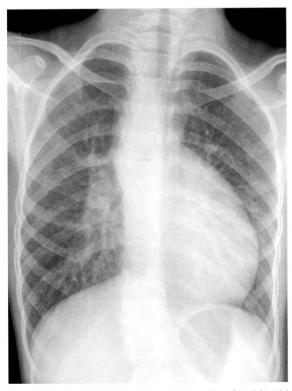

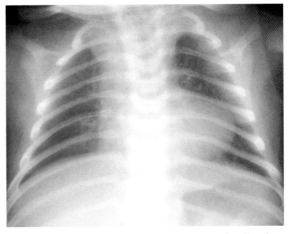

Figure 20-29. Pulmonary atresia with ventricular septal defect. There is no definite cardiomegaly. The main pulmonary artery is not apparent.

Figure 20-28. Double inlet left ventricle with juxtaposition of the right atrial appendage. There is cardiomegaly and increased pulmonary vascular markings.

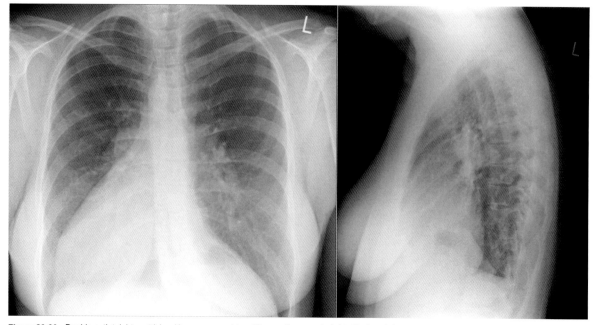

Figure 20-30. Double outlet right ventricle with a common atrium. The cardiac apex is right-sided, and the gastric air bubble is left-sided. There is dextrocardia as well as cardiomegaly with some increase in pulmonary vascularity.

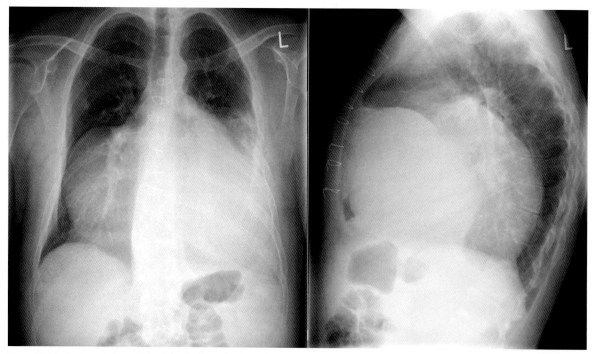

Figure 20-31. Posteroanterior and lateral chest radiographs of a patient with repaired (Fontan) tricuspid atresia. There is massive right atrial enlargement and resultant cardiomegaly.

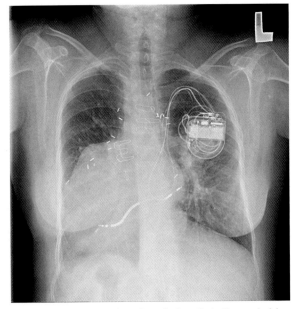

Figure 20-32. Posteroanterior radiograph of a patient with a repaired double outlet right ventricle with a surgical bioprosthetic valved right ventricular to pulmonary artery conduit, as well as a dual chamber pacemaker and implantable cardioverter defibrillator.

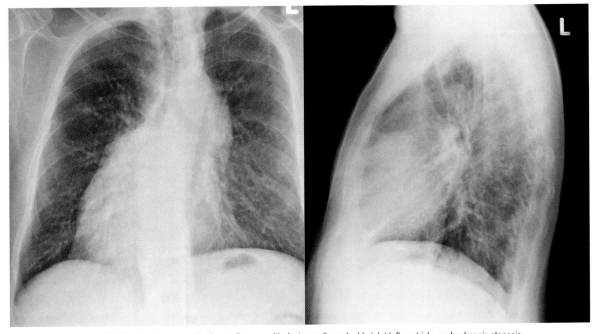

Figure 20-33. Complex congenital heart disease, with dextrocardia, a double inlet left ventricle, and pulmonic stenosis.

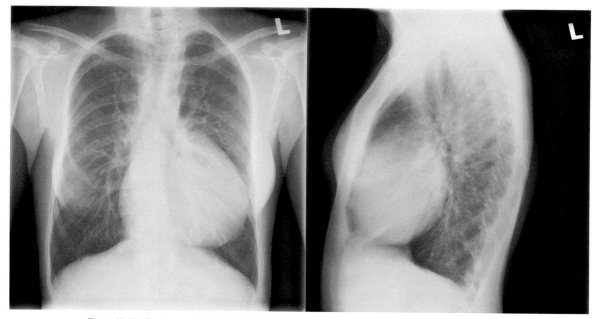

Figure 20-34. Complex congenital heart disease: double inlet right ventricle with prior pulmonary artery banding.

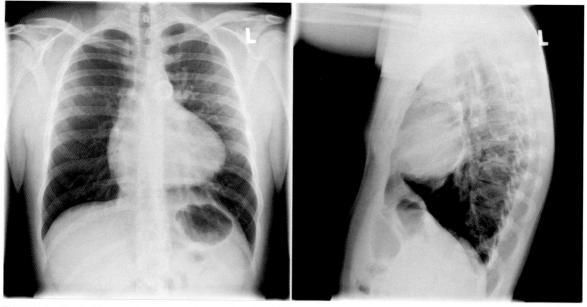

Figure 20-35. Repaired truncus arteriosus with prior sternotomy (conduit insertion) and stenting of the conduit. Note the signs of right heart chamber enlargement.

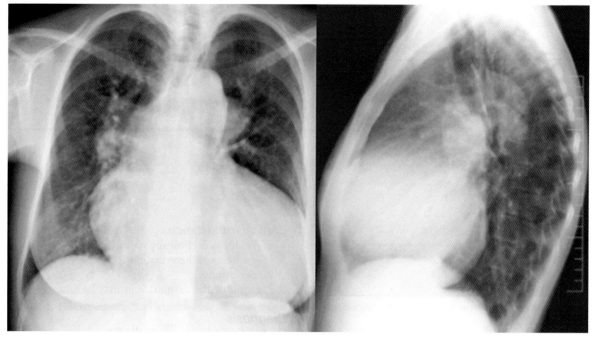

Figure 20-36. Truncus arteriosus. All four cardiac chambers are enlarged (especially the right heart chambers and left ventricle), as are the main and central pulmonary arteries.

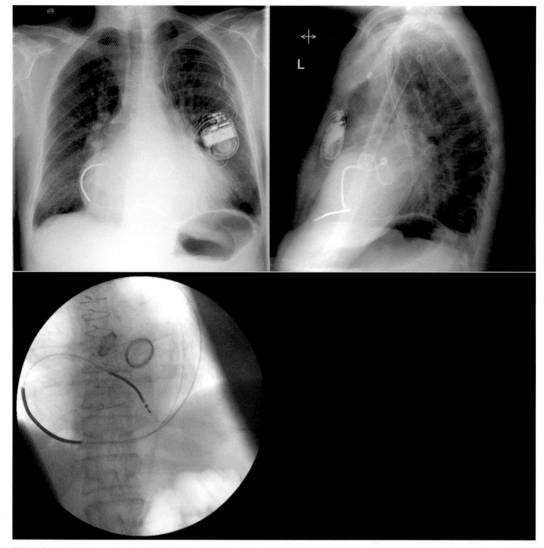

Figure 21-11. An implantable cardioverter defibrillator lead has been inserted into this patient with mechanical aortic and mitral valve prostheses, notably following the course of a persistent left superior vena cava through the coronary sinus and into the right ventricular apex. The lower image is fluoroscopic and corresponds approximately to the anteroposterior chest radiograph.

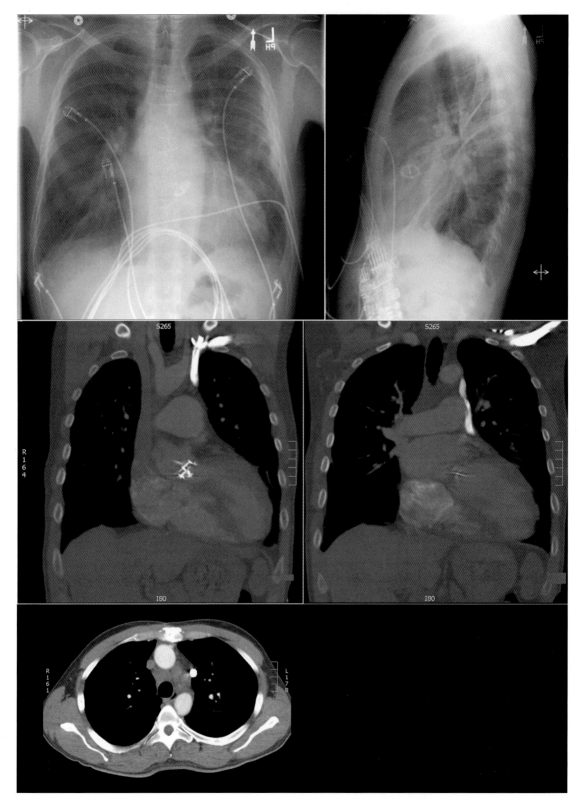

Figure 21-12. Chest radiographs and contrast-enhanced computed tomography (CT) scans with contrast injection from the left arm. The chest radiographs depict cardiomegaly and the Medtronic Hall–type mechanical aortic valve replacement. There is a vertical linear silhouette extending down from the level of the aortic arch alongside the pulmonary artery. The coronal CT scans reveal that this descending vertical silhouette is due to persistence of a left superior vena cava. The left coronal CT scan also depicts a right superior vena cava. The two vena cava are seen on the axial CT scan on the bottom, with the right superior vena cava non–contrast-enhanced in its usual position beside the ascending aorta and with the persistent left vena cava contrast-enhanced to the left side of the aortic arch.

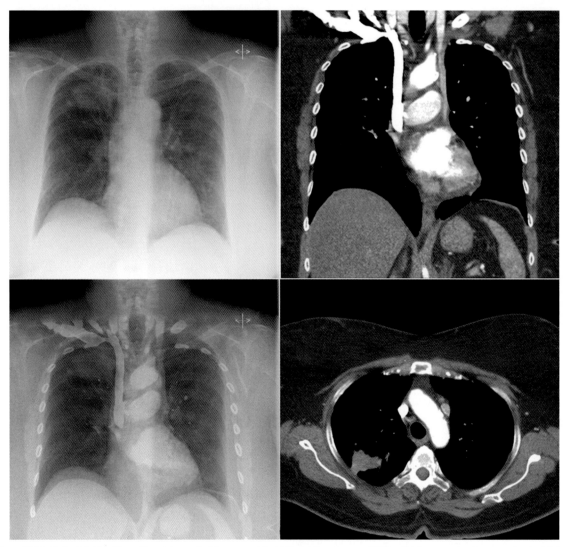

Figure 21-13. To the left side of the aortic arch is a vertical line—a persistent left superior vena cava (SVC), which is apparent on the coronal and axial views as the lesser contrast SVC; the dye is injected via the right arm in this case. The left lower image reflects superimposition of the posteroanterior radiograph and the coronal computed tomography scans. There is a large mass in the right upper lobe, a non–small cell bronchogenic carcinoma.

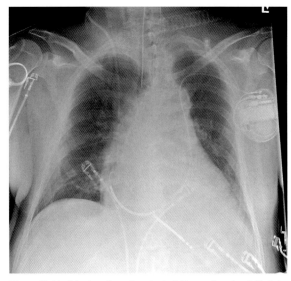

Figure 21-14. Prior insertion of an implantable cardioverter defibrillator (ICD) via the left subclavian vein and a persistent left superior vena cava. Despite the convoluted course, the ICD was inserted without difficulty. There are also several tubes: an endotracheal tube, a central venous line inserted by the right internal jugular vein, and a nasogastric tube.

22 Central Venous and Pulmonary Artery Catheters

Key Points

- Chest radiography has a standard role to assess for the position of central venous lines and pulmonary artery catheters following their insertion.
- Some postinsertion complications can be identified or excluded by chest radiography.

Determining malposition of catheters and tubes constitutes a forte of chest radiography and is mandatory following their insertion and repositioning.

CENTRAL VENOUS LINES
(Figs. 22-1 to 22-13)

To avoid mechanical irritation (from the catheter tip) and chemical irritation (from infusate) of the right atrium, the catheter tip of a central venous line should be further than the junction of the internal jugular vein and subclavian veins (near the level of the first thoracic rib). In addition, the tip should not be further in than the junction of the superior vena cava and right atrium. Central venous catheters that are intended to record central venous pressure should lie distal to the last venous valves (in the subclavian and internal jugular veins, 2.5 cm proximal to the beginning of the brachiocephalic vein) and before the right atrium. The ideal position of the tip of a peripherally inserted central catheter (PICC) line is in the distal superior vena cava.

Complications that are apparent on or may be suggested by a chest radiograph that should be excluded after every central venous line (and pulmonary arterial line) insertion include the following possibilities.

❒ Misplacement into a branch or tributary vessel
  • Via a subclavian stick, into the ipsilateral jugular vein
  • Via a jugular venous stick, into the ipsilateral subclavian vein
  • Via a subclavian stick, into the contralateral subclavian vein
❒ Misplacement into the pleural space
❒ Misplacement into the pericardial space
  • Hemothorax
❒ Pneumothorax or pneumomediastinum
❒ Cardiac tamponade
❒ Catheter knotting/kinking
❒ Superior vena caval thrombosis (progressive dilation of the superior vena cava)

PULMONARY ARTERY CATHETERS
(Figs. 22-14 to 22-31)

The tip of a pulmonary artery catheter should be 5 to 7 cm from the bifurcation of the pulmonary artery, no further than the left or right pulmonary artery, or at most, in the proximal part of a lobar artery. A more distal location of the tip is associated with increased risk of lung infarction. The tip should also be at the level of the left atrium (West zone 3). Following insertion, all of the previously mentioned complications should be excluded and the position of the catheter tip verified. A repeat radiograph should be performed when the catheter is repositioned. The balloon should not be seen to be inflated on a routine radiograph, because this likely indicates that the balloon was left inflated, with high risk of pulmonary infarction. About one fourth of pulmonary artery catheters are seen to be malpositioned on a routine postinsertion radiograph. If correct position has been confirmed and if there is no associated pneumothorax, then follow-up radiographs are indicated only if specific questions arise.

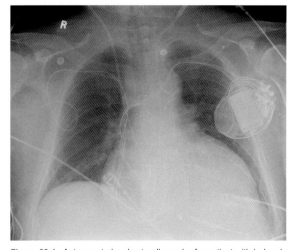

Figure 22-1. Anteroposterior chest radiograph of a patient with ischemic cardiomyopathy with severe heart failure. There is an implantable cardioverter defibrillator lead, dual chamber pacing, leads, and a coronary venous cardiac resynchronization lead. There are old sternotomy wires and left internal thoracic bypass graft clips. A right internal jugular central venous catheter has its tip in the right atrium. An attempt to enter the left internal jugular vein by catheter insertion has instead occurred as a left common carotid artery puncture with the tip of the catheter in the distal aortic arch.

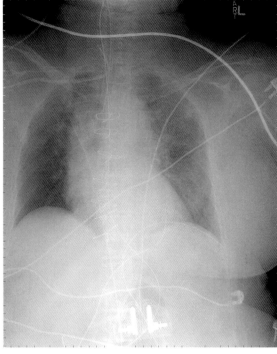

Figure 22-2. Post–aortocoronary bypass. The endotracheal tube, left and right chest tubes, pericardial drainage chest tube, and nasogastric tubes are in their correct positions. A central line inserted via the right subclavian vein has pursued a course into the right internal jugular vein.

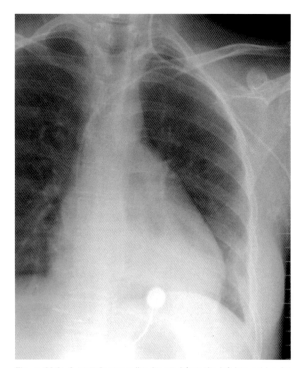

Figure 22-3. A central venous line inserted from the left internal jugular vein is malpositioned in the left subclavian vein. Another central venous line has been inserted via the left subclavian vein.

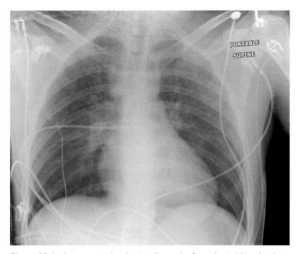

Figure 22-4. Anteroposterior chest radiograph of a patient with an inadvertent intra-arterial insertion of a right central venous line. The line is inserted down the right common carotid artery into the innominate artery and likely into the aortic arch.

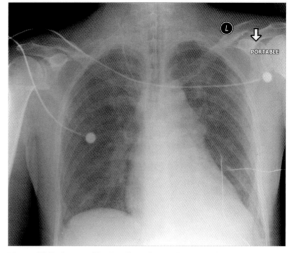

Figure 22-5. A central line has been inserted via the right common carotid artery down the innominate artery into the aorta. There is pulmonary edema.

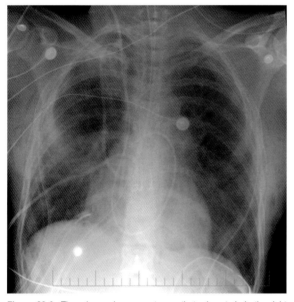

Figure 22-6. There is a pulmonary artery catheter inserted via the right internal jugular vein, in good position, as well as a central venous line inserted via the left subclavian vein, with its tip at the top of the superior vena cava. The patient is intubated and has a nasogastric tube, bilateral chest tubes, and a mediastinal tube, as well as transverse sternotomy wires. There is pulmonary edema and subcutaneous emphysema.

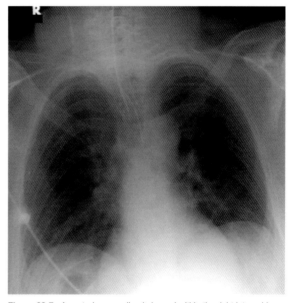

Figure 22-7. A central venous line is looped within the right internal jugular vein. The patient's head is turned to the right, resulting in the different projection of the internal jugular line, the endotracheal tube, and the nasogastric tube.

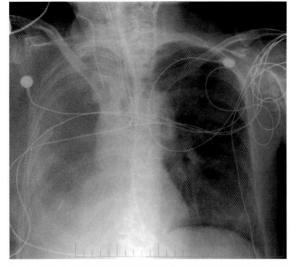

Figure 22-8. Post–right pneumonectomy. There are central venous lines inserted via both internal jugular veins, the endotracheal tube tip is down into the left mainstem bronchus, and the nasogastric tube is in the stomach.

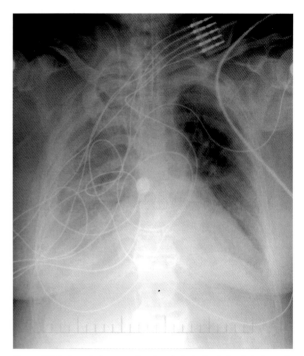

Figure 22-9. A central venous line inserted via the left subclavian vein is located in the left superior intercostal vein. The tip of the central line inserted via the right internal jugular vein is in the superior vena cava. This intubated patient has severe pulmonary edema.

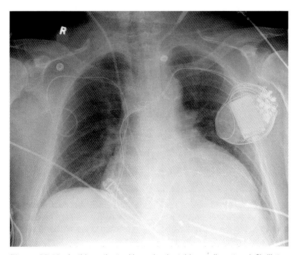

Figure 22-10. In this patient with an implantable cardioverter defibrillator, dual chamber pacer leads, and a coronary sinus lead, with prior left internal mammary artery bypass grafting, the central line inserted via the right internal jugular vein has its tip in the right atrium. The central line inserted in the left neck is in the left common carotid artery, and its tip is in the aortic arch.

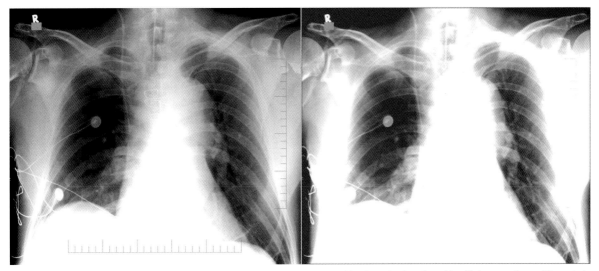

Figure 22-11. In this intubated patient, following catheter insertion into a right internal jugular vein, there is a right-sided pneumothorax. The aorta is enlarged, and there has been a prior median sternotomy.

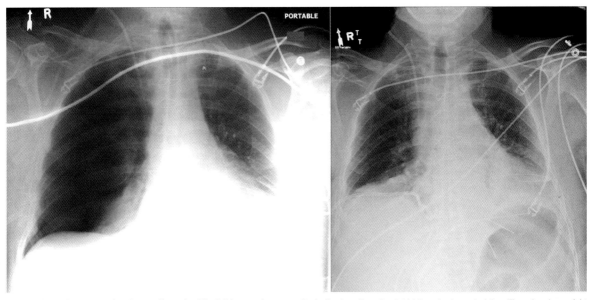

Figure 22-12. Anteroposterior chest radiographs. The left image shows a patient after insertion of a right internal vein central line. There is a large right pneumothorax. The right hemithorax is significantly enlarged, consistent with tension pneumothorax. The right image shows after insertion of a chest tube. The right lung volume has normalized.

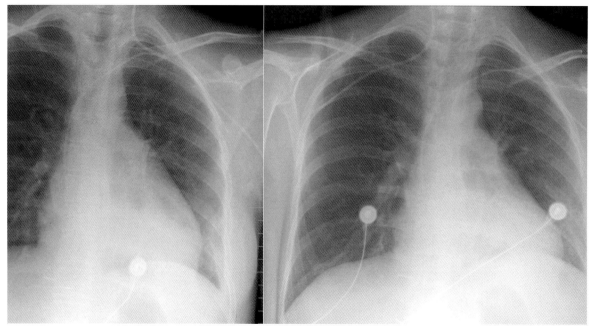

Figure 22-13. Frontal radiographs of the patient as in Figure 22-12. The left image shows a central venous line inserted from the left internal jugular vein malpositioned in the left subclavian vein. Another central venous line has been inserted via the left subclavian vein. The right image shows a central line inserted via the right subclavian vein, now malpositioned up the internal jugular vein.

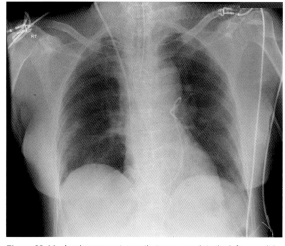

Figure 22-14. A pulmonary artery catheter courses into the left upper lobe pulmonary artery, but its tip is malpositioned inferiorly in the left lower pulmonary artery.

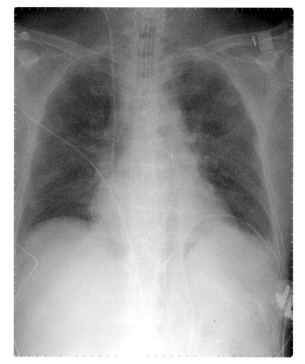

Figure 22-15. Post–aortocoronary bypass. The endotracheal tube, left chest tube, and pericardial tubes are all in the correct position. The tip of the intra-aortic balloon pump is a bit low. The pulmonary artery catheter, whose tip is in the correct position, is looped in the right heart.

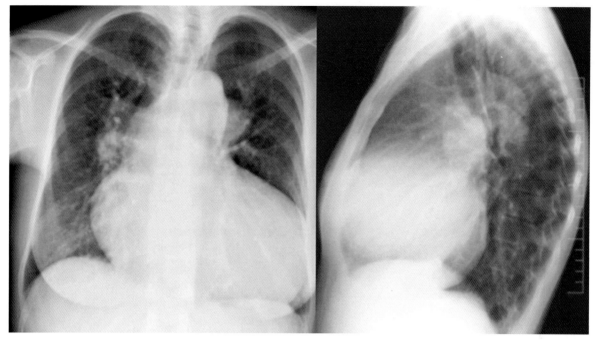

Figure 20-36. Truncus arteriosus. All four cardiac chambers are enlarged (especially the right heart chambers and left ventricle), as are the main and central pulmonary arteries.

21 Radiographic Findings by Diagnosis: Other Congenital Abnormalities

Ebstein's Anomaly

See Figures 21-1 to 21-9. Possible findings are discussed in the following sections.

Cardiac Findings on Chest Radiography
- Massive right atrium (small true right ventricle, large atrialized right ventricle)
- Aneurysmal dilatation of the right ventricular outflow tract
- Enlarged infundibulum
- A flasklike heart that may simulate pericardial effusion

Vascular Findings on Chest Radiography

Pulmonary blood flow may be reduced if there is right-to-left shunting across an atrial septal defect ("pulmonary undercirculation") or if there is right ventricle outlet tract obstruction from a tethered anterior tricuspid valve leaflet.

Cleft Mitral Valve

Cleft mitral valves result in mitral insufficiency.

Congenital Vascular Anomalies: Isolated Right-Sided Aortic Arch

See Chapter 7 for further discussion.

Interruption of the Inferior Vena Cava with Azygous Continuation

Note the following characteristics:
- This condition is rare in otherwise normal patients.
- This condition can be associated with heterotaxy/situs abnormality.
- It accounts for 3% of cases of congenital heart disease.

Clinical Importance

This condition is clinically significant.
- Right heart catheterization from the groin cannot be performed.
- Ligation of the azygous vein may be fatal.

Diagnosis

Diagnostic findings include the following:
- Markedly increased azygous vein on the chest radiograph
- Absence of the inferior vena cava shadow on the lateral chest radiograph

Persistent Left Superior Vena Cava

A persistent left superior vena cava (Graphic 21-1; Figs. 21-10 to 21-14) is suggested by an abnormally vertical vascular border (caused by the persistent left superior vena cava) where the gently curving left subclavian vein is normally seen. When a catheter or pacer wire discloses the anomaly (superior vena cava enters the coronary sinus, then enters the right atrium through the coronary sinus ostium), the abnormality is obvious.

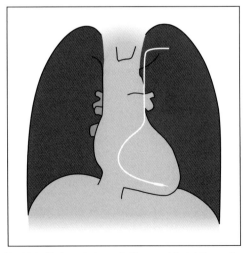

Graphic 21-1. Posteroanterior projection: persistent left superior vena cava (revealed by the pacemaker lead course).

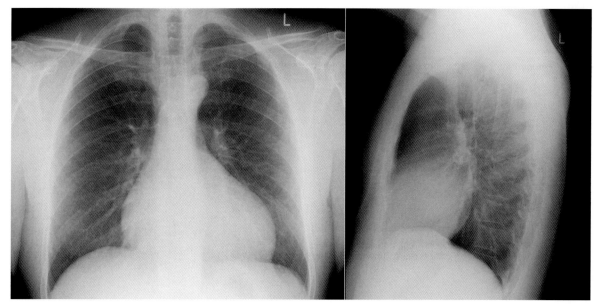

Figure 21-1. Ebstein's anomaly. There is cardiomegaly with prominence of the right heart chambers. The appearance of the main pulmonary artery is small.

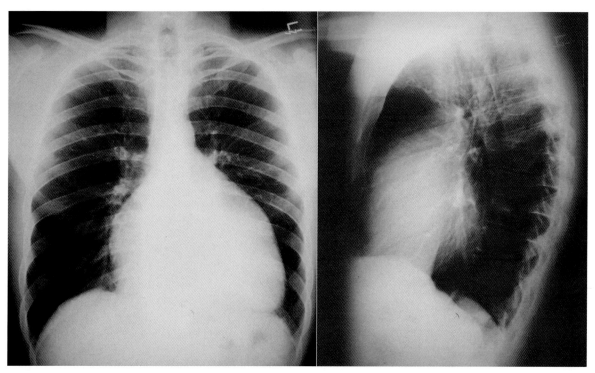

Figure 21-2. Ebstein's anomaly. There is cardiomegaly with prominence of the right heart chambers. The appearance of the main pulmonary artery is small.

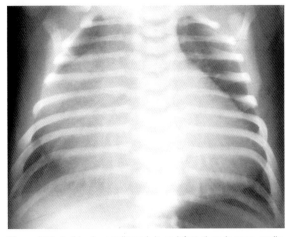

Figure 21-3. In this chest radiograph in an infant, there is gross cardiomegaly, particularly of the right-sided contours due to Ebstein's anomalies.

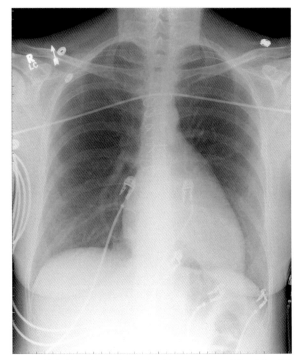

Figure 21-4. There is cardiomegaly with prominence of the right atrial contour, a small main pulmonary artery due to rotation of the heart due to Ebstein's anomalies. The patient had previously undergone surgical repair of an associated atrial septal defect.

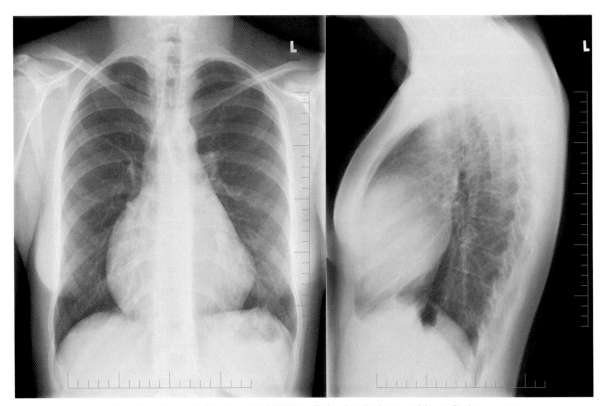

Figure 21-5. Ebstein's anomaly. Note the marked right heart dilation, the raised apex, and the small pulmonary artery.

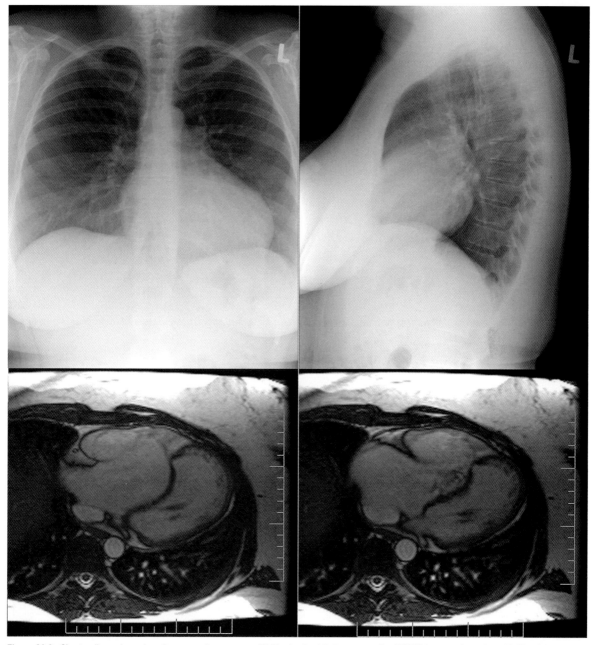

Figure 21-6. Chest radiographs and cardiac magnetic resonance (CMR; steady-state free precession [SSFP]) images of a patient with Ebstein's anomaly. Note the signs of right heart chamber enlargement, the raised apex, and the small pulmonary artery. The CMR images reveal the atrialization of the right ventricle, marked enlargement of the right atrium and atrialized ventricle, and tricuspid regurgitation.

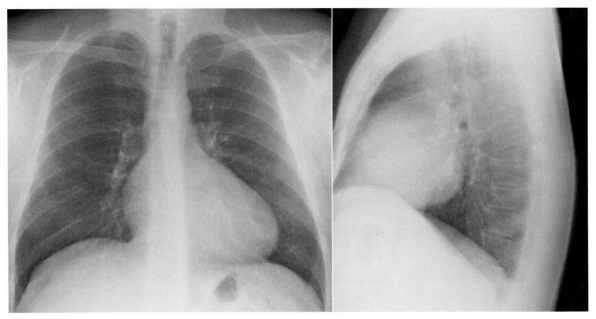

Figure 21-7. Ebstein's anomaly. Note the moderate cardiomegaly, the prominence of the right atrium and right ventricle as well as the small main pulmonary artery.

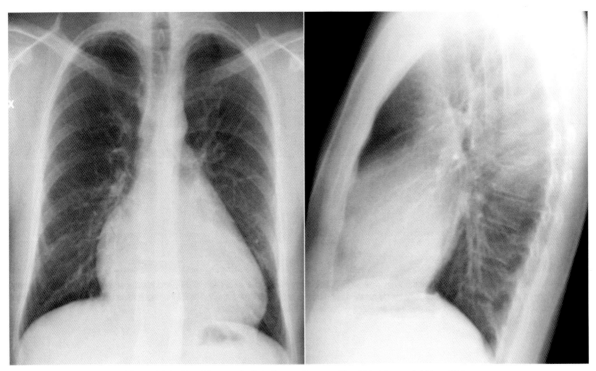

Figure 21-8. Ebstein's anomaly. Note the prominence of the right atrium and right ventricle.

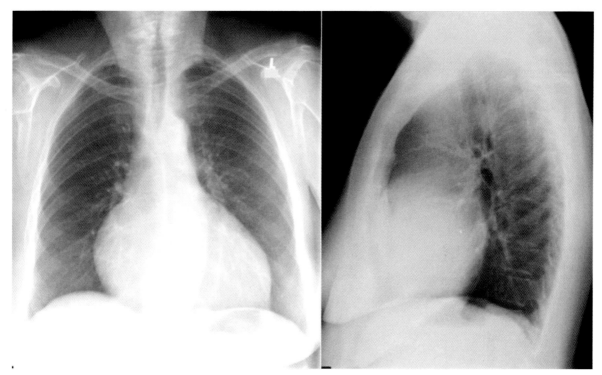

Figure 21-9. Ebstein's anomaly. Note the obvious cardiomegaly, the prominence of the right atrium and right ventricle as well as the small main pulmonary artery.

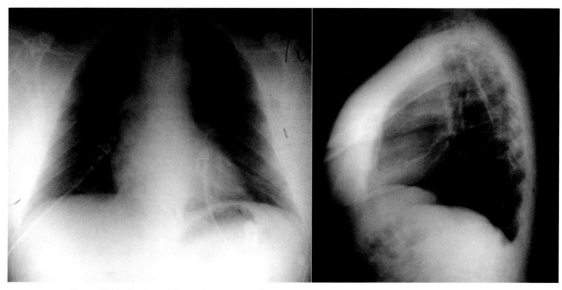

Figure 21-10. Persistent left superior vena cava. There is a vertical silhouette running to the left side of the spine.

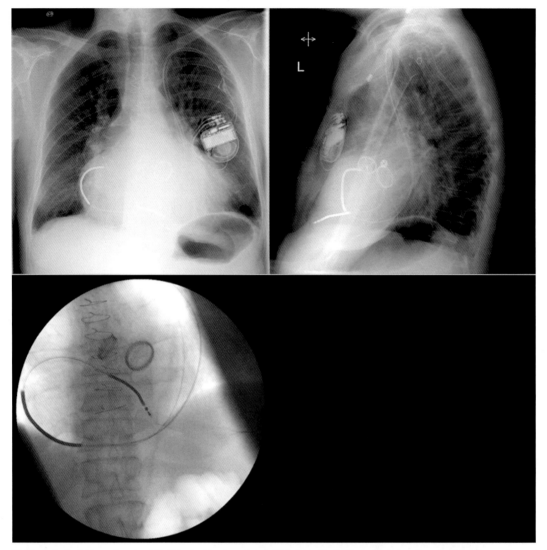

Figure 21-11. An implantable cardioverter defibrillator lead has been inserted into this patient with mechanical aortic and mitral valve prostheses, notably following the course of a persistent left superior vena cava through the coronary sinus and into the right ventricular apex. The lower image is fluoroscopic and corresponds approximately to the anteroposterior chest radiograph.

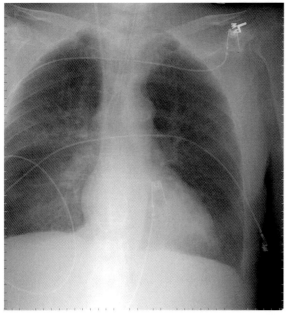

Figure 22-16. The endotracheal tube is in the correct position. The pulmonary artery catheter is looped in the right heart, and its tip is still within the right heart. There is pulmonary edema and extensive aortic intimal calcification.

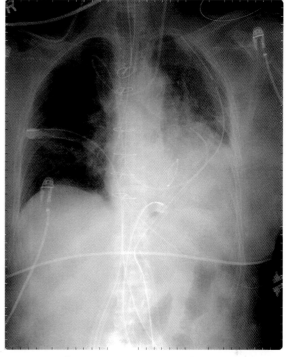

Figure 22-17. Post–mitral valve replacement. The endotracheal tube, left and right chest tubes, and pericardial drainage chest tube are in the correct position. The sewing ring of the mitral bioprosthesis is apparent. The cardiothoracic ratio is increased, and there are some "mitral" features to the heart silhouette. The pulmonary artery catheter, inserted via the left jugular vein, has looped in the brachiocephalic vein. The course of the catheter through the right heart is more toward the left side than usual because of right heart cavitary dilation associated with the mitral disease.

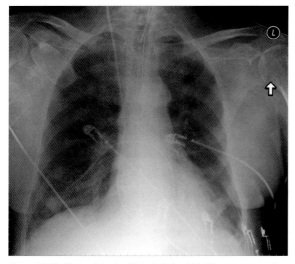

Figure 22-18. The endotracheal tube tip is too high. The pulmonary artery catheter is too far lateral and distal. It has substantially surpassed the superior vena cava.

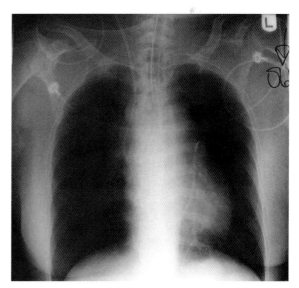

Figure 22-19. The endotracheal tube is in good position. A pulmonary artery catheter has been inserted. The lung fields are clear and overinflated. There is borderline cardiomegaly, and the superior aspect of the heart shadow/mediastinum is widened. The course of the catheter along the right margin of the mediastinum is deviated/displaced to the right by mediastinal bulk. Massive mediastinal adenopathy from lung carcinoma within the mediastinum caused respiratory failure by compressing the mainstem bronchi, which are not radiographically evident due to their compression.

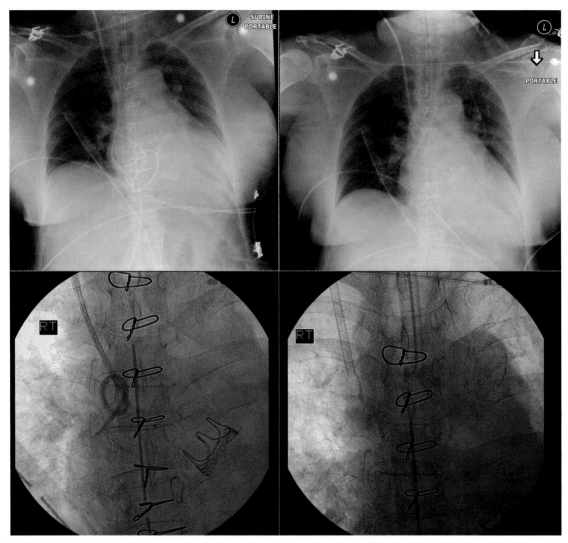

Figure 22-20. Chest radiographs and fluoroscopy of a patient in whom the pulmonary catheter had knotted in the right heart. This is seen in the left upper image. The right upper image shows attempted withdrawal of the catheter, which has tightened the knot. The left lower image is a fluoroscopic view of the tightly knotted catheter. With manipulation of the knot by a wire introduced from the groin, the catheter was straightened and, as can be seen, was withdrawn successfully.

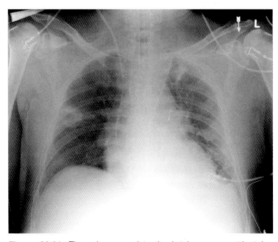

Figure 22-21. There is an endotracheal tube, nasogastric tube, sternal wires, and a pulmonary artery (PA) catheter. The tip of the PA catheter has crossed the line of the superior vena cava (SVC), which is delineated by the PA catheter within the SVC. Lateral to the tip of the PA catheter there is a pleural-based opacity, a pulmonary infarction due to the PA catheter.

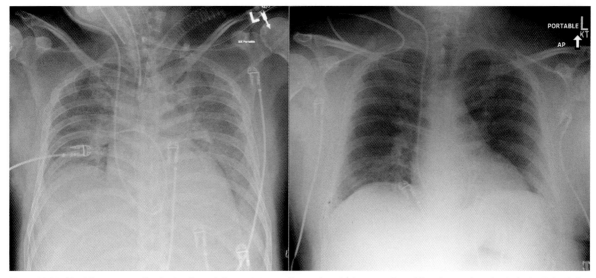

Figure 22-22. The left anteroposterior chest radiograph demonstrates cardiomegaly and pulmonary edema. There is an endotracheal tube that is borderline high as well as a nasogastric tube and a pulmonary artery (PA) catheter, whose tip is in the ideal position, not past the superior vena cava. The right chest radiograph shows that there has been interval resolution of most of the pulmonary edema and also removal of the endotracheal and nasogastric tubes. The tip of the PA catheter is slightly more distal than ideal.

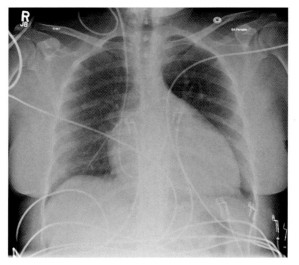

Figure 22-23. There is gross cardiomegaly with a globular or flasklike appearance to the heart and mild interstitial pulmonary edema. The pulmonary artery catheter tip is much too far distal.

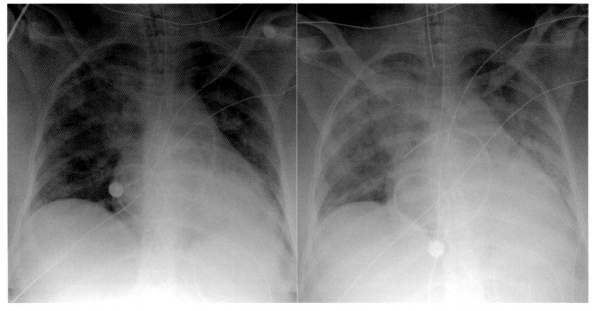

Figure 22-24. Intubated patient with severe heart failure. On the left anteroposterior radiograph, a pulmonary artery catheter appears to loop in the right heart but is probably just following a rolling course. Its tip is within the main pulmonary artery. On the right anteroposterior radiograph, subsequently, it has migrated and its tip is too far laterally, possibly within the interlobar artery.

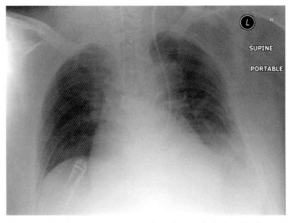

Figure 22-25. A pulmonary artery catheter inserted via the right internal jugular vein follows a course via a persistent left superior vena cava, into the right heart and into the main pulmonary artery.

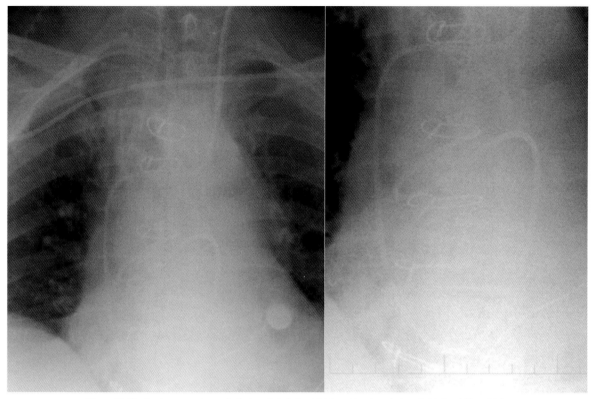

Figure 22-26. A pulmonary artery catheter inserted via the left internal jugular vein is curled in the right ventricle.

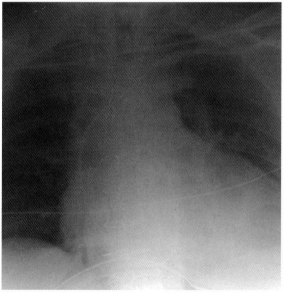

Figure 22-27. A pulmonary artery catheter inserted via the left subclavian vein has its tip likely within the right ventricular outflow tract.

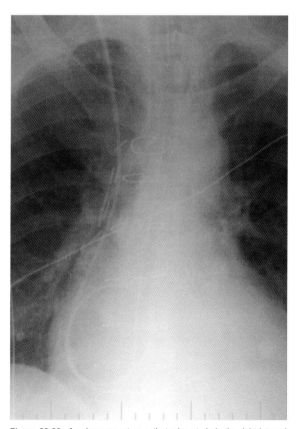

Figure 22-28. A pulmonary artery catheter inserted via the right internal jugular vein is curled in the right atrium.

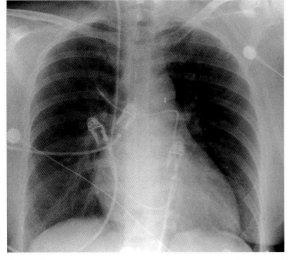

Figure 22-29. A pulmonary artery catheter inserted via the right internal jugular vein has migrated too far and is in the right upper pulmonary artery. Note the tip of the intra-aortic balloon pump in the distal aortic arch as well.

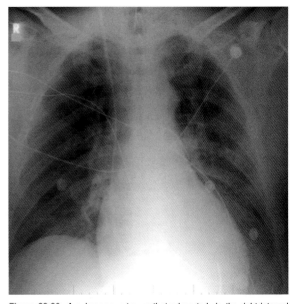

Figure 22-30. A pulmonary artery catheter inserted via the right internal jugular vein has migrated too far and is in the pulmonary artery to the left lower lobe. The endotracheal tube is too high.

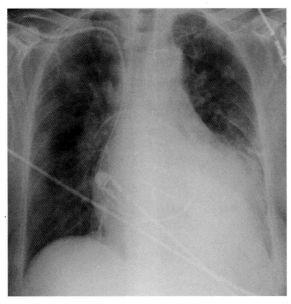

Figure 22-31. A pulmonary artery catheter inserted via the right subclavian vein has migrated slightly too far and is probably in the interlobar pulmonary artery. The pulmonary arteries appear enlarged, and the balloon may have been advanced further than usual to "wedge" (occlude) more distally within the enlarged artery.

23 Pacemakers and Implantable Cardioverter Defibrillators

Key Points

■ Chest radiography has a standard role in the identification of several potential complications such as pneumothorax, hemothorax, and several forms of malposition after insertion of pacemakers, implantable cardioverter defibrillators (ICDs), and cardiac resynchronization therapy devices.

■ Pacemaker leads are apparent, and ICDs are more obvious because of their larger coils. Coronary sinus leads for cardiac resynchronization therapy are finer leads.

ENDOCARDIAL PACER LEADS

The position and integrity of endocardial pacer leads should be verified, especially when pacemaker dysfunction is clinically suspected (Graphics 23-1 to 23-4; Figs. 23-1 to 23-15). The most common cause of pacemaker dysfunction that is apparent on the chest radiography is distal lead displacement/misplacement.

❒ With a **right atrial lead**, the tip should be in the right atrial appendage.

❒ With a **right ventricular lead**, the tip should lie anteriorly at the apex of the heart.

Every conceivable misplacement and displacement of pacer leads has occurred, especially of temporary transvenous pacers inserted in emergency situations. It is necessary to scrutinize the posteroanterior and lateral radiographs for signs of possible placement/migration of the lead:

❒ Into the coronary sinus

❒ Across an atrial septal defect or patent foramen ovale, into the left atrium, left ventricle, or pulmonary veins

❒ Into the pericardial space, as may occur following any insertion, but especially following an inferior wall myocardial infarction, complicated by complete heart block and associated with right ventricular necrosis. A normal appearance does not exclude pericardial misplacement.

❒ Into the right ventricular outflow tract

❒ Displacement of ventricular leads into the right atrium or superior vena cava, or displacement of atrial leads into the superior vena cava or ventricle

❒ Other misadventure

Lead fracture should be excluded, especially when pacemaker dysfunction is suspected. Lead fracture is usually seen near the site of attachment to the pulse generator but may also be seen at the venipuncture site.

Radiographically evident complications of insertion (pneumothoraces, hemothoraces) are always to be sought postinsertion. Increasingly, endocardial pacer leads are inserted via the axillary vein to lessen the chance of pneumothoraces, although the chance still exists.

EPICARDIAL PACER LEADS

Epicardial pacer leads may be temporary (post–open heart surgery) or permanent (Graphics 23-5 to 23-7; Figs. 23-16 to 23-19) Temporary leads are fine wires. Permanent leads have a fixation screw.

CARDIAC RESYNCHRONIZATION LEADS
(Figs. 23-20 to 23-22)

A third lead, inserted via the coronary sinus into a left lateral cardiac vein to pace dyssynchronous ventricles simultaneously, is used to achieve cardiac resynchronization. The coronary sinus lead appearance is thinner and finer than a ventricular lead. Usually, but not always, there is an ICD coil as part of the package.

IMPLANTABLE CARDIOVERTER DEFIBRILLATORS (Graphics 23-8 to 23-10; Figs. 23-23 to 23-34)

An ICD lead is similar in appearance to a right ventricular pacemaker lead, but most are considerably larger or thicker. Current ICD leads are inserted endovascularly. Older ones included pericardial patches or screws (also of variable appearance). An ICD also has pacemaker capability and is often in the company of an atrial pacemaker lead for dual chamber capability.

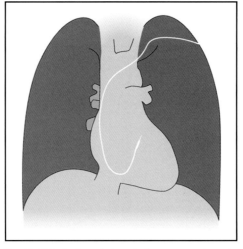

Graphic 23-1. Posteroanterior projection: coronary sinus misplacement of a ventricular pacemaker lead.

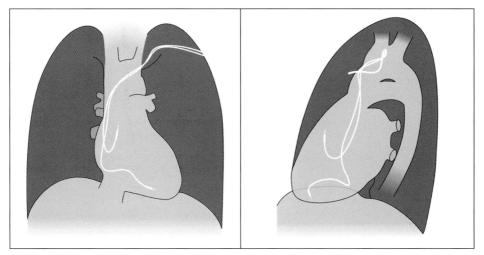

Graphic 23-2. Posteroanterior and lateral projection graphics of dual chamber (atrial and ventricular)/atrioventricular sequential endocardial pacer leads. Note the respective positions of the atrial lead in the atrial appendage and the ventricular lead.

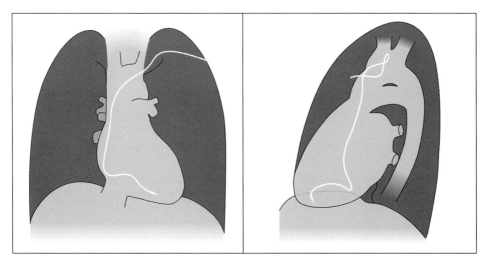

Graphic 23-3. Posteroanterior and lateral projection graphics of a single ventricular endocardial pacer lead.

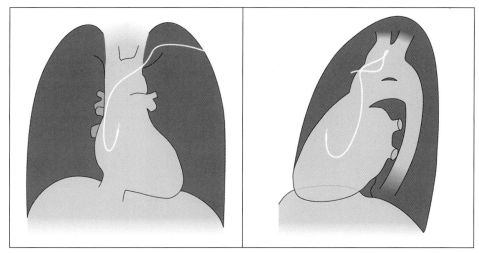

Graphic 23-4. Posteroanterior and lateral projection graphics of a single atrial endocardial pacer lead.

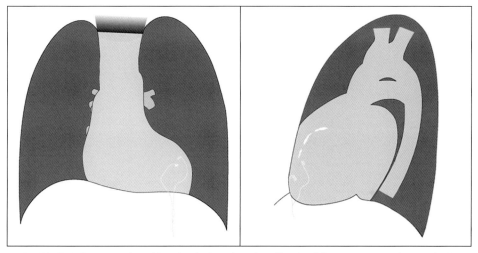

Graphic 23-5. Posteroanterior and lateral projections of a patient with epicardial screw-type ventricular pacer leads.

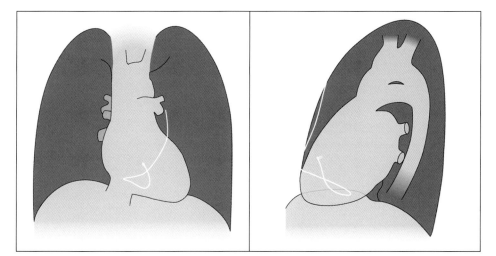

Graphic 23-6. Posteroanterior and lateral projections of a patient with a single permanent epicardial screw-type pacer lead.

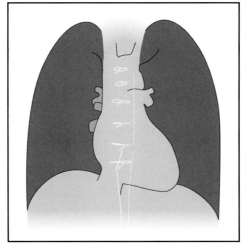

Graphic 23-7. Anteroposterior projection: a patient poststernotomy, with a chest tube and a temporary epicardial pacer lead.

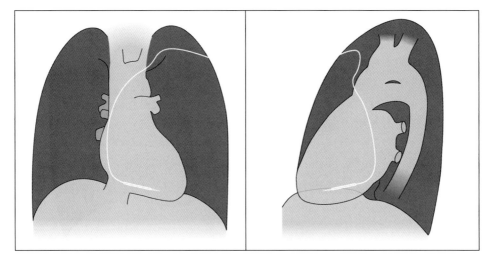

Graphic 23-8. Posteroanterior and lateral projections: a unipolar implantable cardioverter defibrillator (ICD) lead. Note the coil component of the ICD lead.

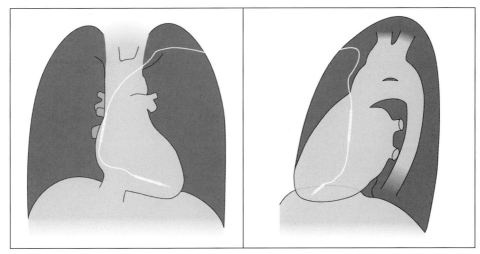

Graphic 23-9. Posteroanterior and lateral projections: a patient with a bipolar implantable cardioverter defibrillator lead. Note the two thick coil components.

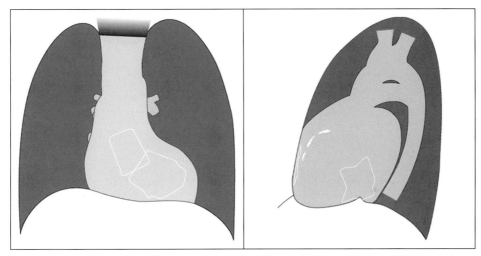

Graphic 23-10. Posteroanterior and lateral projections: old patch type implantable cardioverter defibrillator electrodes.

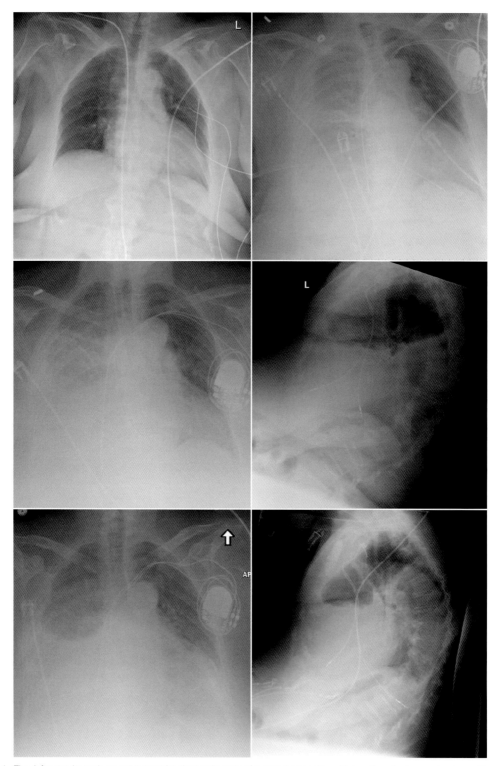

Figure 23-1. The left upper image is an anteroposterior chest radiograph of a patient presenting with symptomatic sinus node pauses. Transcutaneous pacer leads are present over the left chest. The right upper image is a chest radiograph several weeks after insertion of a dual chamber pacemaker. A very large right-sided pleural effusion has evolved. The ventricular endocardial pacemaker lead may be in the correct position, but the right atrial endocardial lead appears to be extracardiac. The middle images are posteroanterior (PA) and lateral chest radiographs at the time of re-presentation, again showing the right ventricular endocardial lead likely in the right position but the right atrial lead appearing too far inferior (PA radiograph) and too far posterior (lateral radiograph). The lower images (a few days later) show that the left pleural effusion has further enlarged and the right atrial lead has migrated further inferiorly and posteriorly. The site of perforation of the right atrial lead was the inferior aspect of the superior vena cava.

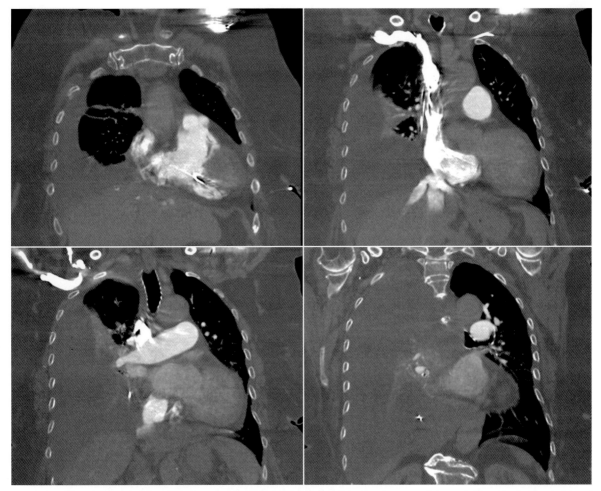

Figure 23-2. Same patient as in Figure 23-1. Contrast-enhanced computed tomography scans along coronal planes at different levels. The study is not electrocardiography-gated, and therefore there are motion artifacts. In the left upper image, the right ventricular endocardial lead is within the right ventricular cavity. In the right upper image, one of the pacemaker leads is external to the superior vena cava on the right side. In the lower images, the right atrial pacemaker lead is external to the heart, inferiorly and posteriorly located within the left pleural effusion.

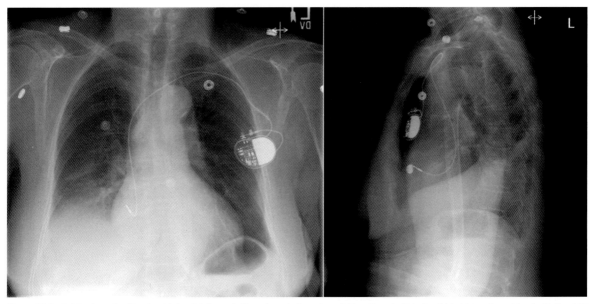

Figure 23-3. Atrial-only pacing (for sinoatrial nodal disease). There is a single endocardial lead inserted into the right atrial cavity and located in the right atrial appendage.

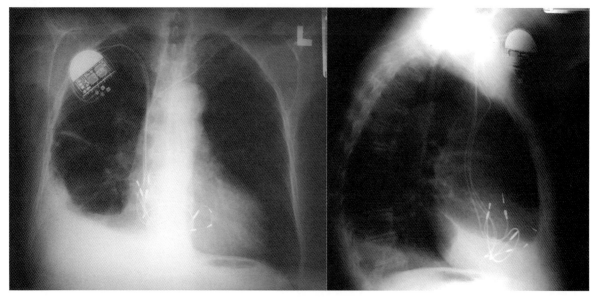

Figure 23-4. A dual chamber pacing system had previously been inserted via the left subclavian vein. The system was changed to the right subclavian side and the old leads cut, enabling the old ventricular lead to migrate into the right ventricle, resulting in prominent tricuspid insufficiency as the lead held the tricuspid valve open. The resulting right-sided heart failure was responsible for the right pleural effusion.

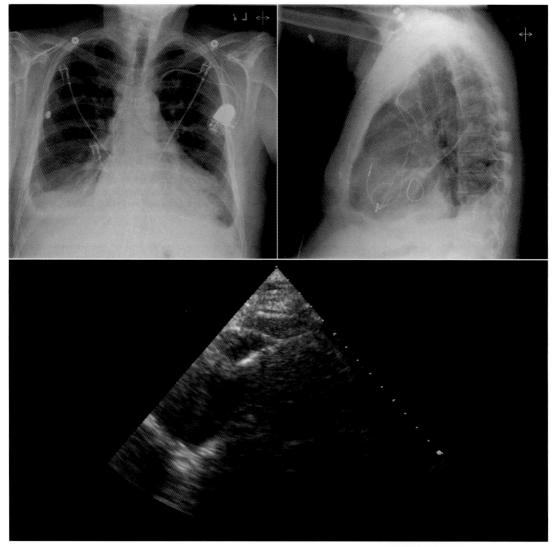

Figure 23-5. Following mitral and tricuspid valve repairs (mitral and tricuspid annuloplasty rings), the patient developed complete atrioventricular block and underwent insertion of a dual chamber pacemaker. The position of the ventricular lead tip is unremarkable on the chest radiographs, but by transthoracic echocardiography the ventricular lead is seen to have migrated through the right ventricular apex into the epicardial fat over the left ventricular apex.

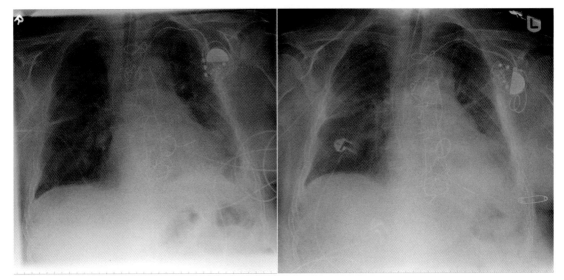

Figure 23-6. Ventricular lead insertion through a patent foramen ovale (PFO) and also across a mechanical mitral prosthesis. The left image shows post-ventricular pacemaker lead insertion, inadvertently through the PFO and mitral prosthesis. The right image is after revision and reinsertion. The pacer had functioned well when pacing via the left ventricle, with a right bundle branch block pattern at that time, as expected. The lower position of the right heart chambers compared with the left heart chambers is denoted by the differing position of the lead at the two times.

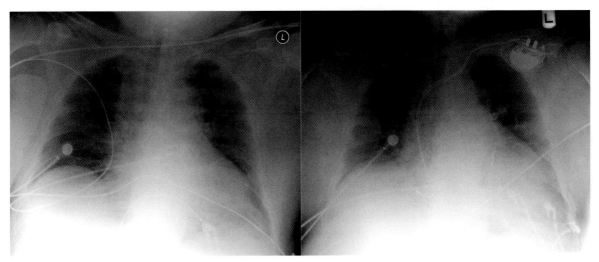

Figure 23-7. Ventricular lead insertion into the right ventricular outflow tract. Preinsertion and postinsertion images.

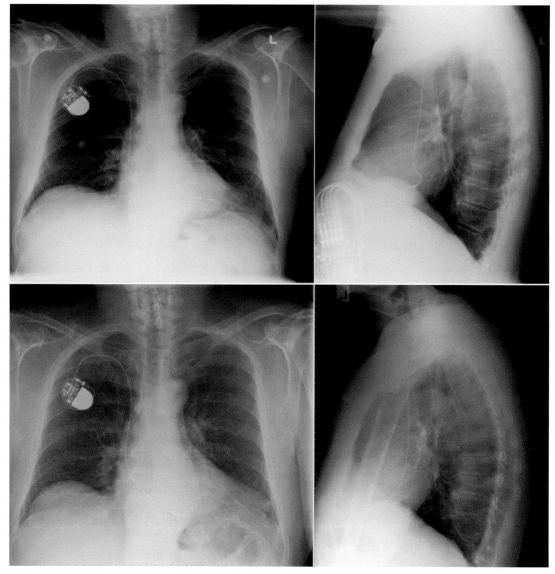

Figure 23-8. Pacer lead into the coronary sinus (*upper images*), and after revision and (*lower images*). The curvature of the pacer lead when in the coronary sinus is not strikingly abnormal on the posteroanterior (PA) radiograph; however, the lateral radiograph reveals the posterior location of the lead and in where the atrioventricular groove would plausibly be. When repositioned, the curvature is only slightly different on the PA radiograph, but far more anterior on the lateral radiograph.

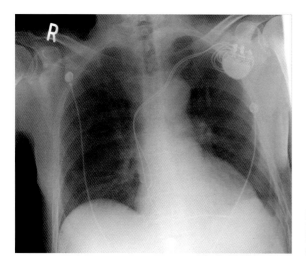

Figure 23-9. Right ventricular perforation. The atrial lead is in the correct position. The distal position of the ventricular lead, which is somewhat more inferior than usual but not clearly abnormal, has perforated the right ventricular apex, resulting in tamponade.

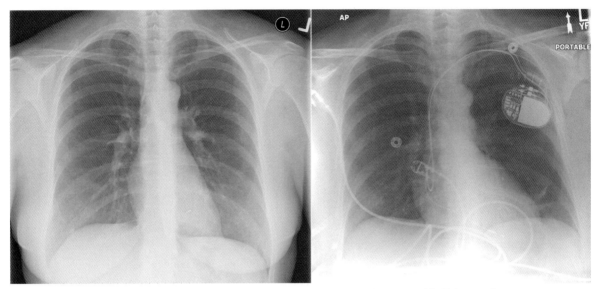

Figure 23-10. *Left:* Pre–pacemaker insertion. *Right:* Post–pacemaker insertion. Note the left-sided pneumothorax.

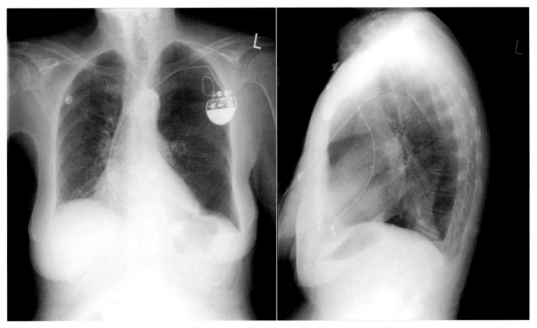

Figure 23-11. A large left-sided pneumothorax developed ipsilateral to a pacemaker lead insertion. A chest tube was required to drain it.

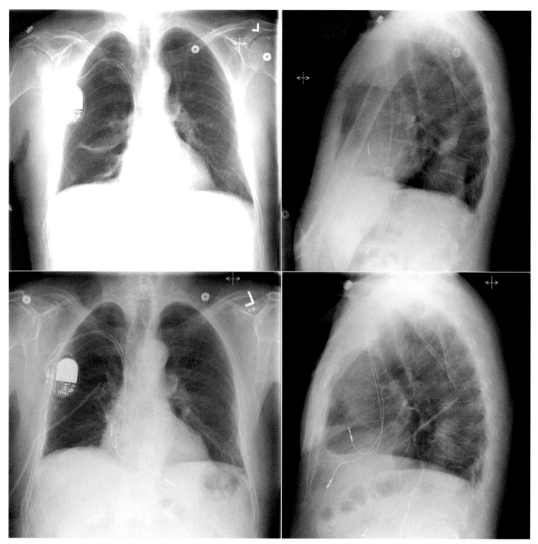

Figure 23-12. The upper radiographs show a moderate-sized right-sided pneumothorax due to insertion of a dual chamber pacemaker. Notably, the insertion was via the axillary vein, where pneumothoraces are rarely associated. The lower radiographs reveal resolution of the pneumothorax following insertion of a pleural catheter.

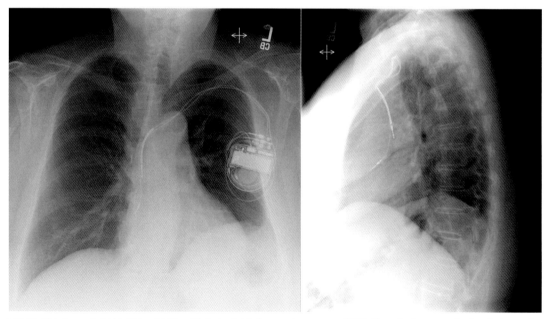

Figure 23-13. Dislodgement of right atrial and right ventricular leads into the superior vena cava (SVC). The patient was experiencing diaphragmatic pacing due to the stimulus of the vagus nerve in proximity to the ventricular lead in the SVC.

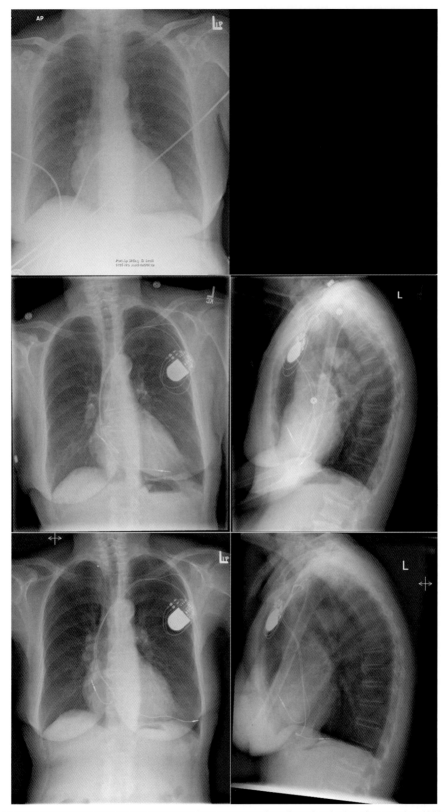

Figure 23-14. The evolving position of a pacer lead. The upper image is an anteroposterior radiograph at the time of presentation with high-degree atrioventricular block. The middle images are after insertion of a permanent dual chamber pacemaker, with the lead position correct. The lower images (taken 2 weeks later) are at the time of failure of the ventricular lead to capture. The ventricular lead has migrated though the right ventricular free wall and pericardium and is located against the pleura. There was no pericardial effusion or pneumothorax.

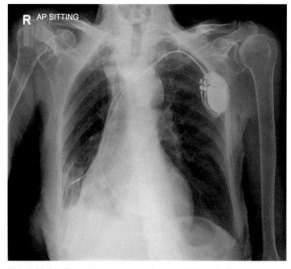

Figure 23-15. Frontal (anteroposterior) chest radiograph of a patient post–dual chamber pacemaker insertion. The right ventricular endocardial lead position is plausibly correct. The right atrial lead has migrated extravascularly or extracardiac into the left pleural space or lung. Note the associated left pleural effusion.

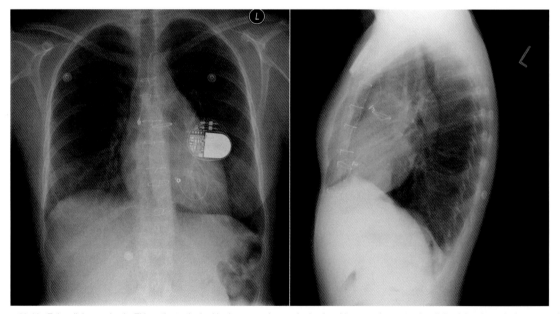

Figure 23-16. Epicardial pacer leads. This patient, who had had many endovascular lead problems, underwent epicardial atrial and ventricular pacemaker insertion at the time of a Bentall procedure. The sewing ring of the mechanical aortic valve prosthesis is apparent on the posteroanterior radiograph, and the sewing ring and occluders (in the closed position) are apparent on the lateral radiograph. The pacemaker box has migrated inferiorly through its pocket.

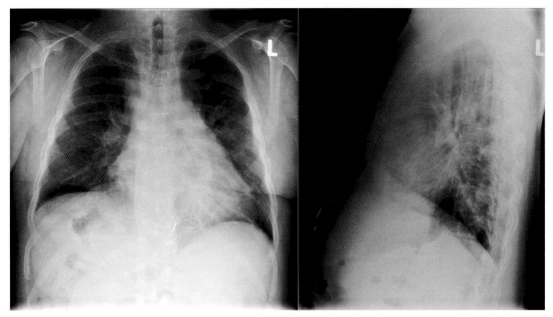

Figure 23-17. Poststernotomy posteroanterior and lateral chest radiographs of a patient with temporary epicardial pacer leads.

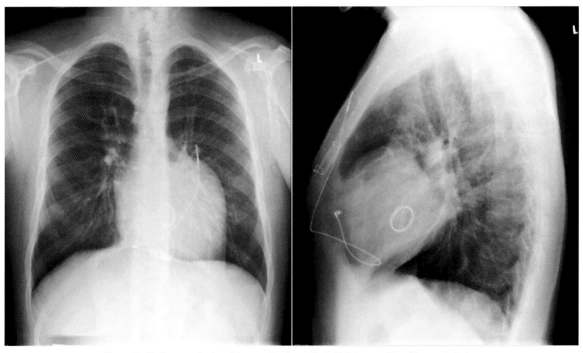

Figure 23-18. Permanent epicardial pacemaker in a patient with L-transposition of the great arteries.

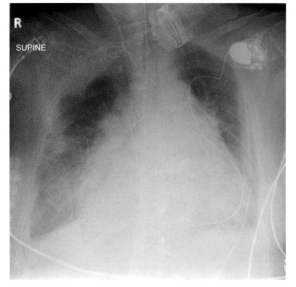

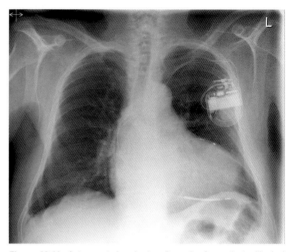

Figure 23-20. Anteroposterior chest radiograph of a patient with dual chamber and biventricular (coronary sinus lead seen along the anterolateral border of the heart) cardiac resynchronization pacing and without an implantable cardioverter defibrillator lead.

Figure 23-19. Anteroposterior chest radiograph of a postoperative patient with sternotomy wires, an endotracheal tube, chest tubes, a pulmonary artery catheter, and temporary epicardial pacemaker leads.

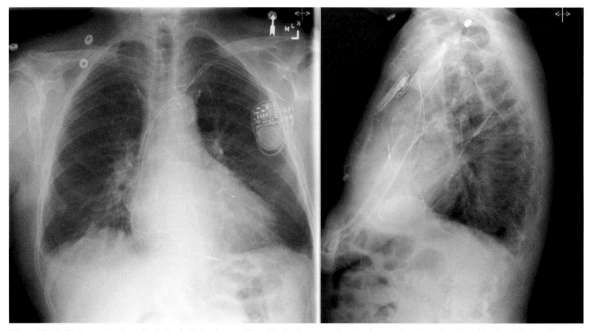

Figure 23-21. Radiographs of a patient with dual chamber and biventricular (coronary sinus lead seen along the anterolateral border of the heart) cardiac resynchronization pacing leads and also an implantable cardioverter defibrillator lead.

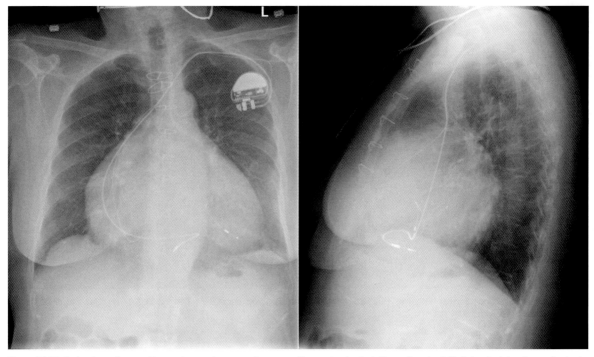

Figure 23-22. Ischemic cardiomyopathy, previous aortocoronary bypass grafting, and an implantable cardioverter defibrillator, dual chamber pacing leads, and a cardiac resynchronization therapy lead.

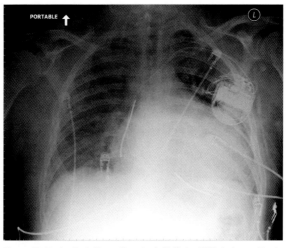

Figure 23-23. Implantable cardioverter defibrillator (ICD) device and leads. As is very common, given the indications for ICD insertion, there is associated significant cardiomegaly and left ventricular dysfunction bespoken by the presence of pulmonary edema.

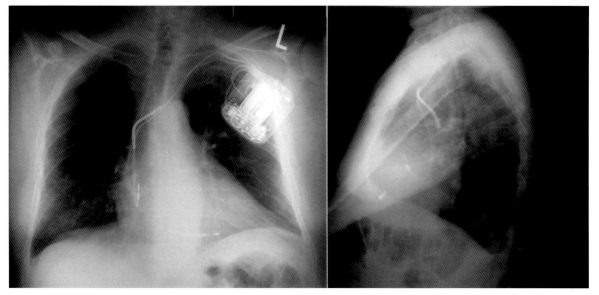

Figure 23-24. Implantable cardioverter defibrillator (ICD)/dual chamber pacer. The older era of the ICD is apparent by the large size of the device. The thicker shadow of one lead is the coil.

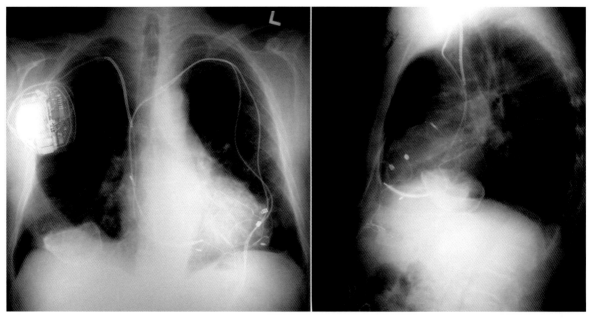

Figure 23-25. Implantable cardioverter defibrillator (ICD) with epicardial patch leads, epicardial pacer leads, and endocardial leads. The patient had previously undergone ICD insertion of patch electrodes via a small left thoracotomy with the leads tunneled from an upper abdominal site. The patches are apparent on both the posteroanterior and lateral views. The epicardial leads are the corkscrew-shaped devices. The system was subsequently revised with endovascular leads that were replaced from the left to the right subclavian site.

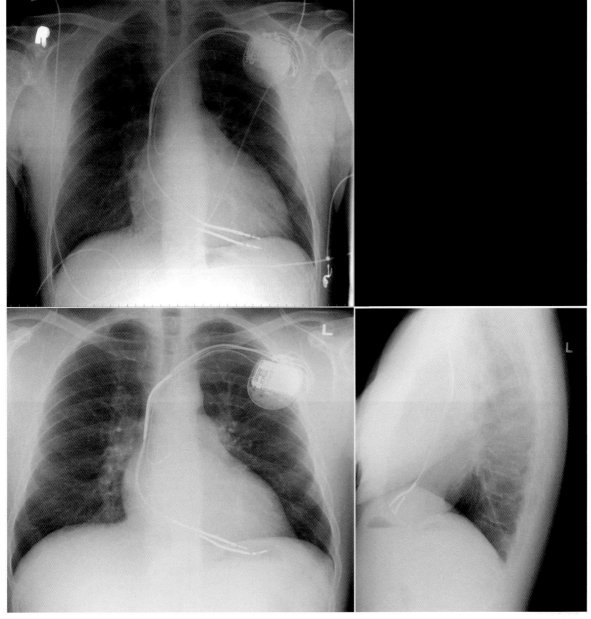

Figure 23-26. Implantable cardioverter defibrillator ventricular lead perforation into the pericardial space. In the upper image, the right atrial and right ventricular leads are in the correct position following ventricular lead revision (insertion of a second lead prompted by defectiveness of the first lead). In the lower images, a few weeks later, the ventricular pacing lead is dysfunctioning and the QRS capture pattern has changed. The ventricular lead had perforated the right ventricular apex and migrated 2 cm further through the pericardial space, without causing a pericardial effusion.

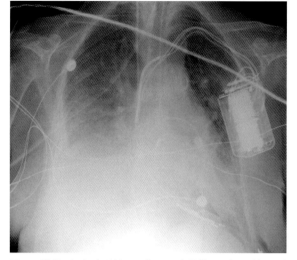

Figure 23-31. An implantable cardioverter defibrillator of an older and larger design. There is one atrial lead and two ventricular leads. The patient, in severe heart failure, is intubated for ventilatory support with a pulmonary artery line.

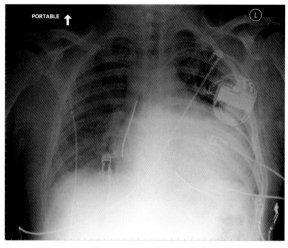

Figure 23-32. A typical implantable cardioverter defibrillator–related chest radiograph, with cardiomegaly due to the underlying heart disease, dual chamber pacing leads, and obvious coils on the ventricular lead. There is radiographic evidence of left-sided heart failure as well.

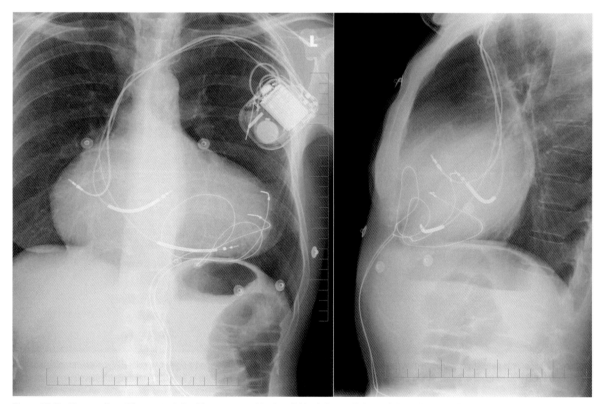

Figure 23-33. Transposition of the great arteries. There are two old epicardial leads inserted via an abdominal pocket. There is a dual chamber pacemaker/implantable cardioverter defibrillator (ICD) and an old ICD lead that has been displaced.

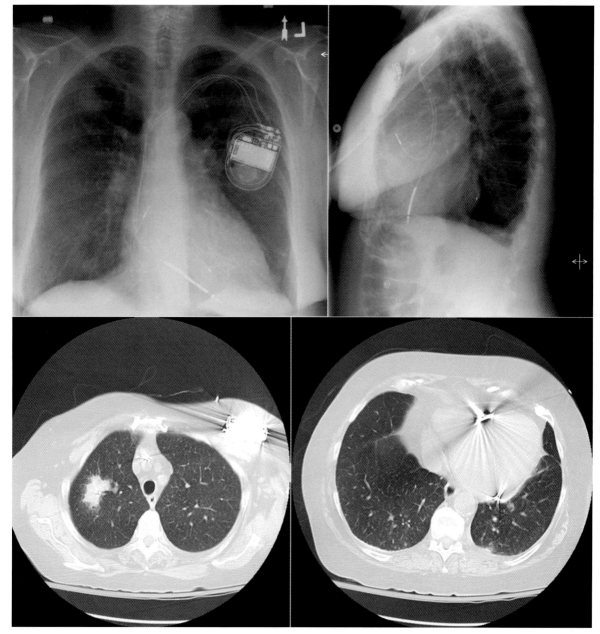

Figure 23-34. In addition to the cardiomegaly, implantable cardioverter defibrillator (ICD), dual chamber pacer, and cardiac resynchronization therapy leads, there is generalized prominence of the interstitium of the lungs and pulmonary infiltrates, the most obvious of which is in the right upper lobe. The interstitial prominence and infiltrates are well depicted on computed tomography scanning. In the context of the enlarged heart, ICD, and pulmonary markings, amiodarone lung disease was probable given the pre-ICD use of amiodarone.

24 Percutaneously and Surgically Inserted Ventricular Assist Devices

Key Points

- Intra-aortic balloon pump position is readily verified by chest radiography, because the tip is radiopaque. The tip should be located at the very distal aortic arch or proximal descending aorta.
- Percutaneously inserted ventricular assist devices are radiographically apparent, and at least in a comparative sense, their position can be verified by chest radiography.
- The positions of cannulae of extracorporeal membrane oxygenation (ECMO) systems can be verified by abdominal and chest radiography.
- The cannulae of ventricular assist devices are also radiographically apparent.

PERCUTANEOUS DEVICES

Pulsatile Devices: Intra-aortic Counterpulsation Balloon (Figs. 24-1 to 24-7)

The tip of an intra-aortic balloon (which is highly visible because of its metallic marker) should be at least 4 cm below the "knuckle" of the aorta (i.e., below the left subclavian artery). The balloon appears as a cylindrical lucency if the radiographic exposure happened to be while it was inflated in diastole. Widening or haziness of the aorta suggests aortic dissection as a complication of the catheter. Incorrect insertion into the inferior vena cava is suggested by the shadow of the catheter lying to the right of the patient's vertebral column.

Continuous Flow Devices: Impella 2.5

The Impella 2.5 (2.5 L/minute support), a continuous flow ventricular assist device, provides continuous flow assist comparable to that of intra-aortic balloon pump. It is percutaneously inserted from the groin. Radiographically and fluoroscopically, the pigtail tips are apparent, the mechanical intake device and the mechanical output device are obvious and the conduit between the two is fairly obvious, and the more proximal catheter is marked by a faint radiopaque stripe. The pigtail tip holds the intake back from the apical wall; the intake housing draws ventricular cavity blood into it, and the output housing with the impeller pump draws blood through the intake housing and

ejects it into the aortic root on the far side of the aortic valve, offloading and resting the left ventricle. On a frontal radiograph, the pigtail is directly left inferiorly and the conduit initially follows the same line before it angulates vertically or vertically/leftward up the aortic root.

SURGICALLY INSERTED VENTRICULAR ASSIST DEVICES

There are several models of surgically inserted (left and right) ventricular assist devices with widely different designs and radiographic appearances.

Impella 5.0

The Impella 5.0 (5.0 L/minute support) is inserted by surgical cutdown or via sternotomy (Graphic 24-1; Figs. 24-8 to 24-13). There are two models. The Impella 5.0 is similar to that described previously. The Impella 5.0 LD is similar but without the pigtail component.

Extracorporeal Membrane Oxygenation

ECMO is a means of temporarily providing blood oxygenation and cardiac output supplementation (Figs. 24-14 and 24-15). It is used to provide oxygenation support during expected to be reversible syndromes of acute lung injury where mechanical ventilation either is not able to provide adequate oxygenation or airway pressures are prohibitive.

The usual configuration supplies continuous venovenous flow:

- Two afferent cannulae (28F via the right and left femoral veins; one of the two may be advanced into the right atrium)
- One afferent cannula (28F inserted via the left subclavian vein into the innominate vein or superior vena cava)
- Extracorporeal membrane oxygenator and roller pump

The cannulae are radiographically obvious in the femoral, iliac, and subclavian veins. They may be somewhat obscured by attenuation by the spine and heart in the right atrium.

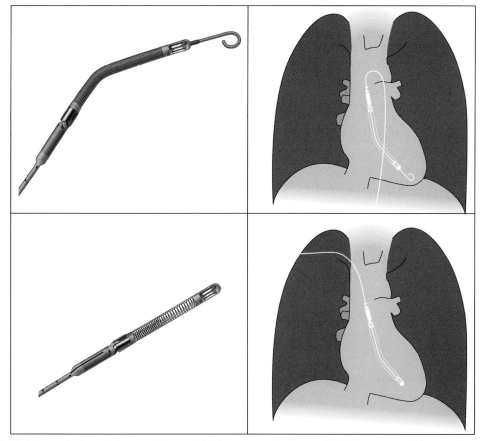

Graphic 24-1. Illustrations and schematic diagrams of the Impella 5.0 (*upper images*) and the Impella LD (*lower images*). Note that the Impella 5.0, like the Impella 2.5, has a distal pigtail component. The position of the Impella devices involves straddling the aortic valve such that the intake and output components are on either side of the valve.

Thoratec HeartMate XVE

The Thoratec HeartMate XVE left ventricular assist device is an earlier device (first inserted in 1991) that consists of a blood chamber, inflow and outflow conduits each containing a 25-mm porcine valve within a Dacron tube, and a blood chamber/pulsatile pump capable of delivering more than 80 mL of stroke volume at variable rates (Graphics 24-2 and 24-3; Figs. 24-16 to 24-18). The blood chamber pump is powered via an electrical cable. The afferent intake is typically via a Dacron tube graft from the left ventricular apex and it connects directly to the blood chamber/pump. The blood is returned via a longer Dacron tube graft, usually to the ascending aorta.

Thoratec HeartMate II

The Thoratec HeartMate II is a contemporary model of ventricular assist device that uses a magnetic levitating impeller that delivers variable continuous flow (Figs. 24-19 to 24-23). Smaller and lighter than the Thoratec XVE model, the HeartMate II is more portable.

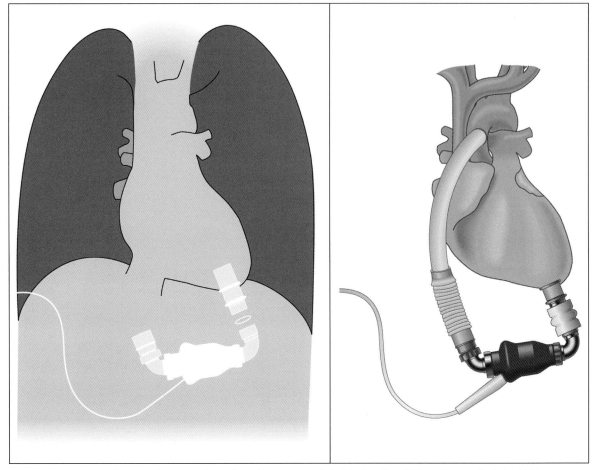

Graphic 24-2. Schematic illustrations of the radiographic appearance (*left*) of the HeartMate II left ventricular assist device (*right*).

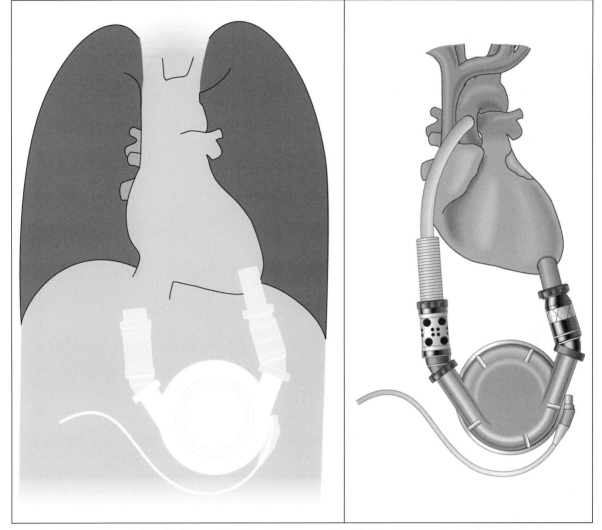

Graphic 24-3. Schematic illustration images of the radiographic appearance (*left*) of the HeartMate XVE left ventricular assist device (*right*).

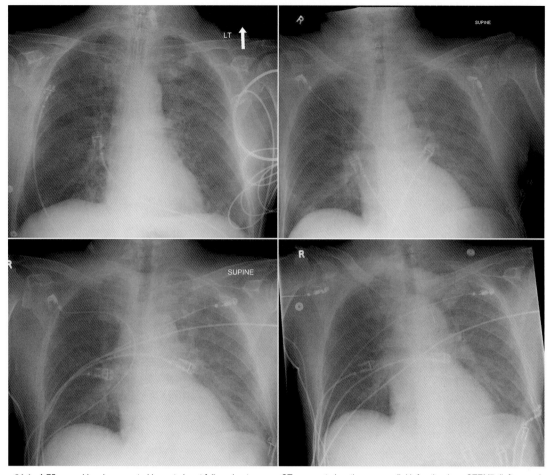

Figure 24-1. A 75-year-old male presented in acute heart failure due to a non–ST-segment elevation myocardial infarction (non-STEMI) *(left upper image)*. He underwent coronary angiography, which revealed an occluded right coronary artery and 95% left mainstem stenosis. An intra-aortic balloon pump was inserted, with the radio-opaque tip verified to be in the correct position *(right upper image)*, and cardiac surgery consulted. The patient stood up at the bedside, despite the inserted balloon pump. Chest radiography revealed its acquired malposition with the radio-opaque tip visualized in the lower thoracic aorta *(left lower image)*; it was repositioned at the bedside. Follow-up chest radiography demonstrated that the tip is slightly high in the aorta and deflected medially by the aortic wall *(right lower image)*. Note the difference in the upper and lower right images with respect to the balloon pump tip marker position.

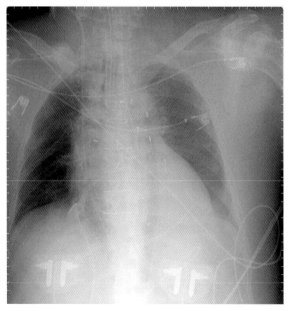

Figure 24-2. The radiographically apparent intra-aortic counterpulsation balloon catheter tip is in the correct position. By chance occurrence, the radiograph was obtained in early or mid-diastole when the balloon was inflated, and the size and length of the balloon are apparent. The endotracheal, nasogastric, and chest tubes are in the correct positions.

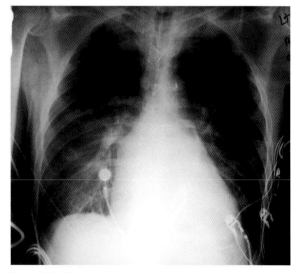

Figure 24-3. The intra-aortic counterpulsation balloon catheter tip is too high, as the marker is at the top of the distal arch.

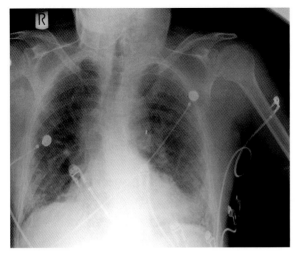

Figure 24-4. The intra-aortic counterpulsation balloon catheter is slightly low; the tip of the marker is a few centimeters lower than the aortic arch.

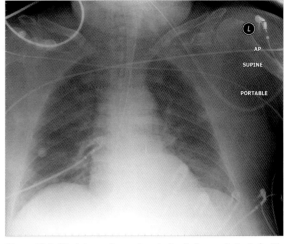

Figure 24-5. The intra-aortic counterpulsation balloon catheter is frankly low; the tip of the marker is multiple centimeters lower than the distal aortic arch. The endotracheal and nasogastric tubes are in the correct positions.

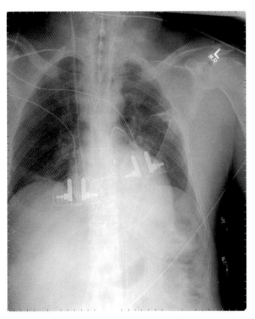

Figure 24-6. The intra-aortic counterpulsation balloon catheter tip is low; the tip of the marker is multiple centimeters lower than the distal aortic arch. The endotracheal, nasogastric, and chest tubes, as well as the pulmonary artery catheter are in the correct positions.

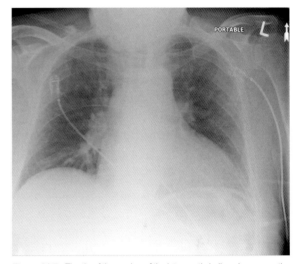

Figure 24-7. The tip of the marker of the intra-aortic balloon is seen on the right side of the heart, and the aortic arch is left-sided. The tip lies in the right atrium due to misinsertion into the femoral vein, not the femoral artery.

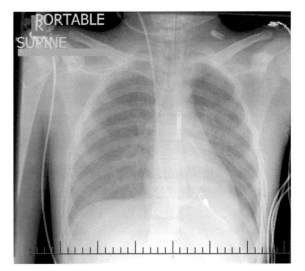

Figure 24-8. Impella left ventricular assist device, as well as an endotracheal tube and pulmonary artery catheter.

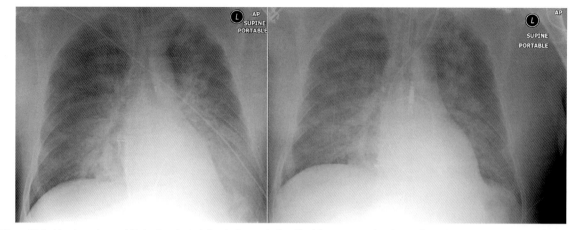

Figure 24-9. Massive anteroseptal infarction due to left mainstem occlusion. The left anteroposterior chest radiograph reveals normal heart size, severe interstitial and airspace pulmonary edema, and an intra-aortic balloon tip marker in good position. The right anteroposterior chest radiograph reveals the same cardiac findings and some improvement of pulmonary edema infiltrates. A pulmonary artery catheter has been inserted, and its tip is in good position. There has been insertion via the groin of an Impella 5.0 left ventricular assist device, whose tip crosses the aortic valve into the left ventricular outflow tract.

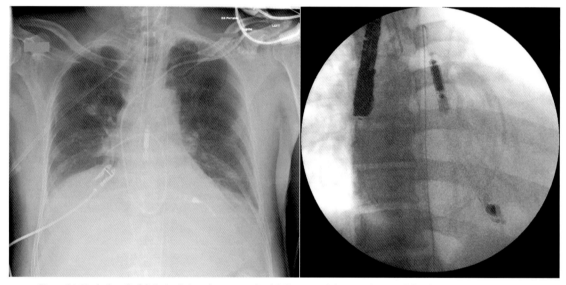

Figure 24-10. An Impella 5.0 device that can be seen on the right fluoroscopic image to have partially migrated back into the aorta.

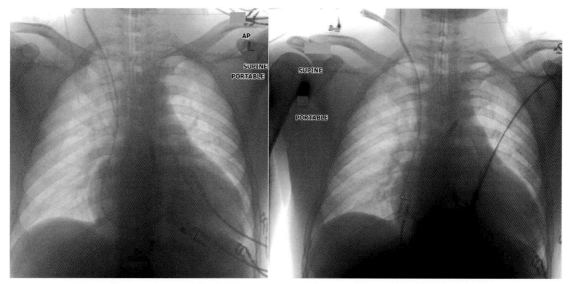

Figure 24-11. An Impella 5.0 device well into the left ventricular cavity, resulting in partial flexion of the pigtail tip.

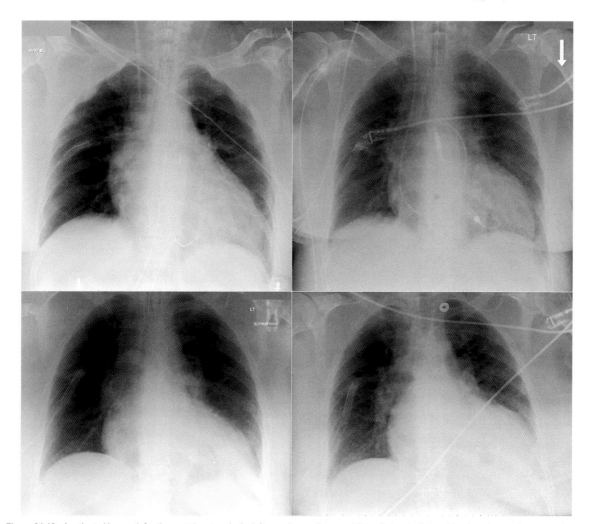

Figure 24-12. A patient with a postinfarction septal rupture. In the left upper image, there are bilaterally inserted internal jugular vein central venous catheters and a left subclavian vein inserted catheter, all in good position. The patient is intubated, in heart failure, and with bilateral chest tubes. The tip of the intra-aortic balloon pump (IABP) is a bit low. In the right upper image, the IABP, left chest tube, and left subclavian and internal jugular central venous catheters have been removed. An Impelia 5.0 left ventricular assist device has been inserted via the right subclavian artery, and a pulmonary artery catheter has been inserted and is properly positioned in the main pulmonary. The lower images show post–Amplatzer device closure of the ventral septal rupture. Unfortunately, the heart failure is seen to have continued to progress.

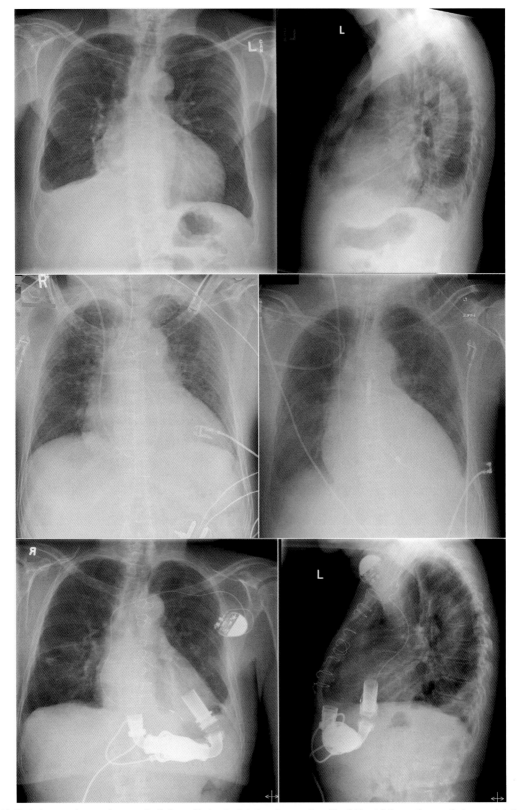

Figure 24-13. In the upper images, there are the findings of ischemic dilated cardiomyopathy with mild heart failure, subsequently bypassed. In the middle images, there is much worsened heart failure, resulting in admission. In the left middle image, there is congestive heart failure, endotracheal intubation, a pulmonary artery catheter, and an intra-aortic balloon pump (IABP) as hemodynamic support. There has been little improvement in the heart failure. In the right middle image, an Impella 5.0 device has replaced the IABP as hemodynamic support. There has been improvement in the heart failure. In the lower images (same admission), hemodynamic support now involves a HeartMate II device, and further significant improvement in the left-sided heart failure has occurred.

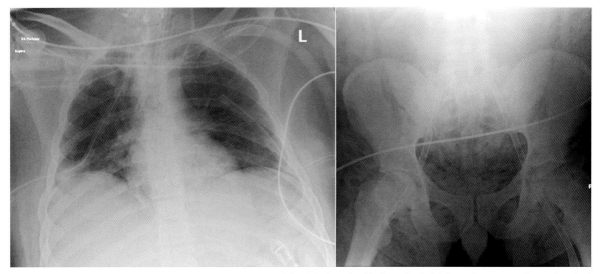

Figure 24-14. Extracorporeal membrane oxygenation catheters via the left subclavian vein, right femoral vein, left femoral artery, as well as endotracheal tube, bilateral chest tubes, and extensive subcutaneous emphysema are present.

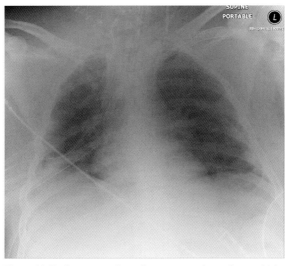

Figure 24-15. Extracorporeal membrane oxygenation catheters via the left subclavian vein and via a femoral vein into the right atrium, as well as endotracheal tube, bilateral chest tubes, and a central line via the left jugular vein are present.

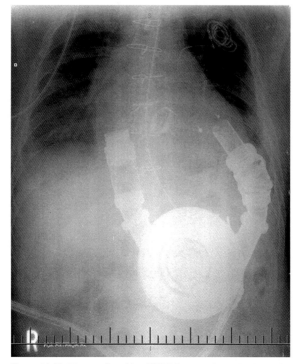

Figure 24-16. Thoratec HeartMate XVE left ventricular assist device following implantation of a Perimount mitral valve bioprosthesis.

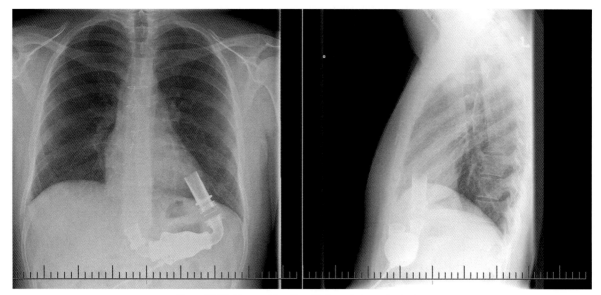

Figure 24-17. Thoratec HeartMate II left ventricular assist device.

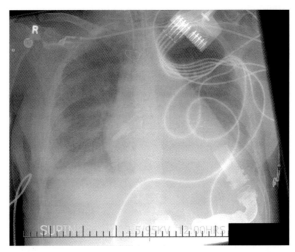

Figure 24-18. HeartMate II and Impella RD right ventricular assist devices. There are also sternotomy wires, and endotracheal and nasogastric tubes.

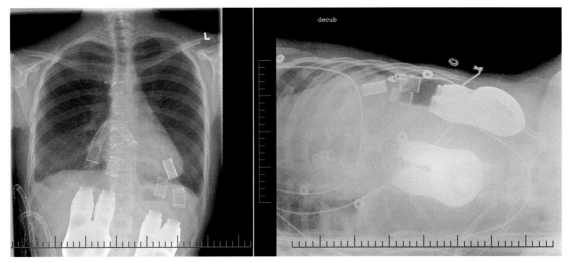

Figure 24-19. Cannulae and pumps of Thoratec biventricular assist devices.

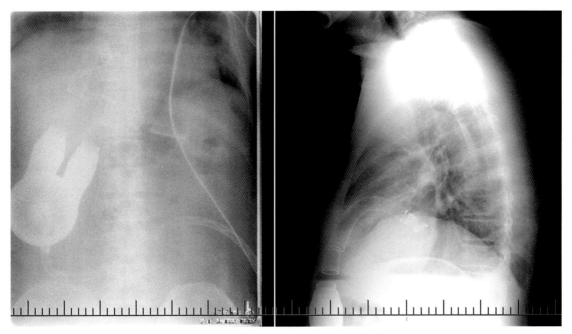

Figure 24-20. Thoratec right ventricular assist device.

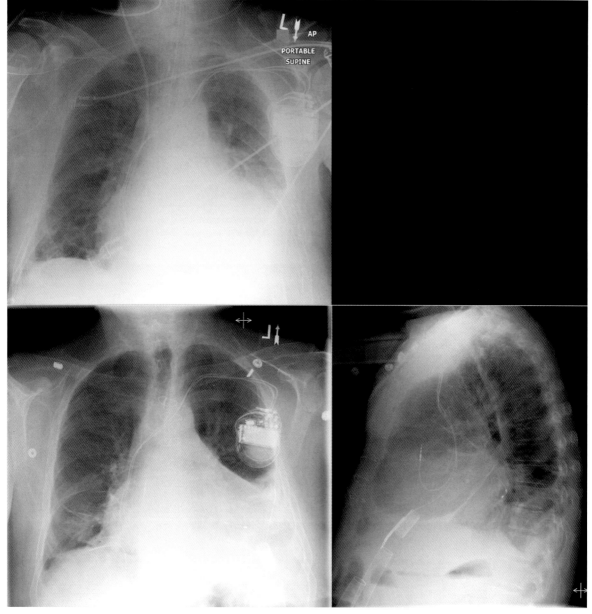

Figure 24-21. Before (*upper image*) and after (*lower images*) insertion of a Thoratec left ventricular assist device. With the assist device in situ, the heart failure findings have improved. As well, there are an implantable cardioverter defibrillator and biventricular/three-chamber pacemaker.

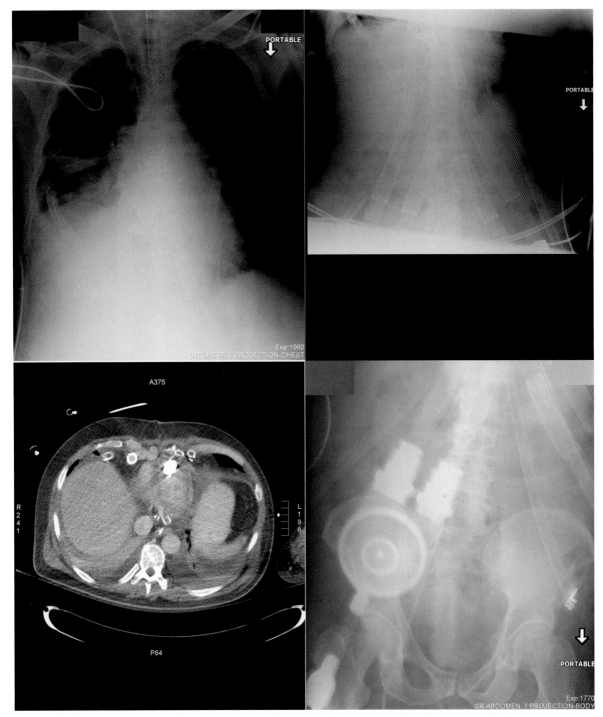

Figure 24-22. The anteroposterior chest radiograph and abdominal flat plate reveal the cannulae of a left ventricular assist device. The computed tomography scan reveals the cannulae within the heart.

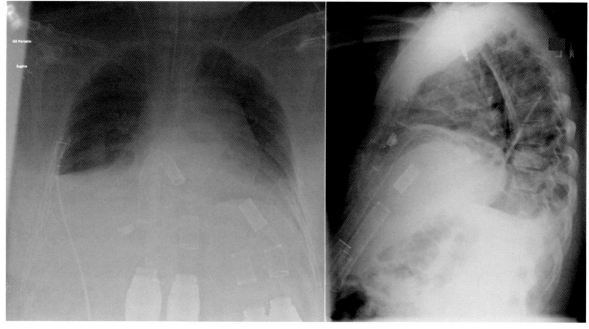

Figure 24-23. Biventricular assist devices.

Tubes and Drains

ENDOTRACHEAL TUBE

Because correct positioning of the endotracheal (ET) tube is of such major clinical importance, there is a radiopaque stripe along the length of the tube to facilitate visualization. The other aspect of the ET tube that is easily visualized is the air cuff, which confers a rounded lucency several centimeters proximal to the tip. The ideal position of the tip of the ET tube is 5 cm proximal to the carina, so that the balloon cuff is safely beyond the vocal chords and the tip is safely away from the carina. The position of the tip of the ET tube is dependent on the position of the chin/neck and varies by about 2 cm, depending on the amount of flexion/extension of the neck, and by up to 1 cm, depending on the rotation of the neck (Table 25-1).

Therefore, the tip of the ET tube should be at least 2 cm proximal to the carina. Overinsertion of the ET tube may selectively intubate the right mainstem bronchus with the risk of overinflating the right lung and hypoventilating the left lung.

Complications of Endotracheal Intubation
Complications of intubation (Figs. 25-1 to 25-10) and ventilation that are apparent on a chest radiograph are often potentially life-threatening and should be excluded on every radiograph, both immediately following intubation and with each subsequent radiograph. These possibilities are listed in the following sections.

Right Mainstem Bronchus Intubation
❐ Location of the tip of the ET tube
❐ Possible overinflation of the right lung
❐ Possible volume loss of the left lung

Bronchus Intermedius Intubation
(This involves deep intubation of the right mainstem bronchus with the tip beyond the take-off of the upper lobe bronchi.)
❐ Location of the tip of the ET tube
❐ Possible volume loss of the right upper lobe

❐ Possible overinflation of the right lower and middle lobes
❐ Possible volume loss of the left lung

Barotrauma
❐ Pneumothorax
❐ Pneumomediastinum
❐ Pneumopericardium
❐ Subcutaneous emphysema

Hypopharyngeal Tear (Traumatic Intubation)
❐ Subcutaneous emphysema of the neck
❐ Possible pneumomediastinum
❐ Pneumothorax

Esophageal Intubation
❐ Distension of esophagus and stomach with air
❐ Location of ET tube to the side of the trachea

Cuff Overinflation
❐ The walls of the trachea should not be distended outward by the cuff. Distension is overinflation.
❐ Width of the ET tube two thirds of the width of the trachea

TRACHEOSTOMY TUBES

Tracheostomy tubes are placed to maintain airway adequacy over the long term. Advantages of tracheostomy tubes over ETs include avoidance of vocal cord complications, maintenance of the ability to eat, and the fact that the neck position does not influence the tip of the tube within the trachea. The tip of the tracheostomy tube should be one half to one third of the distance between the carina and the tracheostomy ostia. The tracheostomy tube cuff should hug, but not distend, the walls of the trachea. A chest radiograph is indicated after insertion to exclude complications. After that, a chest radiograph is indicated only to address specific suspected complications.

CHEST TUBES

All chest tubes have a radiopaque strip on the side to aid in their visualization (Figs. 25-11 and 25-12). They have a hole at the tip and side perforations that are apparent on a chest radiograph as interruptions of the radiopaque strip. All the side holes should be within the chest cavity.

Pleural tubes and drains (Fig. 25-13) that are placed through a subxiphoid approach normally lie inferiorly and posteriorly in the recesses of the chest cavity, beside the vertebral column, to evacuate fluid that will accumulate in the dependent part of the chest cavity in a supine or semisupine patient. Pleural tubes that are placed through an intercostal incision should similarly lie inferiorly and superiorly. Most chest tubes work well even away from the standard position. An increasing pneumothorax, or one that fails to resolve with a pleural tube in place, suggests failure of the chest tube system or a persistent air leak.

Pericardial tubes and drains (Figs. 25-14 to 25-21) may be placed after open heart surgery or after percutaneous drainage. A small amount of pneumopericardium may be seen following either procedure. An increasing pneumopericardium suggests failure of

the tube system, persistent air leak within the chest cavity, or gas-forming bacterial pericarditis.

Mediastinal tubes (Fig. 25-22) are placed routinely at the end of cardiac surgery. Usually, one or two tubes are used: a straight tube placed anteriorly and an angled tube placed over the diaphragm.

NASOGASTRIC AND FEEDING TUBES (Figs. 25-23 to 25-31)

Malposition of a nasogastric tube is common. The most distal side hole (about 10 cm proximal to the tip) should be within the stomach itself. Malposition of small feeding tubes is common. Malposition within the bronchus intermedius or left lower lobe bronchus is common. Pressure on the nasogastric tube while within a bronchus may cause it to migrate through the lung into the pleural space, resulting in a pneumothorax and bronchopleural fistula.

TABLE 25-1	Neck and ET-Tube Tip Positions	
NECK POSITION	**INFERIOR BORDER OF MANDIBLE**	**DISTANCE FROM CARINA (cm)**
Extension	At or below C4 vertebra	7 ± 2
Neutral	At C5 or C6 vertebra	5 ± 2
Flexion	At or below T1 vertebra	3 ± 2

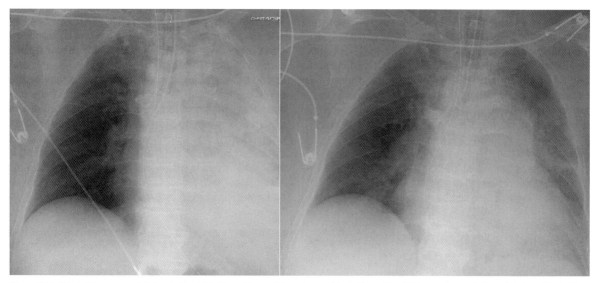

Figure 25-1. The left image reveals left mainstem intubation, with complete collapse of the left lung. The right image demonstrates reinflation of the left lung following withdrawal of the endotracheal tube (tip) into the trachea.

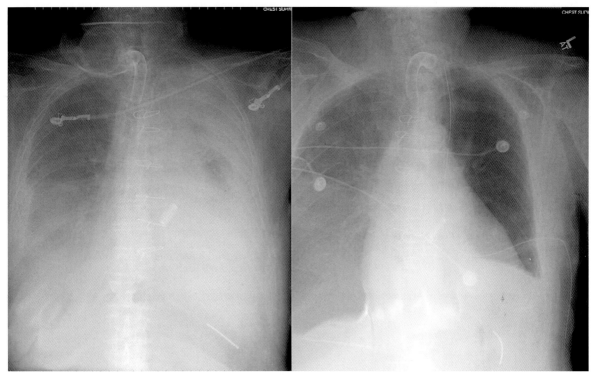

Figure 25-2. The left anteroposterior chest radiograph is post–aortic valve replacement, showing endotracheal intubation via tracheostomy for chronic respiratory failure. The left lung has collapsed due to bronchial plugging. The right anteroposterior chest radiograph is following chest tube insertion and reexpansion of the left lung.

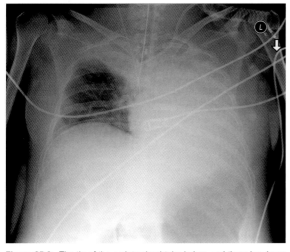

Figure 25-3. The tip of the endotracheal tube is low, and there has been complete collapse of the left lung. The volume of the right lung is small due to the intubation of the bronchus intermedius to the exclusion of the right upper lobe.

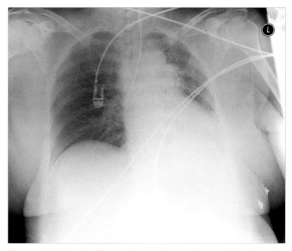

Figure 25-4. The tip of the endotracheal tube is low, and there is partial collapse of the left lung as well as leftward displacement of the heart and mediastinum.

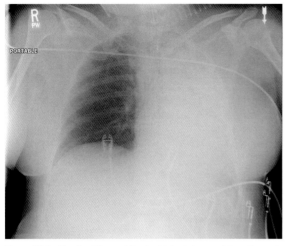

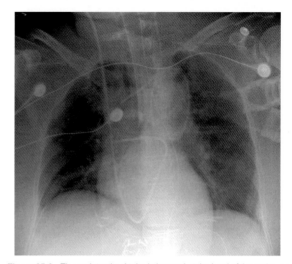

Figure 25-5. The tip of the endotracheal tube is low, and there is nearly complete collapse of the left lung with shift of the heart and great vessels into the left hemithorax.

Figure 25-6. The endotracheal tube is low and at the level of the carina or just into the right mainstem bronchus. The patient is severely rotated, but the positions of the pulmonary artery line and the left internal jugular central venous lines appear to be correct.

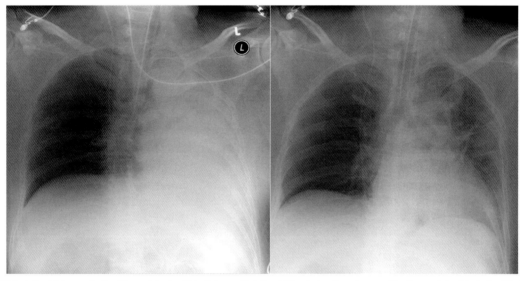

Figure 25-7. In the left image, the tip of the endotracheal tube is low and into the right mainstem bronchus, resulting in complete atelectasis of the left lung. In the right image, the left lung is again ventilated and has reexpanded after withdrawal of the endotracheal tube.

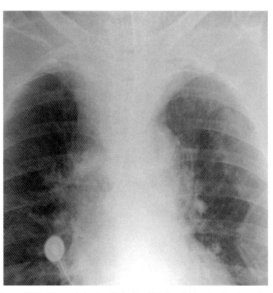

Figure 25-8. The endotracheal tube is within the right mainstem bronchus.

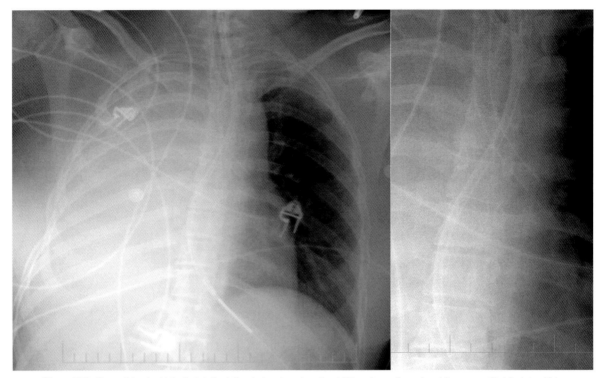

Figure 25-9. The endotracheal tube tip is in the left mainstem bronchus, the right lung has collapsed, and the nasogastric tube is too high.

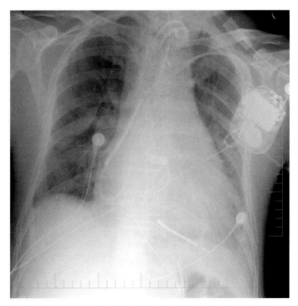

Figure 25-10. Tracheostomy tube, sternotomy wires, implantable cardioverter defibrillator and atrial pacemaker leads, mechanical mitral and aortic valve prostheses, right subclavian central venous line, chest tube, and a nasogastric tube.

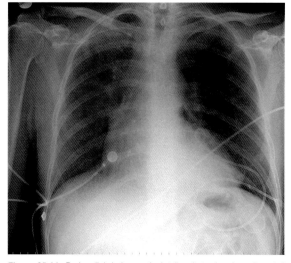

Figure 25-14. Pericardial drainage. A pigtail catheter has been inserted via an anterior intercostal approach into the pericardial cavity, uncomplicated by pneumothorax or left pleural effusion.

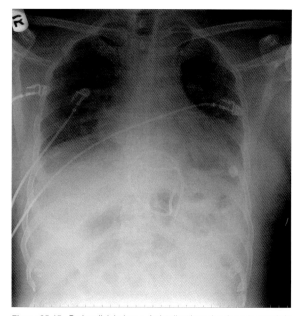

Figure 25-15. Pericardial drainage. A pigtail catheter has been inserted via the traditional xiphocostal approach into the pericardial cavity.

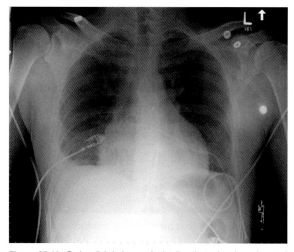

Figure 25-16. Pericardial drainage. A pigtail catheter has been inserted via an anterior/apical intercostal approach into the pericardial cavity, uncomplicated by pneumothorax or left pleural effusion.

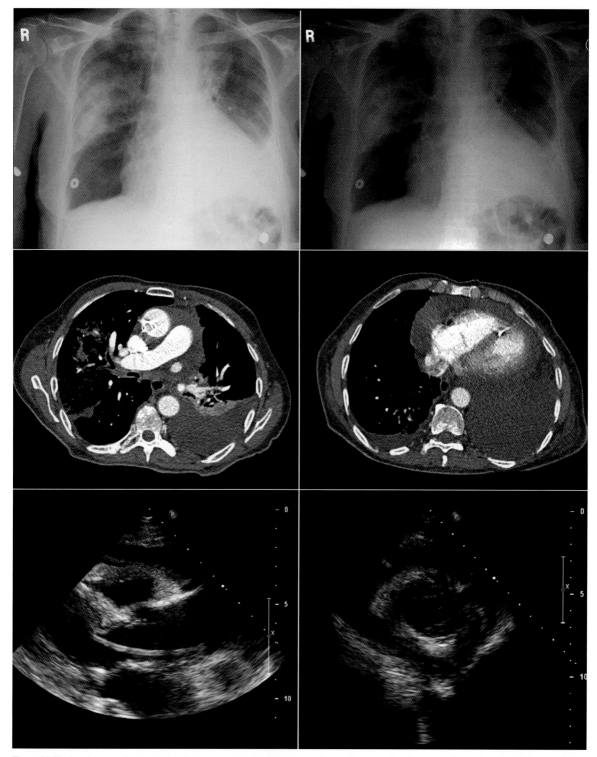

Figure 25-17. A patient with disseminated malignancy and a pericardial drain inserted to alleviate pericardial tamponade. On the chest radiographs (*upper images*) and with "windowing," the position of the pericardial drain is unremarkable. On the axial contrast-enhanced computed tomography scans (*middle images*), the drain pigtail is within the ascending aorta and has entered the left ventricle via the apical interventricular septum. On the transthoracic echocardiographic long axis (*lower left*) and short axis (*lower right*) images, the drain is seen to be within the ascending aorta and to be oriented on the short axis view too directly toward the heart, because it was indeed perforating it.

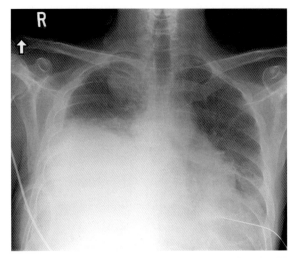

Figure 25-18. An 8-Fr pigtail drain has been inserted within the pericardial space. There is a large right pericardial effusion.

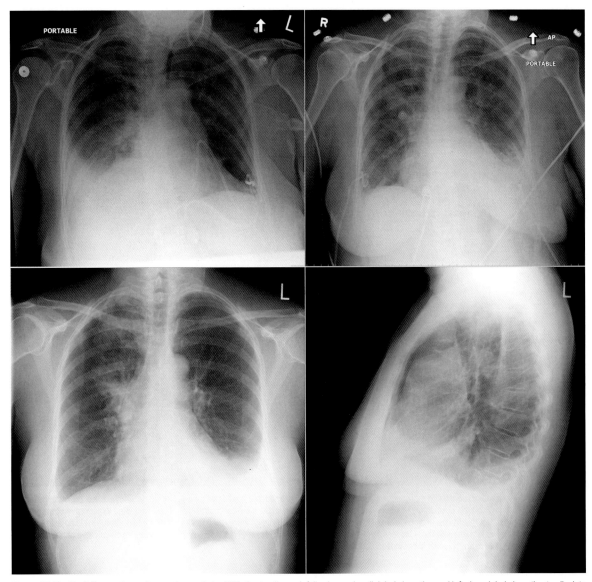

Figure 25-19. The left upper image is an anteroposterior (AP) chest radiograph following pericardial drain insertion and left pleural drain insertion to alleviate (1) the hemodynamics of tamponade due to metastatic adenocarcinoma and (2) dyspnea due to a large left pleural effusion. A right pleural effusion persists. The right upper image is an AP chest radiograph following insertion of a right pleural drain and after withdrawal of the pericardial drain. The lower images are posteroanterior and lateral chest radiographs following removal of all drains, with the right upper lobe mass lesion and the origin of the pleural and pericardial and other metastases evident.

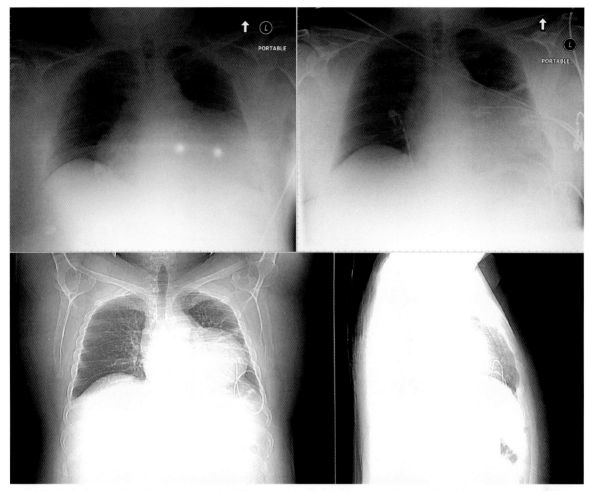

Figure 25-20. The left upper image is an anteroposterior (AP) chest radiograph of a patient presenting with pericardial tamponade. Note the markedly enlarged and globular shape of the heart, with normal lung fields. The right upper image is an AP chest radiograph following insertion of a pericardial drain via an apical approach. The lower images are computed tomography scout views that reveal the pericardial drain somewhat better.

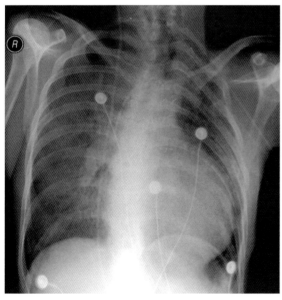

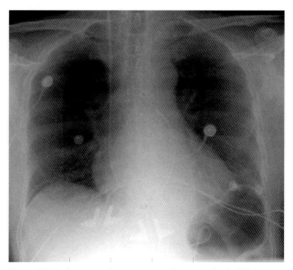

Figure 25-22. Post–open heart surgery, with two mediastinal drains and epicardial pacer wires.

Figure 25-21. There is a ventriculoperitoneal shunt and a central venous line in proper position. The chest wall is dysplastic, and there has been a prior sternotomy and pulmonary valve replacement.

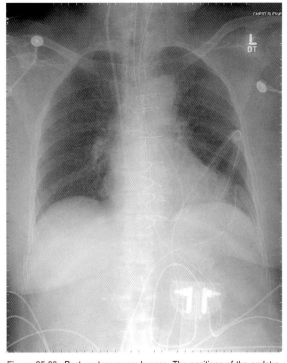

Figure 25-23. Post–aortocoronary bypass. The positions of the endotracheal tube, nasogastric tube, pulmonary artery catheter, and chest tube are all normal.

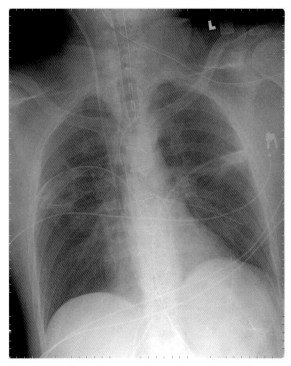

Figure 25-24. Post–aortocoronary bypass. The positions of the endotracheal tube, pulmonary artery catheter, and chest tube are all normal. The nasogastric tube, however, has been inserted down the trachea, and the tip is down the left bronchi into the left lower lobe.

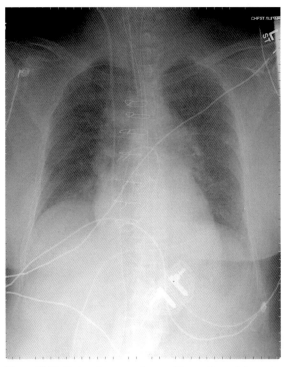

Figure 25-25. Post–aortocoronary bypass. The positions of the endotracheal tube, pulmonary artery catheter, and chest tube are all normal. The nasogastric tube, however, has looped within the esophagus.

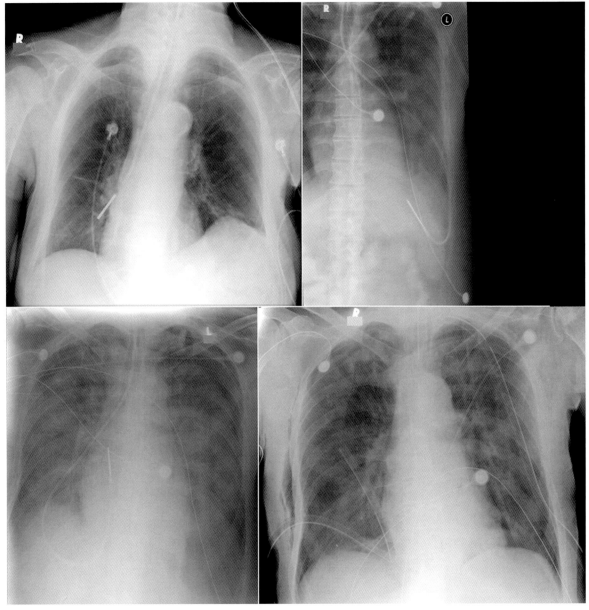

Figure 25-26. Feeding tube misadventures. In the right upper image, the feeding tube has been inserted into the right mainstem/right lower lobe bronchus. In the left upper image, the feeding tube has been repositioned and is now in the left pleural space. In the left lower image, the feeding tube has again been repositioned and is in the right pleural space. In the right lower image, bilateral chest tubes have been inserted to rectify the bilateral pneumothoraces that ensued from the feeding tube malpositions.

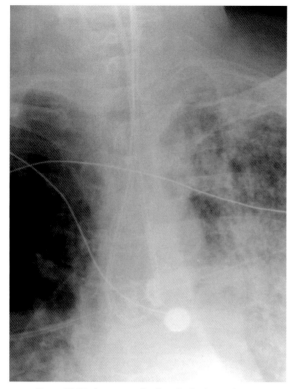

Figure 25-27. An nasogastric tube coiled in the esophagus.

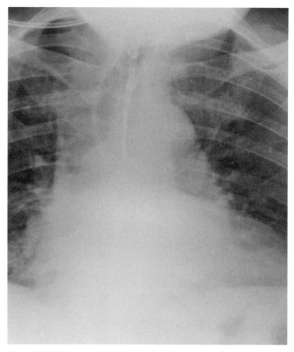

Figure 25-28. A nasogastric tube in the esophagus, although it appears to be in the trachea.

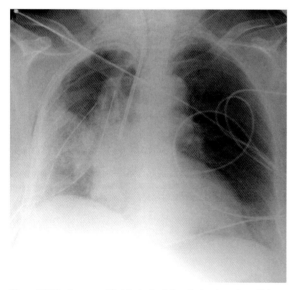

Figure 25-29. A nasogastric tube in the left mainstem bronchus. Note as well the central venous line inserted via the left subclavian vein, into a small systemic vein rather than the innominate vein. Two right-sided chest tubes are also present.

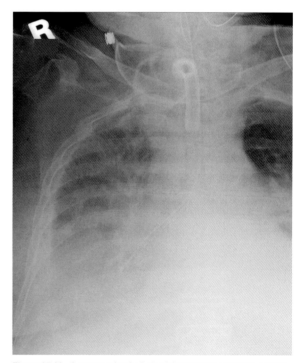

Figure 25-30. A nasogastric tube in the right mainstem bronchus. A tracheostomy tube is present as well.

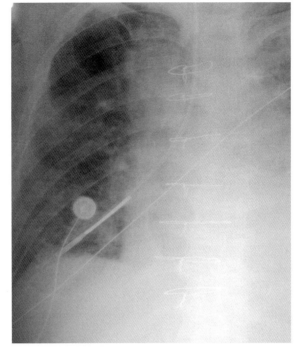

Figure 25-31. A feeding tube well into the right lower lobe bronchus.

26 Postoperative Patients in the Intensive Care Unit

Key Points

- Chest radiography is a key diagnostic test in the coronary care unit (CCU) and intensive care (ICU) unit.
- Chest radiography is a standard admission test in both venues.
- Chest radiography plays an important role in the following:
  - Identifying and monitoring pulmonary parenchymal and pleural sequelae to surgery and complications of heart disease
  - Identifying and monitoring the position of central venous lines and cannula, the endotracheal tube, chest drains, and pacemaker leads
- Common chest radiographic findings in patients in the CCU or ICU include the following:
  - Atelectasis
  - Pleural effusions
  - Pulmonary edema
  - Air collections
  - Diaphragmatic paralysis

CHEST RADIOGRAPHY IN THE CORONARY CARE AND INTENSIVE CARE UNITS

Routine Use of Chest Radiography

A chest radiograph on admission to the CCU is appropriate, if not mandatory. Subsequent radiographs are performed according to the clinical evolution of the patient and the need to monitor treatment effect.

The benefit of routine (i.e., daily, morning) chest radiography in the ICU is controversial. Several studies have described unexpectedly high detection rates of clinically unsuspected findings that have resulted in changes in management. Other studies have reported higher rates of therapeutic management, altering findings when the study was performed because of a change in a patient's condition. More recent studies have seriously challenged the belief that routine chest radiography makes a contribution, citing that the only scenarios where important observations are made with any frequency were in patients post–Swan-Ganz insertion, in those post–endotracheal intubation, and in those with suspected new pathophysiologic slates.

COMMON CHEST RADIOGRAPHIC FINDINGS IN PATIENTS IN THE CORONARY CARE AND INTENSIVE CARE UNITS

Atelectasis

Atelectasis is less common in the CCU setting than in the ICU setting, unless the patient is bedridden, has lung disease, is elderly, or is mechanically ventilated. The likelihood and severity of atelectasis is proportional to the amount of time the patient is in bed. The left lower lobe is most frequently affected (67% of cases) compared with the right lower lobe (about 25%) and the right upper lobe (10%). Left lower lobe atelectasis following cardiac surgery may result from (left) phrenic nerve paralysis as a result of the surgery, or from compression by the heart in the opened chest of the left lower lobe.

Atelectasis is commonly seen following surgery and may be seen in any patient in the ICU. Thoracic (especially cardiac) and upper abdominal surgery are common backgrounds for development of atelectasis. Underlying chronic lung disease, a smoking history, obesity, increasing ventilation time, and advanced age are all risk factors for the development of atelectasis. More than several days of atelectasis increases the risk of pneumonia.

The chest radiograph is much less sensitive than a computed tomography scan for the detection of atelectasis postcardiac surgery. Therefore, normal appearing lungs on chest radiography do not exclude clinically relevant atelectasis. Chest radiographic findings on atelectasis are as follows:

- Normal-appearing lung (which is the most common appearance)
- Linear/platelike/patchy infiltrates
- Lobar consolidation
- Volume loss

Pleural Effusions

Pleural effusions are commonly seen in patients with congestive heart failure, following surgical (thoracic and abdominal surgery) interventions and in the general ICU population.

Enlarging effusions suggest ongoing congestive heart failure, hemorrhage, or infection. Late-developing pleural effusions may be seen with the postpericardiotomy syndrome. Moderate and large effusions are readily appreciated on an anteroposterior or posteroanterior chest radiograph. Very small effusions (i.e., about 150 mL) are seen better by lateral decubitus radiographs than by erect or supine radiographs, and they are best detected by ultrasound or cardiac magnetic resonance imaging.

Pulmonary Edema (Fig. 26-1)

The portable chest radiograph may be unreliable in depicting the usual signs of pulmonary edema and distinction of cardiogenic and noncardiogenic edema is often difficult. In a supine patient, venous redistribution is normal and therefore, is not a useful sign. Portable chest radiographs are usually anteroposterior, therefore increasing the depiction of heart size and rendering assessment of true heart size more difficult.

Air Collections (Fig. 26-2)

Patients on positive end-expiratory pressure (PEEP) ventilation run the risk of barotrauma that may result in abnormal air collections within the chest cavities and chest wall (pneumomediastinum, pneumothorax, pneumopericardium, and subcutaneous emphysema). An erect radiograph should be taken whenever a pneumothorax is suspected. The size of a pneumothorax correlates fairly well with its clinical importance.

It is noteworthy that in the supine patient air collections in the pleural space collect superiorly and anteriorly, making radiographic depiction difficult because the collection is seen en-face and not edge-on.

Mechanical ventilation often rapidly increases the size of a pneumothorax, culminating in a tension pneumothorax in many patients. It is important to recall that tension pneumothorax is a clinical diagnosis as the radiographic findings in ventilated patients are not sufficiently reliable. Pleural adhesions and PEEP may annul apparent shift of the mediastinum (which otherwise would be a good sign of tension pneumothorax). Depression of the ipsilateral hemidiaphragm, flattening of the heart border, and compression of vascular structures (such as the superior and inferior vena cava) are probably superior signs of tension pneumothorax. Air collection at the base of the lung may produce a prominent visualization of the diaphragmatic sulcus—the "deep sulcus sign."

Diaphragmatic Paralysis

Diaphragmatic paralysis (Fig. 26-3), which may occur because of disease or as a complication of sternotomy, results in persistent elevation of the hemidiaphragm. Absence of motion of the diaphragm is not well detected by routine chest radiographs, and its confirmation requires fluoroscopy or ultrasound.

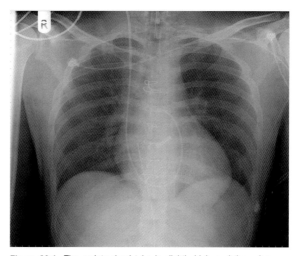

Figure 26-1. The endotracheal tube is slightly high, and the pulmonary artery catheter is in the correct position. A bileaflet occluder aortic mechanical prosthesis is seen projecting partially over the spine, but the Dacron tube graft of the composite aortic valve/root replacement (Bentall procedure), for acute dissection in Marfan syndrome, is not. There is very mild left-sided heart failure.

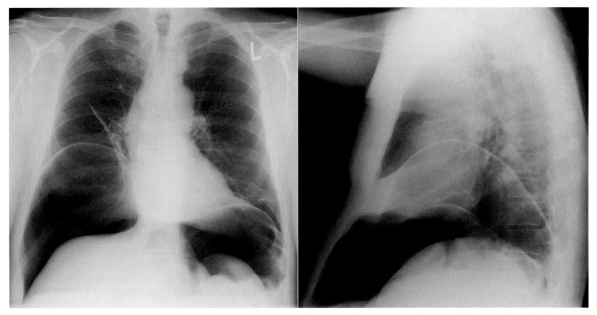

Figure 26-2. A large amount of pneumoperitoneum (seen as lucent air over the liver and under the diaphragm) has resulted in elevation of the diaphragms, especially the right one, resulting in volume loss of the right lung.

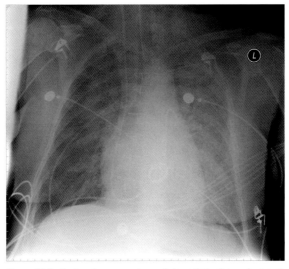

Figure 26-3. Post–aortocoronary bypass/prior mitral valve replacement. The endotracheal tube is slightly high, and the pulmonary artery catheter and chest tube in the pericardial space are in the correct position. A single tilting disk Björk-Shiley mechanical prosthesis in the mitral position is seen projecting to the left of the spine. There is pulmonary edema and a left pleural effusion.

27 | Cardiac and Vascular Calcification

TECHNICAL ISSUES

Cardiac and vascular calcifications are always signs of disease and are therefore noteworthy.

Cardiac and vascular calcification is often better appreciated with an overexposed radiograph and is best appreciated when seen on a tangential plane, thus rendering the calcification very dense and therefore visually more obvious. When seen en-face, a layer of calcification is visible at its thinnest and is therefore least apparent. Superimposition of other shadows (the heart itself, or in particular, the spine) often, if not usually, obscures calcification that would be apparent if projected free of other structures. Areas to scrutinize are those with greater likelihood to calcify (the aortic and mitral valves and annuli, the left ventricular walls, the diaphragmatic pericardial surface, and atrioventricular grooves), and those areas where calcification is most readily appreciated.

SITES OF CARDIAC CALCIFICATION

Pericardial Calcification
Pericardial calcification (Figs. 27-1 to 27-4) is most prominent in the interventricular and atrioventricular grooves, and lateral to the right atrial and ventricular walls (Graphic 27-1). When looking for pericardial calcification, it is necessary to scrutinize the lateral chest radiograph well, particularly the diaphragmatic surface.

Pericardial calcification does not usually involve the left heart as much the right heart, and it does not often involve the apex (which, if calcified, is far more often due to prior infarction). Pericardial calcification should prompt serious consideration of the diagnosis of constrictive pericarditis, and clinicians should seek other radiographic and clinical features of constriction.

Myocardial Calcification (Figs. 27-5 to 27-9)
A calcified ventricular aneurysm is seen as a fine dense line when viewed on edge and is consistent with an old transmural infarction. On the frontal chest radiograph, an anterolateral, or apical, calcified aneurysm may be visible. Rarely, a calcified septal aneurysm may be seen on a lateral chest radiograph. Myocardium may calcify following traumatic injury as well as postinfarction.

Left Ventricular Apical Calcification
This finding suggests a calcified old infarction or calcified organized intraluminal apical thrombus within the aneurysm.

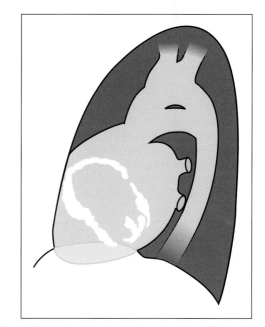

Graphic 27-1. Lateral chest projection: pericardial calcification. Note the extensive plaquelike calcification, depicted principally in the atrioventricular grooves.

Mitral Annular Calcification (Figs. 27-10 to 27-15)

On the frontal chest radiograph, mitral annular calcification (MAC), also referred to as submitral calcification, is generally seen as a crescentic reverse C or occasionally as an O. Calcification of the annulus may occur as a primary abnormality and not extend onto the mitral valve leaflets; thus, the presence of MAC correlates poorly with functional disturbances of the mitral valve. It is most common in elderly female patients and in individuals with renal failure and causes little associated functional disturbance. However, MAC may be associated with, or occasionally cause, mitral insufficiency. The greater the circumference of the annulus that is calcified, the greater the likelihood of an associated functional disturbance.

Left Atrial Mural Calcification

Left atrial mural calcification is an uncommon finding (Figs. 27-16 and 27-17). It is seen as a thin line on the roof of the left atrium when viewed tangentially on the lateral chest radiograph. Left atrial wall calcification nearly always occurs in the setting of severe mitral stenosis with chronic marked left atrial dilation. The atrium is thereby noncompliant, and tolerates mitral insufficiency poorly.

Calcified Left Atrial Thrombus

A calcified left atrial thrombus is seen as a rocklike structure, appearing as a mass, in the left atrium. It is an uncommon finding of advanced mitral stenosis and usually appears as a lobulated rounded mass.

Left Atrial Appendage Calcification

Left atrial appendage calcification is exceedingly rare but may be seen on the frontal chest radiograph. It occurs again in the setting of chronic mitral valve disease (usually stenosis).

Valves

See Chapter 8 for identification of valves by location on the lateral chest radiograph.

Radiographic evidence of aortic valve calcification strongly suggests obstruction at the level of the aortic valve in patients (particularly females) younger than 60 years of age. Calcification most commonly affects the aortic valve but may also involve the mitral apparatus and annulus. On the frontal chest radiograph, the aortic valve projects onto the spine and is easily missed unless the lateral chest radiograph is scrutinized. The mitral valve projects partially onto the spine on the frontal chest radiograph and again should be sought on both the frontal and lateral radiographs. An imaginary line drawn from the left mainstem bronchus to the sternodiaphragmatic angle usually distinguishes the aortic valve (above this line) from mitral (beneath this line). The right-sided valves have little, if any, tendency to calcify in a radiographically apparent way.

Mitral Valve Calcification

Calcification of the mitral valve itself is usually caused by rheumatic disease. It appears as a lumplike mass.

Aortic Valve Calcification

Aortic valve calcification is not uncommon in older individuals and may or may not be associated with aortic stenosis in patients older than 65 years of age, In younger patients (i.e., 40 years of age), aortic valve calcification is often associated with aortic stenosis (Graphic 27-2).

Coronary Artery Calcification

Coronary artery calcification is increasingly common with advancing age, and it has a fair, but not strong, association with obstructive disease of the coronary arteries (except in patients younger than 50 years of age, where the association is stronger). The proximal coronary arterial segments calcify the most frequently. The left anterior descending artery is the most frequently calcified of the three coronary arteries. It is necessary to look for "train tracks" (parallel lines) when the artery is projected side-on and for "rings" when the artery is seen end-on.

SITES OF VASCULAR CALCIFICATION

See Figures 27-18 to 27-23 and refer back to Figures 27-14 to 27-17 and Graphic 27-2.

Aortic Calcification

See Chapter 7 for further discussion of the thoracic aorta. Age-related calcification of the aorta is very common and is seen as a fine thin arc within the aortic "knob." Plaquelike and denser calcification of the aorta is usually caused by atherosclerosis but may also be caused by syphilis or aortic vasculitis. Calcification due to atherosclerosis is most often appreciated on the frontal chest radiograph and is seen in the distal aortic arch and proximal descending aorta (see Graphic 27-2). Calcification due to atherosclerosis resides in intimal plaques and therefore serves as a marker of the inner surface of the aorta, such that aortic wall thickness can be estimated when the diagnosis of aortic dissection is sought (see Graphic 7-3).

Aortic Annular Calcification

Aortic annular calcification generally occurs in older individuals and appears as an irregular ring. It is often associated with calcification of the aortic leaflets.

Pulmonary Artery Calcification

Pulmonary artery calcification (Figs. 27-24 and 27-25) is seen only in the presence of severe pulmonary hypertension and often in association with atherosclerosis of the pulmonary arteries. Calcification of the pulmonary arteries may also occur after reparative surgery.

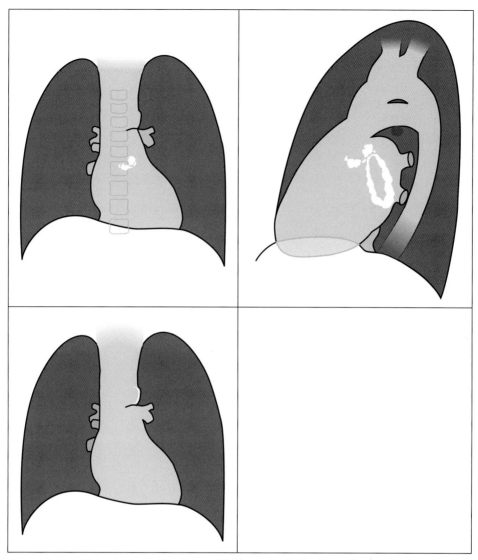

Graphic 27-2. Posteroanterior and lateral chest projections. *Upper left:* Aortic valve calcification (may project over the spinal column). *Upper right:* Aortic valve and mitral annular calcification. The shadow of the right mainstem bronchus is included. *Lower left:* Aortic intimal calcification is best seen in the lateral wall and floor of the aortic "knob."

Calcification of a Patent Ductus Arteriosus

Calcification of a patent ductus arteriosus is a common finding when a ductus arteriosus is detected in adulthood, because the ductal tissue has an avid tendency to calcify. Calcification of a ductus implies patency of the ductus (see Chapter 7).

Rare Causes of Cardiac Calcification

These causes include the following:
- ❏ Calcified myxoma (10% of myxomas)
- ❏ Calcified thrombus in the left atrium or left ventricle
- ❏ Calcified echinococcal cyst
- ❏ Calcified myocardial or pericardial tuberculoma
- ❏ Calcified left ventricular wall from Loeffler eosinophilic fibroelastosis
- ❏ Calcified sinuses of Valsalva

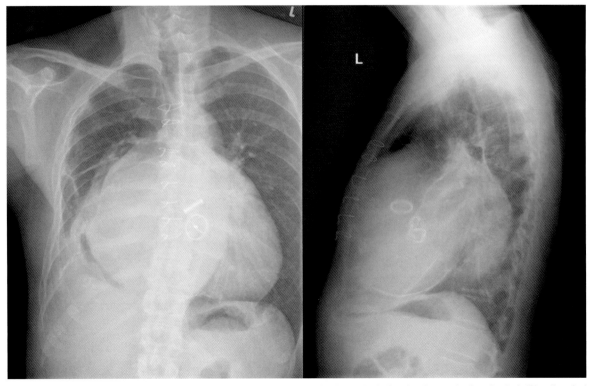

Figure 27-1. Posteroanterior (PA) and lateral chest radiographs of a patient with a bileaflet mechanical aortic valve prosthesis and a single tilting disc mitral prosthesis of the Medtronic-Hall type. There is marked cardiomegaly in particular with massive enlargement of the left atrium, right atrium, and right ventricle. Somewhat visible on the PA radiograph, but much more visible on the lateral chest radiograph, is a peel of pericardial calcification best seen tangentially along the diaphragmatic surface of the heart. The patient was subsequently proven at surgery to have pericardial constriction as a result of having multiple previous valvular surgeries. As well, there is right pleural calcification.

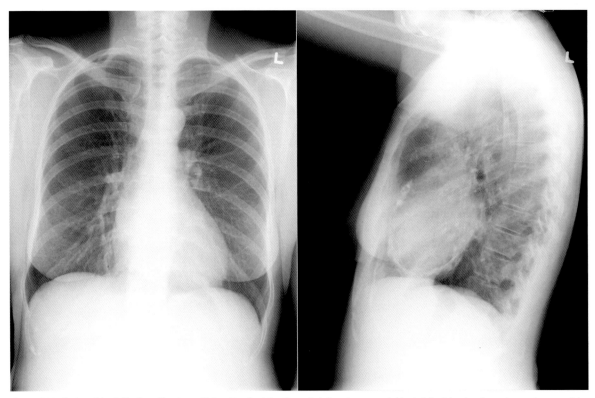

Figure 27-2. Pericardial calcification without constriction. The frontal radiograph is largely unremarkable, but the lateral radiograph reveals a surprising amount of pericardial calcification. The patient, despite having this degree of pericardial calcification, did not have constrictive physiology.

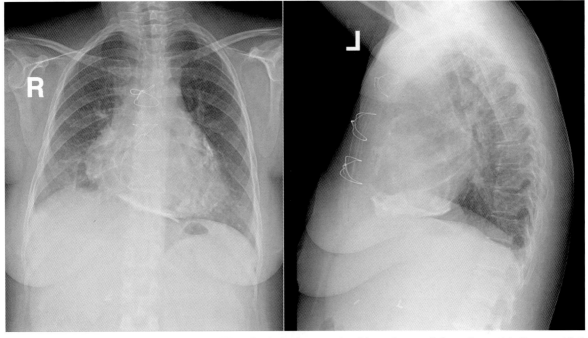

Figure 27-3. Residual calcification postpericardiectomy. This patient had undergone pericardial resection years before and presented with recurrent findings. There was prominent pericardial calcification, particularly under the heart, where pericardiectomy is often incomplete.

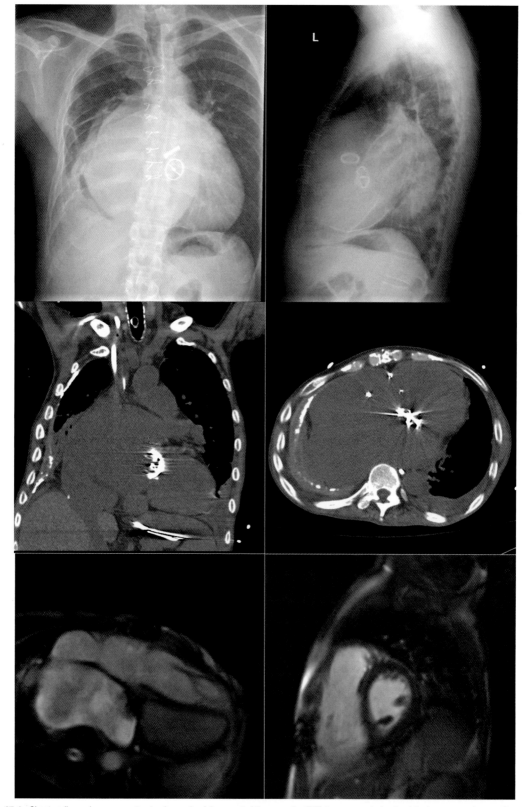

Figure 27-4. Chest radiographs, non–contrast-enhanced axial computed tomography (CT) images, and steady-state free precession cardiac magnetic resonance (CMR) images of a patient with an aortic bileaflet occluder prosthesis and a Medtronic-Hall mitral prosthesis. There are multiple signs of left atrial dilation: a bump at the left upper heart border from left atrial appendage dilation, gross splaying of the carina, a displaced right heart border, and narrowing of the main bronchi. Apparent on the lateral radiograph and non–contrast-enhanced CT scan images is pericardial calcification, a result presumed to be from three prior cardiac surgeries. The calcification is low signal and virtually inapparent on CMR imaging.

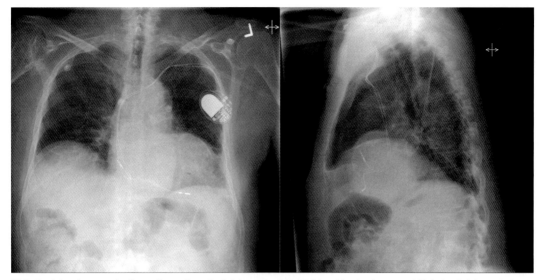

Figure 27-5. Dual chamber pacer leads, cardiomegaly, and a bulging and calcified left heart border due to a calcified chronic left ventricular aneurysm. As are often associated with left ventricular aneurysms, there are signs of heart failure.

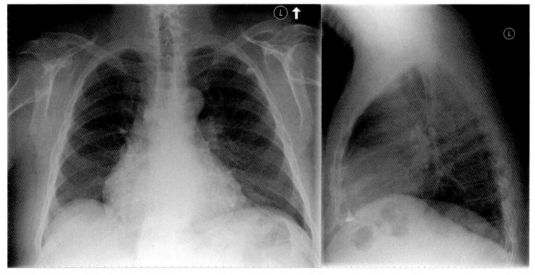

Figure 27-6. A calcified postinfarction left ventricular aneurysm. The cardiothoracic ratio is increased and there is pulmonary vascular congestion with indistinct hila and peribronchial cuffing. On both the frontal and lateral radiographs, a mostly fine thin "shell" of calcification is visible—a calcified left ventricular apical aneurysm. The left upper heart border is straightened by left atrial appendage enlargement, consistent with the pulmonary venous congestion from the left ventricular failure.

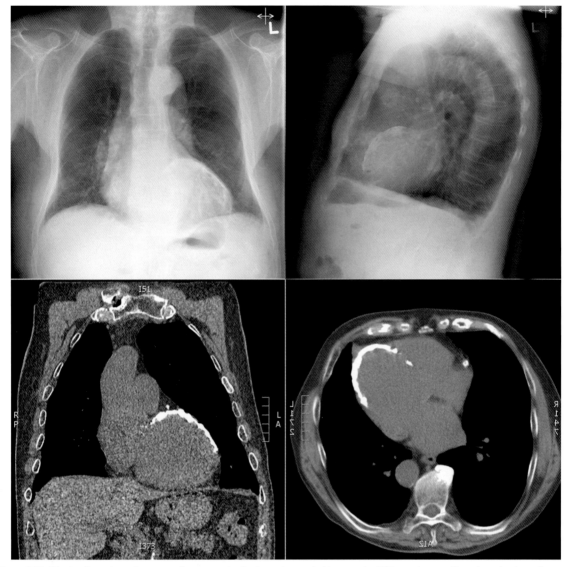

Figure 27-7. Chest radiographs and corresponding non–contrast-enhanced computed tomography (CT) scan images. There is moderate cardiomegaly and a very prominent shell of calcification of an aneurysm of the left ventricle over its anterior and lateral walls. The calcification is faintly and elegantly seen on the chest radiographs and rather heavily and coarsely seen on the non–contrast-enhanced CT scan images due to partial volume averaging CT artifact.

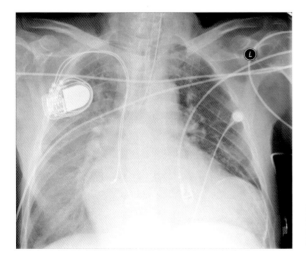

Figure 27-8. There is a right-sided dual chamber pacemaker, and endotracheal tube lying low at the carinal level, with electrocardiogram electrodes over the heart. There is moderate cardiomegaly and a faintly but definitely visible rounded left ventricular calcified apical aneurysm.

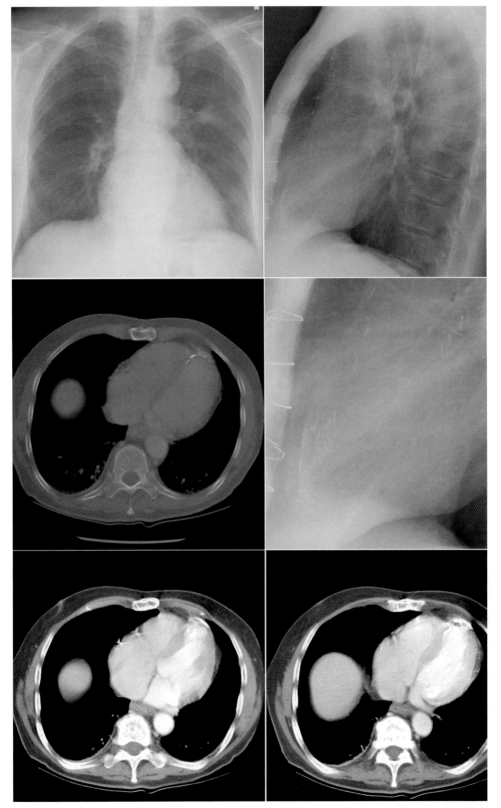

Figure 27-9. The posteroanterior chest radiograph is notable for sternotomy wires and a long length of vascular clips along a mobilized left internal thoracic artery. Only on the lateral chest radiograph is calcification of a left ventricular apical aneurysm apparent; it is seen on the zoomed image (*middle right image*). The computed tomography scans corroborate the calcification of the chronically infarcted myocardium.

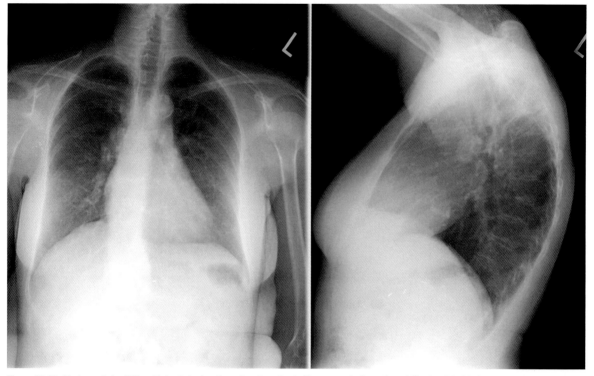

Figure 27-10. Posteroanterior (PA) and lateral chest radiographs of a patient with severe mitral annular calcification. It is faintly seen on the PA radiograph projecting slightly to the left of the spine. It is better seen on the lateral radiograph (as an upward oriented C shape), because it does not project over the spine on the lateral projection.

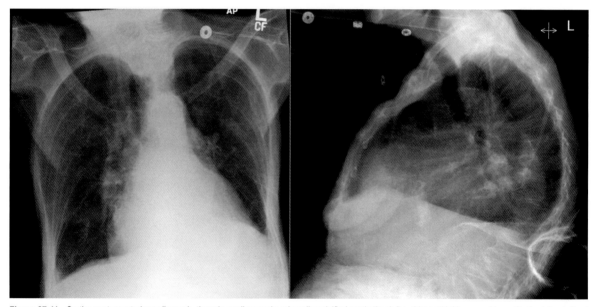

Figure 27-11. On the posteroanterior radiograph, there is cardiomegaly, a heavily calcified aortic "knob," and interstitial lung markings. On the lateral chest radiograph, the extensive calcification of the aorta is seen as well, as is a striking band of mitral annular calcification.

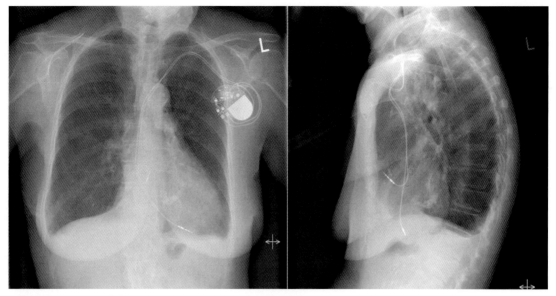

Figure 27-12. Posteroanterior (PA) and lateral views postinsertion of a dual chamber pacemaker. Note the lack of an implantable cardioverter defibrillator coil. The distal aortic arch is extensively calcified. To the left of the vertebral column on the PA radiograph is a reverse C-shaped calcified mass, typical of submitral/mitral annular calcification. It is also well seen on the lateral radiograph and appears again with a reverse C shape.

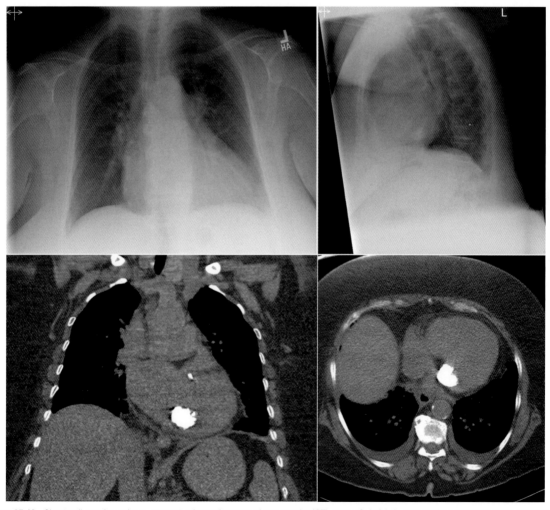

Figure 27-13. Chest radiographs and non–contrast-enhanced computed tomography (CT) scans. Only faintly seen on the posteroanterior radiograph, but better seen on the lateral chest radiograph, is a pin-pong ball–sized radiopaque mass in approximately the position of the mitral annulus but without the crescent shape typical of submitral calcification (mitral annular calcification). The radiopacity of the cardiomegaly and, due to obesity, is partially obscuring the calcified lesion on the radiographs. There is calcified plaque at the distal aortic arch. The CT views corroborate the calcium content of the mass and its location at the left atrioventricular groove level. There is nodular submitral calcification. The coronal CT scan also detects a stent in the proximal left circumflex artery.

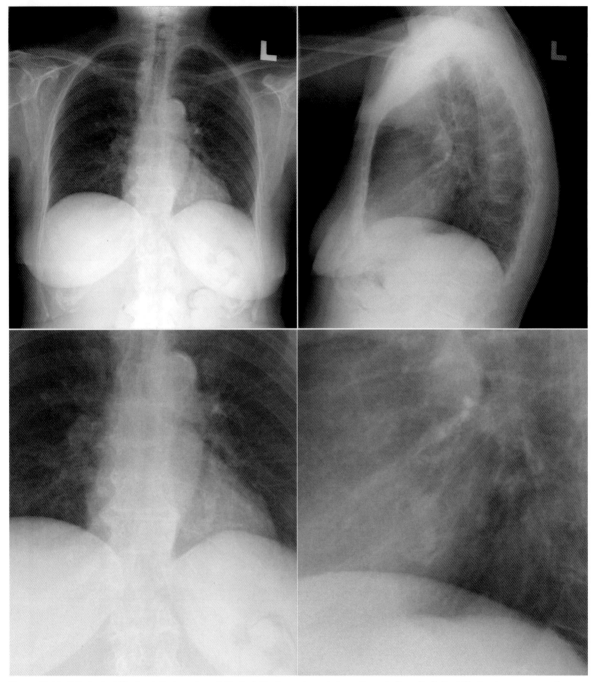

Figure 27-14. Submitral calcification (mitral annular calcification). On the posteroanterior radiograph, the submitral calcification is seen as a radiopaque curving pearl necklace–like structure that is even more evident on the lateral radiograph as an upward open C-shaped structure.

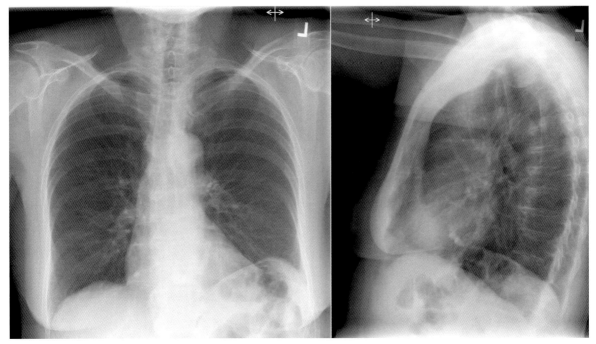

Figure 27-15. On the frontal radiograph, extensive submitral annular calcification in a reverse C pattern is apparent because it is projecting clear of the spine. On the lateral radiograph, it appears as more of a horseshoe.

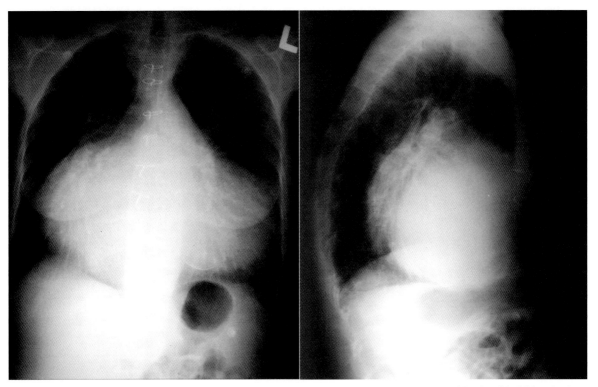

Figure 27-16. Left atrial calcification. There is gross cardiomegaly with a multichamber pattern of carinal splaying, straightening of the left heart border, a "double contour" at the right heart border, and posterior displacement of the left atrium, all due to left atrial enlargement. The patient had previously undergone a mitral commissurotomy. There are signs of right atrial and ventricular enlargement. Best seen on the frontal radiograph, a calcified floor of the left atrium or calcified atrial thrombus is visible.

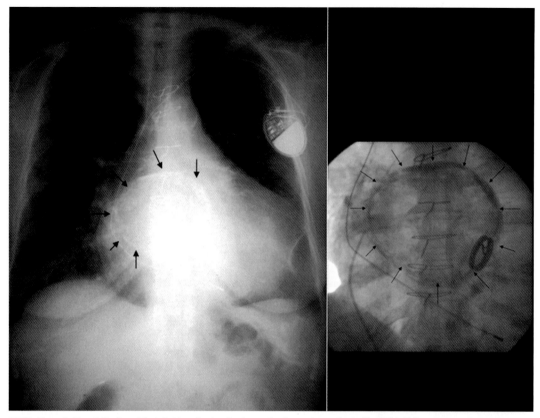

Figure 27-17. Remarkable calcification of the left atrium due to prior rheumatic disease in a patient with a Björk-Shiley mitral prosthesis. There are cardiomegaly and double right heart borders due to biatrial dilation. (From Edwards JM, Chisholm RJ: Porcelain atrium: rheumatic heart disease. *Can J Cardiol* 22:267, 2006, figs. 1 and 2. Used with permission.)

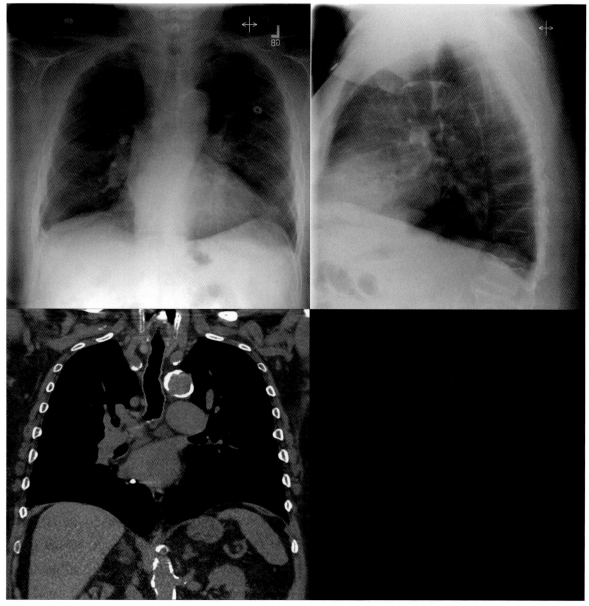

Figure 27-18. Severe calcific aortic stenosis. There is borderline cardiomegaly on the posteroanterior (PA) chest radiograph but more obvious signs of left ventricular enlargement on the PA radiograph. The aortic "knob" seems to be calcified on the PA radiograph, and, in fact, the entire thoracic aorta is calcified on the lateral chest radiograph. The lower image, a non–contrast-enhanced computer tomography (CT) scan that approximately matches the upper PA radiograph, corroborates the calcification of the distal aortic arch. It also demonstrates the more prominent depiction of calcification by CT scanning than by plain film radiography.

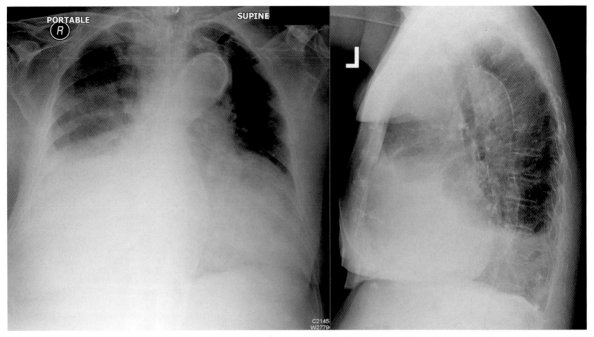

Figure 27-19. There is cardiomegaly with left ventricular enlargement and a left pleural effusion. More striking is the nearly continuous calcification of the aorta—a "porcelain aorta." The patient was diabetic, without renal failure.

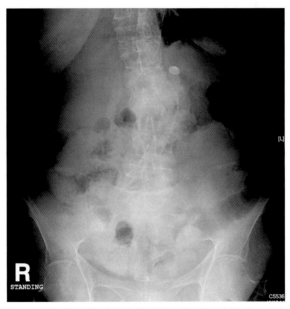

Figure 27-20. The entire abdominal aorta is outlined by calcification, which visibly extends into the iliac arteries.

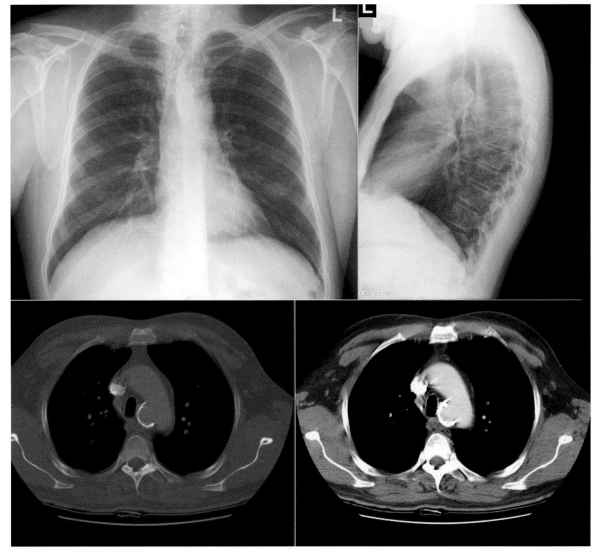

Figure 27-21. The aortic arch is seen to be abnormal on the posteroanterior radiograph. On the lateral radiograph, there is an egg-shaped rim of calcification, which is seen to be located off the underside of the aortic arch. The patient has a history of a remote motor vehicle accident with multiple trauma; the calcified lesion was presumed to be a calcified chronic post-traumatic false aneurysm.

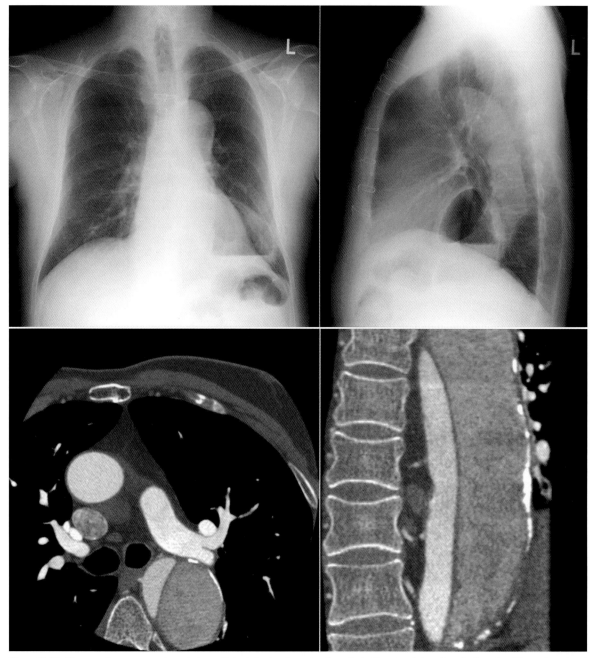

Figure 27-22. The upper images are posteroanterior and lateral chest radiographs of a patient with a chronic type B aortic dissection. The aortic arch and the descending aorta are enlarged. As well, the lateral margin of the aortic arch and descending aorta are more visually prominent than normal. The lower images are contrast-enhanced computed tomography (CT) scans taken in the axial plane (*left lower image*) and in the coronal plane (*right lower image*). The CT scans prominently depict the calcification of the wall of the false lumen. The false lumen remains patent in this case. Note as well the hiatal hernia.

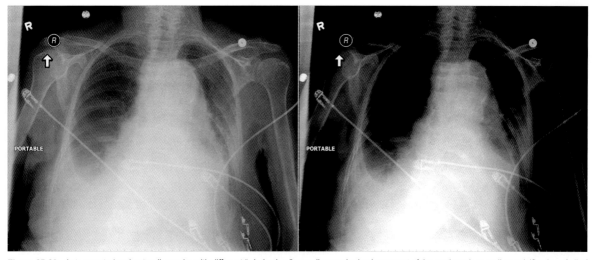

Figure 27-23. Anteroposterior chest radiographs with different "windowing," revealing marked enlargement of the aortic arch as well as calcification of all of the aortic arch and descending aorta.

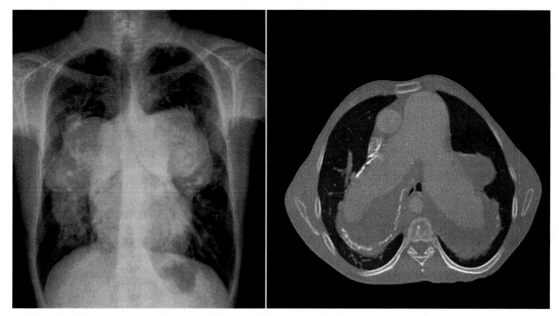

Figure 27-24. The left image is a chest radiograph at admission, which shows massive dilated pulmonary arteries. The right image, an axial contrast-enhanced computed tomography pulmonary angiogram, reveals giant pulmonary arteries with mural thrombosis and calcification. (From Jensen AS, Iverson, K, Vejlstrup NG, Sondergaard L: Pulmonary artery thrombosis and hemoptysis in Eisenmenger syndrome. *Circulation* 115:e632–e634, 2007. Used with permission.)

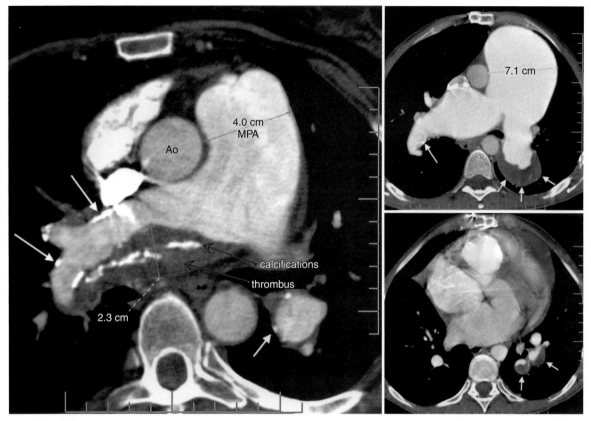

Figure 27-25. *Left:* An axial computed tomography (CT) angiogram at the level of the main pulmonary artery bifurcation that shows dilation of the main pulmonary arteries and an eccentric 23-mm mural thrombus along the posterior wall of the right pulmonary artery. The thrombus is composed of multiple layers of thrombus with embedded linear calcifications, suggesting repeated events during formation. Calcifications are also seen along the anterior free wall of the right pulmonary artery and its main branches (*long arrows*) and in the left interlobar artery (*short arrow*). Ao, ascending aorta; MPA, main pulmonary artery. *Upper right:* Axial CT angiogram at the level of the main pulmonary arteries that demonstrates severe dilation, with the main pulmonary artery measuring 71 mm. There is an associated eccentric irregular thrombus in the left main pulmonary artery (*short arrows*). A tiny focus of calcification is noted in the posterior wall of the right pulmonary artery (*long arrow*). *Lower right:* Axial CT image at the level of lung bases showing extension of the thrombus into the segmental basal arteries of the left lower lobe (*short arrows*). (From Silversides CK, Granton JT, Konen E, et al: Pulmonary thrombosis in adults with Eisenmenger syndrome. *J Am Coll Cardiol* 42:1982–1987, 2003. Used with permission.)

Cardiac and Vascular Trauma

Trauma to the heart and aorta includes blunt and penetrating trauma imparted from widely different directions, resulting in many different forms of cardiac and vascular injury.

Of all traumatic lesions to the thoracic cardiovascular system, the most predictable one is blunt deceleration/acceleration traumatic injury to the thoracic aorta, resulting in a false aneurysm-type lesion, typically of the isthmus proximal descending aorta. It may also involve the ascending aorta, the supradiaphragmatic aorta, or the innominate artery take-off (Figs. 28-1 to 28-13).

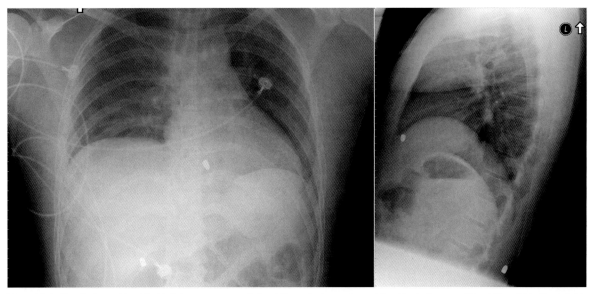

Figure 28-1. The shadows of two intact bullets are seen—one in the right paralumbar region and the other in the apex of the right ventricle. The bullet in the heart was unsuspected, as the entry site was the posterior thigh. The bullet had migrated into the right heart via the deep veins of the leg to the inferior vena cava and then into the heart.

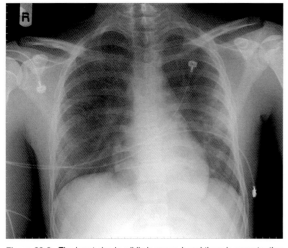

Figure 28-2. The heart size is mildly increased, and there is accentuation of both the pulmonary arterial and venous vasculature. A knife stab wound entering from the apex had resulted in a ventricular septal defect.

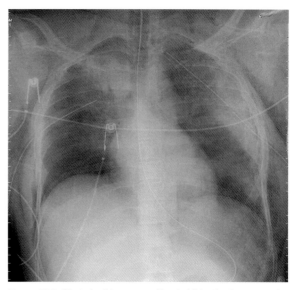

Figure 28-3. Blunt chest trauma resulting in bilateral pulmonary contusions and pneumothoraces (treated with bilateral chest tubes), as well as bilateral rib fractures and a flail chest.

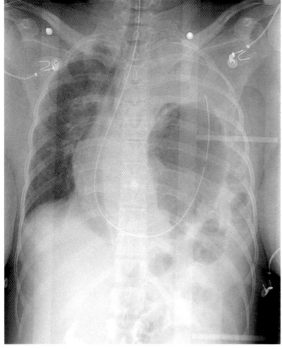

Figure 28-4. Blunt trauma resulting in a left diaphragmatic hernia. The nasogastric tube marks that the stomach has entered the thorax through the hernia.

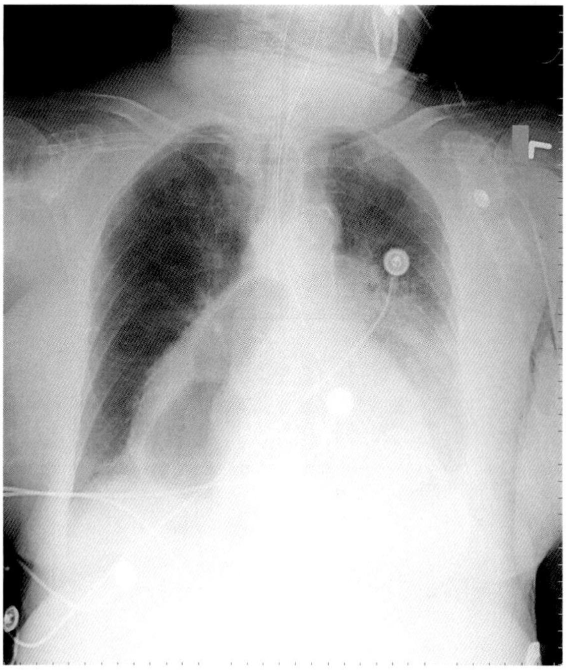

Figure 28-5. Blunt trauma resulting in a right diaphragmatic hernia extending into the pericardial space.

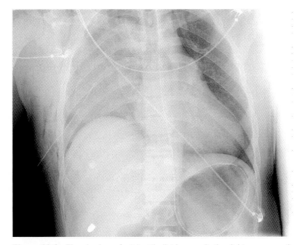

Figure 28-6. The shadow of a intact bullet is seen in the right upper quadrant of the abdomen. The entry had been in the chest, resulting in a hemothorax—hence the chest tube.

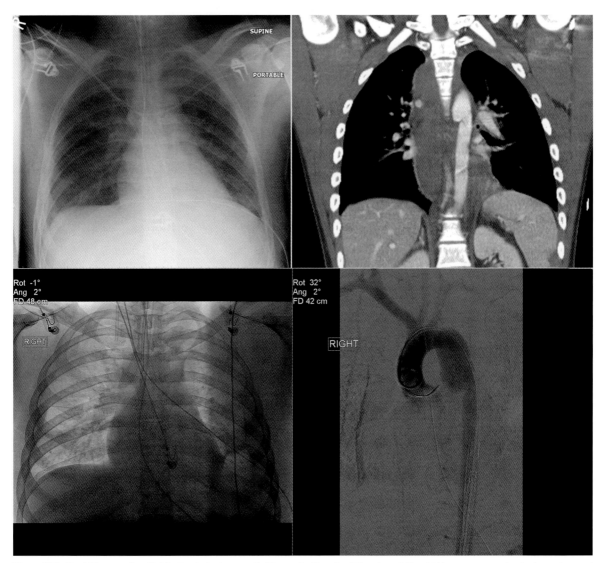

Figure 28-7. The left images show that the heart size is normal but the mediastinum is mildly enlarged. The right images are a contrast-enhanced coronal projection computed tomography scan *(above)* and an angiogram with slight rightward projection *(below),* which reveal a false aneurysm at the site of traumatic disruption of the proximal descending aorta.

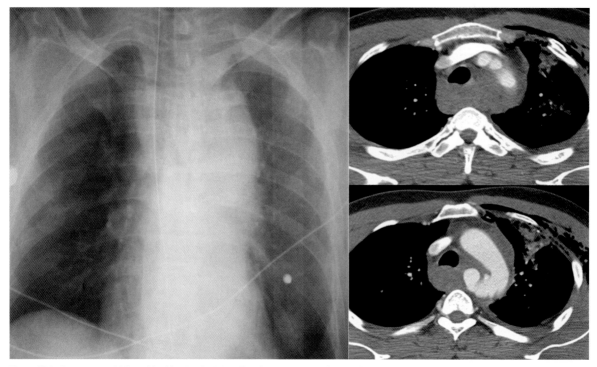

Figure 28-8. Post–motor vehicle accident/deceleration injury. Note the enlargement of the proximal descending aorta and its hazy shagginess due to hemorrhage from a traumatic disruption of the proximal descending aorta, as revealed by the contrast-enhanced axial computed tomography scan images, as well as mediastinal hematoma—the cause of the mediastinal widening.

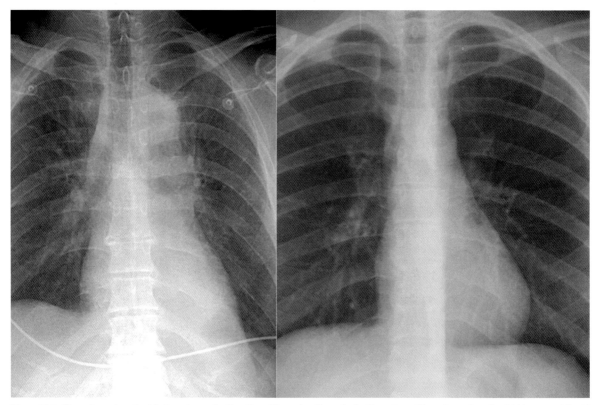

Figure 28-9. The radiograph on the left shows traumatic disruption of the aorta with mediastinal hematoma. The radiograph on the right is a normal frontal radiograph by way of contrast. Note the shagginess of the margins of the traumatically disrupted aorta.

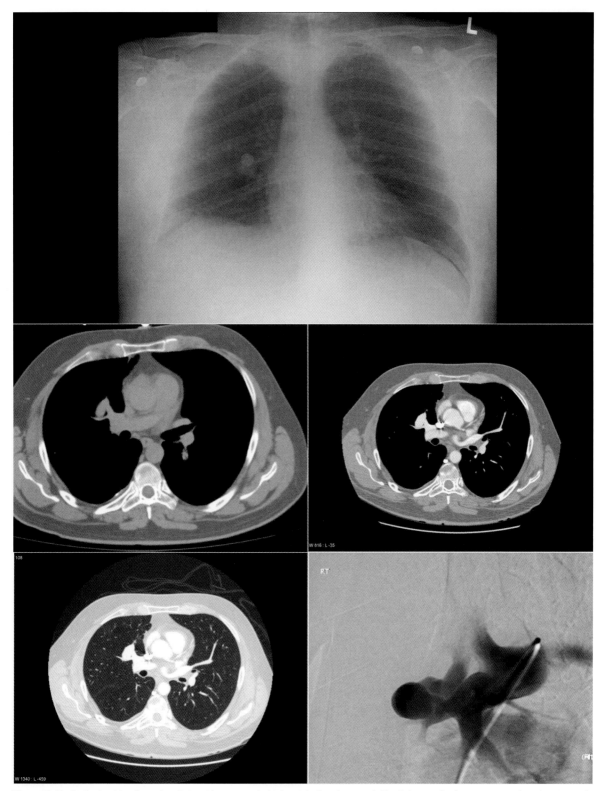

Figure 28-10. On the frontal radiograph, unfortunately near an electrode patch, there is a rounded/oval circumscribed mass, representing a post-traumatic false aneurysm, which is depicted on the computed tomography axial images and on the right pulmonary angiogram.

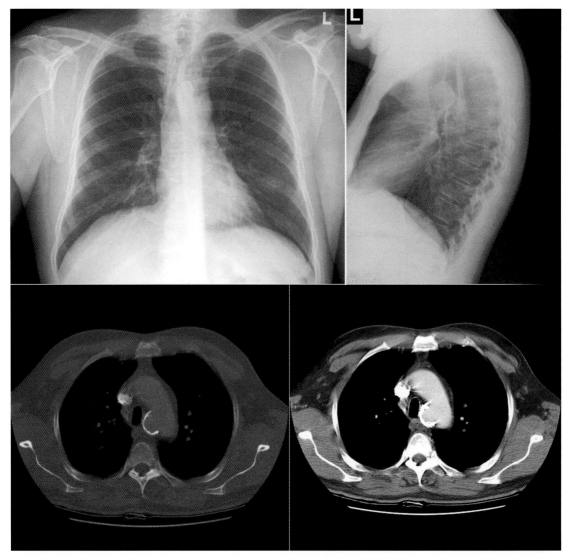

Figure 28-11. Chest radiographs and non–contrast-enhanced and contrast-enhanced axial computed tomography images of a patient with a calcified false aneurysm from prior traumatic disruption of the aorta.

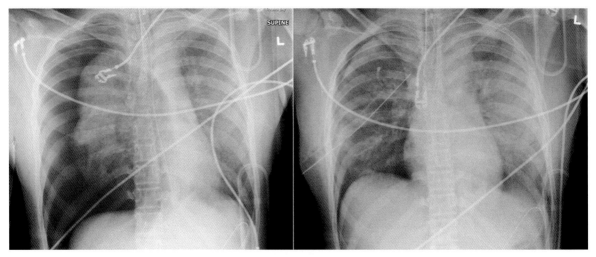

Figure 28-12. Post trauma—note the spine fracture. The left image shows a tension pneumothorax. Note the collapsed lung and the displacement of the heart and mediastinum. The right image is after needle thoracostomy via the second interspace. The pneumothorax has diminished and the "tension" has been eliminated.

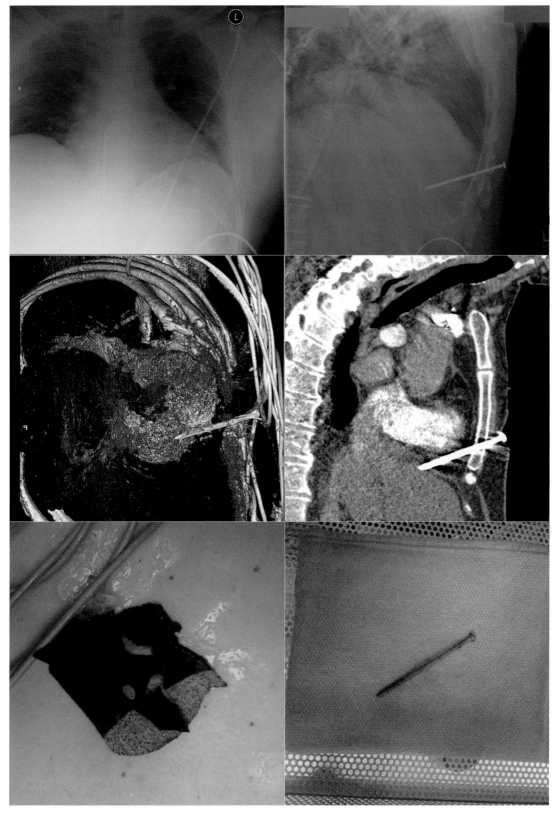

Figure 28-13. Posteroanterior and lateral chest radiographs, 3D volume–rendered and coronal contrast-enhanced computed tomography scans, and surgical photos of a nail, shot by a nailgun through the mid-sternum inferiorly, and passing through the anterior right ventricle and out the diaphragmatic surface of the right ventricle, through the diaphragm, and into the liver. It was extracted uneventfully.

Clinical Uses of the Chest Radiograph

CHEST PAIN

In the workup of a chest pain syndrome, the chest radiograph is useful, if not mandatory, to evaluate the following:
❒ Pleural effusions (supports pleural disease [i.e., inflammation] or congestive heart failure)
❒ Heart size (indicates cardiac disease but does not distinguish pericardial from myocardial, valvular, or other types)
❒ Radiographic signs of congestive heart failure
❒ Aortic size and contour; these may suggest aortic disease
❒ Skeletal disease
❒ Esophageal hernia (hiatal hernia)
❒ Pneumonia

ACUTE CORONARY SYNDROMES

In the workup of a patient with an acute coronary syndrome, the chest radiograph is useful, if not mandatory, to evaluate the following:
❒ Heart size (which indirectly suggests left ventricular dysfunction)
❒ Radiographic signs of congestive heart failure

CONGESTIVE HEART FAILURE

In the workup of a patient with congestive heart failure, the chest radiograph is useful, if not mandatory, to evaluate the following:
❒ Heart size (which indirectly suggests left ventricular dysfunction)
❒ Radiographic signs and severity of congestive heart failure

❒ Valve calcification
❒ Valve prosthesis type and position

HYPERTENSION

In the workup of a patient with hypertension, the chest radiograph is useful to evaluate the following:
❒ Heart size (which indirectly suggests left ventricular dysfunction)
❒ Radiographic signs and severity of congestive heart failure
❒ Aortic size and contour
❒ Coarctation of the aorta (mandatory in a young patient with hypertension or radiofemoral pulse differences)

RESPIRATORY FAILURE

In the workup of a patient with respiratory failure, the chest radiograph is mandatory to evaluate the following:
❒ Presence/absence/severity/type of lung parenchymal disease
❒ Size of lung field
❒ Presence/absence/size of pleural effusions, pneumothoraces, thickening
❒ Heart size (which indirectly suggests left ventricular dysfunction)
❒ Radiographic signs and severity of congestive heart failure
❒ Diaphragmatic height (? paralysis)
❒ Pulmonary vasculature (signs of left heart failure/pulmonary hypertension/pulmonary embolism)
❒ Parenchymal opacities: pneumonia, aspiration, hemorrhage

FOLLOWING PACEMAKER INSERTION

A post–pacemaker insertion chest radiograph is mandatory to verify the following:
❒ Correct position of the pacemaker leads
❒ Absence (or identification) of insertion-related complications (pneumothoraces, hemothoraces, tamponade, pacemaker syndrome with development of heart failure)

PATIENT IN THE INTENSIVE CARE UNIT/CORONARY CARE UNIT

In the workup of a patient with congestive heart failure, the chest radiograph is useful, if not mandatory, to evaluate the following:
- ❏ Post–central venous line insertion chest radiograph (mandatory): to verify the correct position of the central venous line and to exclude (or identify) insertion and line-related complications (pneumothoraces, hemothoraces, tamponade, pulmonary infarction)
- ❏ Post–central venous line repositioning chest radiograph (mandatory): to verify the correct position of the central venous line, and to exclude (or identify) complications
- ❏ Causes of changes in clinical status (cardiac, respiratory, or hemodynamic)

SUSPECTED ADULT CONGENITAL HEART (CARDIOVASCULAR) DISEASE

In the workup of a suspected adult congenital cardiovascular disease, the chest radiograph is a mandatory screening test to determine:
- ❏ Heart size
- ❏ Radiographic signs and severity of congestive heart failure

- ❏ Pulmonary vasculature (signs of reduced or excessive flow, pulmonary hypertension, asymmetry, patent ductus, heart failure)
- ❏ Left-sided or right-sided aorta, aorta size, coarctation of the aorta
- ❏ Side of the gastric air bubble (situs)

SUSPECTED DISEASE OF THE THORACIC AORTA

In the workup of a patient with suspected disease of the thoracic aorta, the chest radiograph is mandatory to evaluate the following:
- ❏ Aorta contour and size
- ❏ Signs of wall thickening
- ❏ Signs of rupture (e.g., pleural effusion, hazy contour)

INDEX

Page numbers followed by f or t indicate figures or tables, respectively.